D0721578

THE
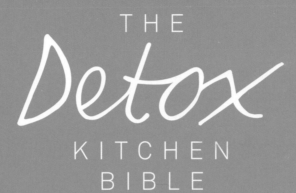
KITCHEN
BIBLE

CALGARY PUBLIC LIBRARY

MAR   2017

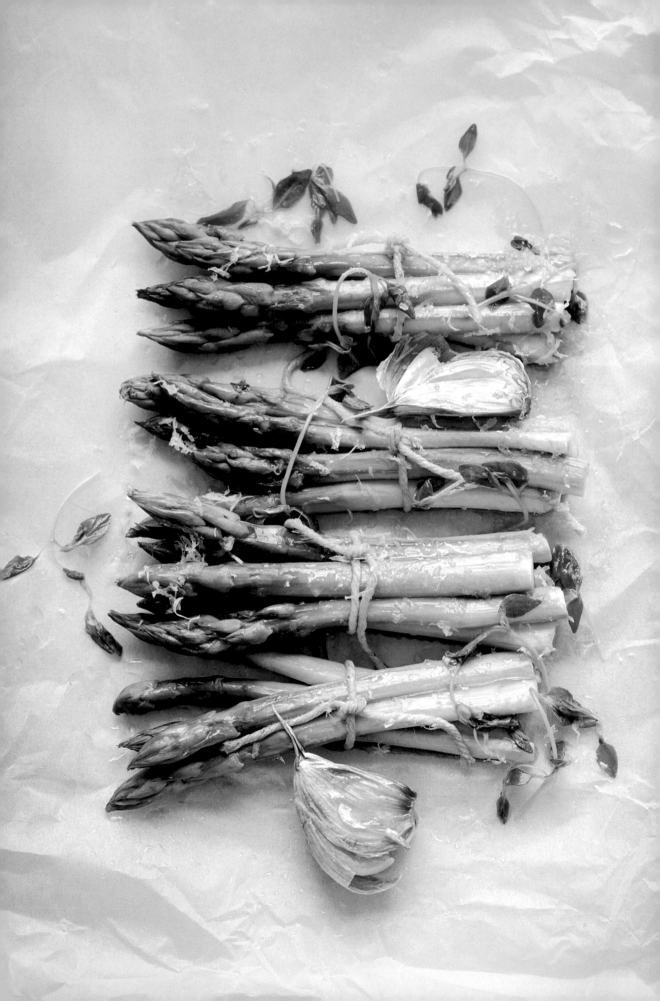

THE
Detox
KITCHEN
BIBLE

200 recipes for glorious health, all free from
wheat, dairy and refined sugar

LILY SIMPSON & ROB HOBSON

BLOOMSBURY
LONDON · OXFORD · NEW YORK · NEW DELHI · SYDNEY

RECIPES

BY LILY SIMPSON

NUTRITION

BY ROB HOBSON

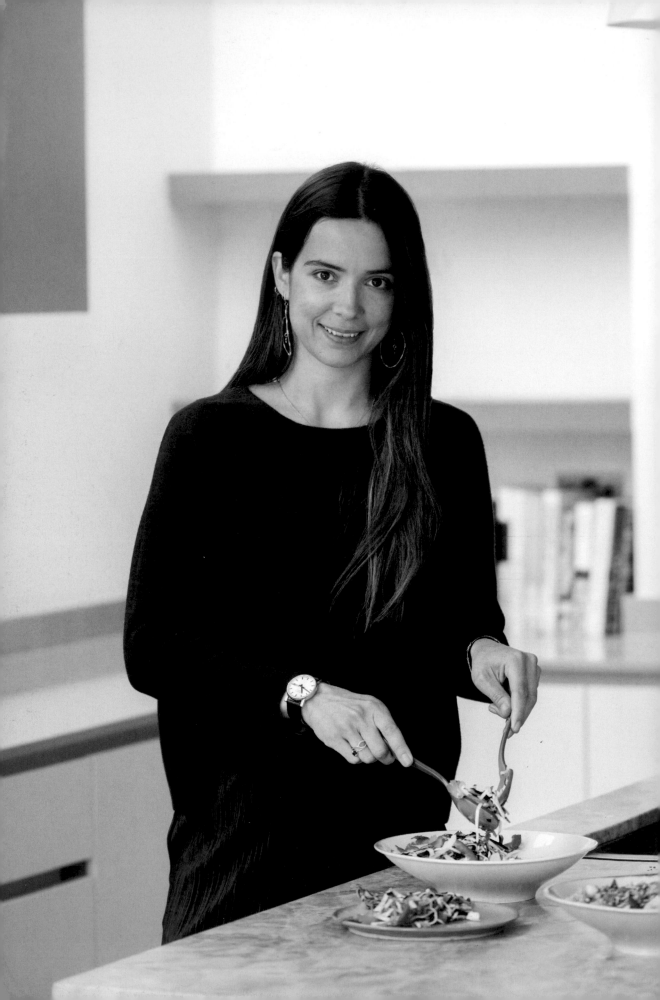

INTRODUCTION

Food should be pleasurable to eat. The key to creating food that is both nourishing and flavourful is simple: you can't go far wrong by starting with fresh fruit and vegetables, lean protein, wholegrains and pulses, and nuts and seeds.

This is why I created the Detox Kitchen, working with nutritionist Rob Hobson. It began as a convenient delivery service with detox plans that were individually designed for our clients, many of whom suffered from digestive complaints, food intolerances, weight maintenance issues, fatigue and other health problems that affected their everyday lives. Now, though, our recipes can offer the perfect diet for anyone looking to improve their health through the food they eat. To achieve this, we put plant-based wholefoods, variety and flavour at the centre of our cooking, and we leave out wheat, dairy and refined sugar. This may sound restrictive, but it really isn't!

Since the Detox Kitchen was launched in 2012, the health food market has grown exponentially. We have branched out, opening two delis and a Selfridges concession in London, and thanks to a wonderfully loyal customer base, the Detox Kitchen now serves delicious, healthy food to thousands of people every day. It's humbling to know that we can help influence the way that people approach their diet – and in turn their lifestyle – in such a positive way.

There have been mixed messages about what 'healthy eating' actually means in recent years. In my mind the definition of a healthy diet is simply that it should be balanced, enjoyable and made up of wholesome, natural food. I feel privileged to have a voice in the health food industry, showing that by eating well and respecting the nutritional needs of your own body, you will look and feel like the best possible version of yourself.

KITCHEN BASICS

Flavour is at the heart of the way I cook. It makes no sense to me to prepare and serve food simply because it is good for you. To have wholesome, healthy food in your life, it is essential that you enjoy eating it.

I am a chef, so when devising a dish, my first aim is to please the tastebuds. But beyond that I want to let the ingredients work their magic on your health and well-being. At the Detox Kitchen we have a simple goal: to create delicious recipes that work with your body, not against it, giving it the best chance to do what it does naturally. In our dishes we limit those elements that can adversely affect health, and maximise the foods that nourish and nurture. Put simply, we believe that our food will make you feel better – from the inside out.

But what exactly do we mean by 'detox'? These days our bodies work harder than ever, using highly regulated processes to rid us of toxins and protect against the damage and stresses caused by modern life. With increased pollution, frenetic lifestyles and diets high in processed foods, it has become even more important to be mindful of what we are putting into our bodies, and to give them a break from the things that can cause unnecessary stress.

My life is busy and I have in the past struggled with my stress levels, often reaching for 'quick fix' foods to keep me going. As a result, I have suffered from the dreaded IBS (irritable bowel syndrome), stomach ulcers and poor skin, frequently having to endure their uncomfortable, energy-draining symptoms on a daily basis. I have also listened to countless friends who have turned to faddy diets to overcome weight issues, leading to poor energy levels and emotional struggles. These in turn often left them lacking in key nutrients, feeling even more tired and developing negative attitudes towards food.

I have seen first-hand how a varied, nutrient-rich diet, free from processed foods, can have a transformative effect on the body, leaving it glowing with health. As soon as you start cooking from this book, you'll see how simple it can be.

RECIPES & PLANS

I tend to dip in and out of our detox programmes, living by an 80/20 split: 80 per cent of the time I eat food that is free of wheat, dairy and refined sugar, and for the other 20 per cent I eat whatever I want. The recipes in this book can be used in the same way: you can dip in and out when you want or you can commit to a week plan. You can even grab the book on a Saturday morning after a Friday night that was a little too indulgent.

Each recipe notes the main nutrients it provides (see right) and highlights an area of health that it may be particularly useful for, which could include a specific condition such as high cholesterol or relieving symptoms associated with the menopause. You can either pick and choose from the recipes or turn to Rob's detailed nutrition section at the back of the book and follow a detox plan. Each of these is tailored for a specific health area, and guides you to build up a targeted menu of recipes that will help you.

SHARING MEALS

The recipes in this book are not intended to be meals eaten alone – we are big believers in the importance of eating with family and friends, sitting down together and taking time to share and appreciate what you have cooked. It's far easier to stick to a healthy eating plan if you do it with others. So most recipes are designed for two or four people, although they can very easily be adapted for one person.

In the pages that follow, I'll show you how to mix herbs, spices, seeds, nuts, wholegrains, pulses, fruit, vegetables, lean meat and fish so that eating healthily becomes one of your greatest pleasures in life – food that you not only enjoy eating, but that you can *feel* is doing good for your whole body.

At the end of most recipes we have given a list of the main nutrients supplied in a serving. To be classed as a 'rich' source for a particular vitamin or mineral, the amount has to comply with recognised guidance; for example, the amount of the nutrient must be at least 30 per cent of the recommended daily allowance (RDA). There may be additional nutrients mentioned in a recipe's introduction, but these are not present in sufficient quantity for the recipe to be classed as a rich source. Where there is no list of nutrients, the dish is still nourishing but contains lower amounts of the beneficial vitamins, minerals and so on.

Following the nutrients is a list of the health issues that may be benefited by including the recipe in your healthy diet, and these are colour coded to relate to the nutritional guides and tailored detox plans at the back of the book.

Heart
① High cholesterol
② High blood pressure
③ Type 2 diabetes

Bones
① Osteoporosis
② Arthritis

Digestion
① Constipation
② Bloating
③ Irritable bowel syndrome (IBS)
④ Indigestion & heartburn
⑤ Food intolerance

Immunity
① Common cold
② Coeliac disease

Skin, hair & nails
① Acne
② Psoriasis
③ Eczema
④ Hair & scalp
⑤ Weak, brittle nails

Mind
① Depression
② Anxiety

Fatigue
① Iron deficiency (anaemia)
② Chronic fatigue syndrome (CFS)
③ Insomnia
④ Headaches
⑤ Migraine

Men
① Prostate
② Fertility
③ Impotence

Women
① Premenstrual syndrome (PMS)
② Urinary tract infections (cystitis)
③ Menopause
④ Polycystic ovary syndrome (PCOS)

There are also detox plans for **Weight** and for **Vegetarians & vegans**.

HOW WE COOK

Cooking without wheat, dairy or refined sugar may at first seem a little daunting, but what it has taught me to do is experiment with flavours by using fresh herbs and spices that really bring vegetables, pulses, fish and meat to life. I promise you that once you have mastered the art of cooking without wheat, dairy or refined sugar, you won't miss them at all.

WHEAT Our daily diets have become heavily reliant on wheat, and most of what we consume is in a highly refined form that includes foods made from white flour, such as white bread, pasta and pastries. Foods like these are quickly digested, causing rapid spikes in blood sugar levels, which can lead to energy slumps and fatigue. Also, along with other refined carbohydrates such as sugar, these kinds of wheat-based foods have been linked to weight gain and other problems when eaten in excess.

Our recipes are not gluten-free (although we do use gluten- and wheat-free flour) because a diagnosed intolerance to gluten is uncommon and avoidance is tricky and restrictive – and it can result in nutrient deficiencies. A specific wheat allergy is rare. Yet many people experience a spectrum of digestive issues when they eat foods made with refined wheat in large amounts daily.

It's becoming more widely accepted that we should be eating a little less carbohydrate (starchy food) in our diets and that this should be coming from fibre-rich wholegrain foods (such as brown rice, oats, barley and quinoa), starchy vegetables (such as sweet potato and butternut squash) and pulses, commonly referred to as complex carbohydrates. These foods not only offer highly nutritious alternatives to refined wheat products but also provide a range of other beneficial nutrients.

At the Detox Kitchen, our love of food means it's not all about nutrition – our attitude is always 'live to eat' and not the other way round. With this in mind, we want to show you the versatility of wholegrains and pulses, which are often at the core of our cooking, and suggest how you can combine their myriad flavours, textures and colours in new and exciting ways.

DAIRY We do not use dairy foods in our recipes, nor any product made from animal's milk, because for some people these can cause digestive upset and in some cases aggravate certain conditions. (Personally, since reducing the amount of dairy in my diet, I have experienced better digestion and seen positive changes in my skin.) Although important for young children and women who are pregnant, dairy foods are not a necessary component of an adult diet.

The main nutrient supplied by dairy foods is calcium, which is primarily associated with healthy bones – especially important for women who are at greater risk of poor bone health after the menopause. Calcium can be obtained from many other wonderful foods, such as fortified rice milk, green vegetables, tofu, almonds, dried fruit, sesame seeds and tahini, and pulses, all of which can easily be added to the diet and offer many other valuable nutrients.

REFINED SUGAR We all eat too much sugar. That is a fact. Refined sugar is addictive and can be the hardest ingredient to give up, but the results are often the most rewarding. Refined sugar has no nutritional value other than calories, and the way the carbohydrates are processed in the body has been strongly associated with weight gain and obesity, as well as other chronic health problems and conditions. Excess sugar also plays havoc with blood sugar levels, which can indirectly affect our hormones, stress levels and mood.

A little sugar is certainly not a bad thing, and sweetness is what makes certain foods so delicious – something we don't want to lose. But at the Detox Kitchen, when we want to sweeten food, we like to keep things as natural as possible, opting for honey and for fruit (the way our ancestors would have done), which can offer a greater range of flavours and nutrients than commercially produced sweeteners. We refer to these kinds of recipes as our sweet treats, and you'll see how easy it is to capture sweetness whilst using only relatively small quantities of natural sugars.

THE DETOX PANTRY

Here you'll find the staple ingredients we have in our pantry that make it easy to knock up fool-proof healthy dishes. There is no need to rely upon stodgy, salty, processed ingredients when you have these seasonings, oils, grains, pulses, nuts and seeds at your fingertips. They will enable you to experiment with new textures and tastes, and will add depth and character to your dishes.

OILS

The oils that we always have on hand are extra virgin olive oil, extra virgin rapeseed oil, extra virgin coconut oil and cold-pressed nut oils. We prefer to use only extra virgin oils that have been cold-pressed because this method produces a cleaner oil of superior nutritional quality. Other methods of extracting oils involve using chemicals and high temperatures, processes that can cause the oil to go rancid and become less healthy.

There are certain oils that are best for certain cooking methods. Generally this is dependent on their flavour and 'smoking point' – some oils are less stable when heated to high temperatures; this causes them to oxidise, forming unhealthy compounds and giving them an unpleasant taste.

EXTRA VIRGIN OLIVE OIL Rich in monounsaturated fats and other naturally occurring compounds that can benefit health, a good extra virgin olive oil is perfect for dressing salads and finishing dishes, giving extra flavour and moisture when needed. High-quality extra virgin olive oil is also fine for light sautéing or drizzling over vegetables to be roasted.

EXTRA VIRGIN RAPESEED OIL The versatility and benefit to health are why we use this oil most often: it's rich in healthy monounsaturated fats and has a good balance of omega 3 and 6 fatty acids. Deep yellow and nutty-tasting, its flavour is less intense than that of olive oil, which makes it perfect for cooking with every day, as well as for drizzling over salads and finishing dishes. Rapeseed oil has a high smoking point, so is ideal for stir-frying or sautéing.

EXTRA VIRGIN COCONUT OIL With its high smoking point, coconut oil is good for tempering or toasting spices, when a high temperature is needed to bring out the aromatic oils and flavours of the spices. For this reason it features heavily in curries. Its sweet flavour also works well in baking. Coconut oil offers properties that may protect us against viruses and bacteria.

GROUNDNUT OIL Typically made by pressing peanuts, this oil has a subtle, nutty flavour. It is good to use when cooking at a high temperature as it does not burn easily.

OTHER NUT OILS We tend not to heat walnut, hazelnut and similar nut oils but rather use them in dressings to emphasise nut flavours. For example, if a salad includes walnuts, we use cold-pressed walnut oil in the dressing. Store these types of nut oils in the fridge as they will keep for longer than at room temperature.

HERBS & SPICES

It's amazing how food will suddenly come alive with the addition of some herbs or spices. My tip for adding them is to use your nose: if I am ever lacking inspiration, I pick up the herb basket and have a good sniff. If ingredients smell good together, they'll taste good together too.

Add herbs with soft leaves, such as basil, coriander and mint, at the *end* of cooking as their flavour can be lost if you heat them; they also add colour and vibrancy as a fresh garnish. Tougher-leaved herbs, such as rosemary and thyme, are best added at the *start* of cooking, because they need time to impart their flavour. The same is true of spices – often the taste of a spice will change over the course of the cooking time.

These are the herbs and spices we use most frequently. They are the backbone of the recipes in this book, adding flavour to all kinds of dishes.

BASIL ① There are many varieties of this soft-leaved herb. In Italian cooking, sweet basil is used most frequently. Its intense aromatic flavour goes perfectly with meat and fish, and the bright green leaves are delicious ripped over a cold gazpacho or blitzed into a vibrant pesto. In Asian cooking, Thai, lemon and holy basil add a peppery sweetness to curries and stir-fries.

CHIVES ② The smallest, most delicately flavoured member of the onion family, chives give salads a sweet onion hit. They are also the perfect quick garnish: simply snip with scissors over any dish.

CINNAMON ③ This is the best spice for bringing out sweetness in a dish and adding an aromatic, warm flavour. Just a sprinkle of cinnamon can do wonders for a boring bowl of porridge. Ground cinnamon is much stronger than stick cinnamon, so use with a delicate touch.

CUMIN ④ Widely used in Indian, Mediterranean and Middle Eastern cuisines, cumin has a powerful smoky flavour and instantly adds a deep aroma to any dish. It's ideal teamed with root vegetables, where the sweetness balances their flavour. If you have a pestle and mortar, grind the seeds; buy the powder if you are short of time.

CORIANDER SEEDS ⑤ Often used in Indian cooking, these little seeds add a citrus flavour. Cook them carefully to enjoy their full potential – if they burn they will taste very bitter and can spoil the dish. Use your nose here: toast them in a dry pan just until their fragrant aroma is released.

FRESH CORIANDER ⑥ You either love this herb or hate it. I love it. So aromatic and full of citrus, peppery and slightly minty flavours, the leaves can bring a dish to life in seconds. I use the roots in the base for curries and stews because the flavour is more intense than that of the leaves and adds an earthy depth.

GARLIC ⑦ This offers a spectrum of flavours, depending on how it is used. I like it raw in Asian-inspired salads and dressings, where it adds a fieriness, and it appears in nearly all of our stews, giving them a lovely mellow flavour. Roasting a bulb whole makes the cloves taste rich and sweet – a brilliant addition to soups or tomato sauce. If you find any green shoots in a garlic clove, remove them as they are bitter and can give you wind.

GINGER ⑧ Pungent, sharp, slightly lemony and peppery, fresh ginger root is one of my favourite ingredients. It adds a lovely freshness to any dish and always features in the base of our curries and broths. Choose a plump-looking root: wrinkly ones will be fibrous and dry. I often don't bother to peel ginger but just grate it with the skin on.

MINT ⑨ Most of our recipes call for spearmint because it is the most widely available mint in supermarkets. I often add a few leaves to a pesto to create a light freshness. It's a nice idea to grow a pot of peppermint so that it is always on hand for making fresh mint tea, perfect for relief from bloating after meals. The best variety for this is Moroccan mint, as it has a smooth, sweet taste.

ROSEMARY ⑩ Traditionally paired with lamb, chicken or robust fish, this intensely aromatic herb is also delicious in hearty bean soups and stews, and complements most root vegetables. It adds a piney, peppery and deeply savoury taste to a dish. Being evergreen, it is available year round.

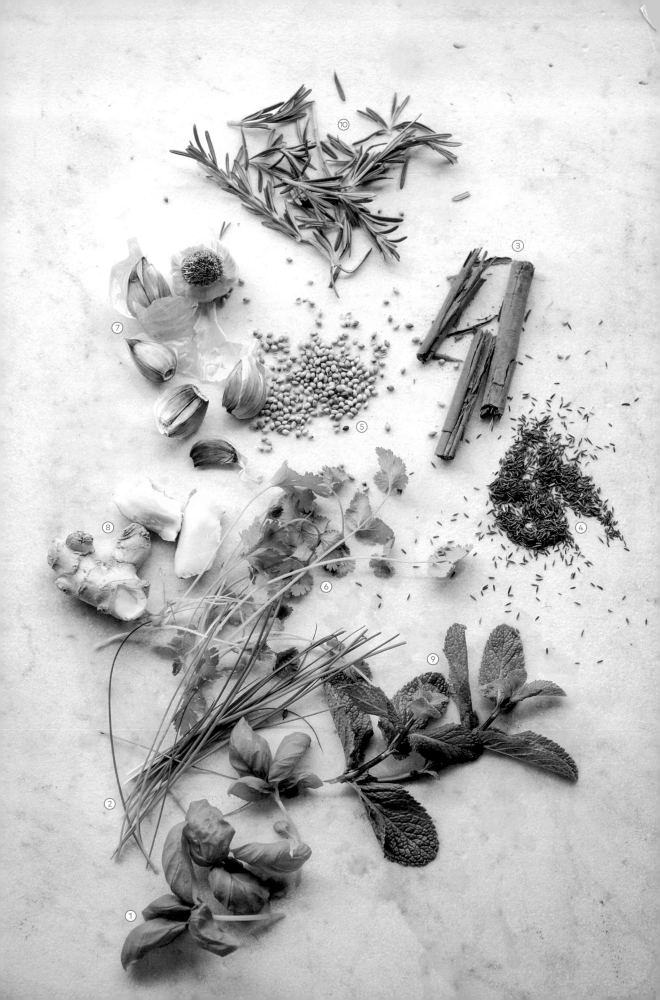

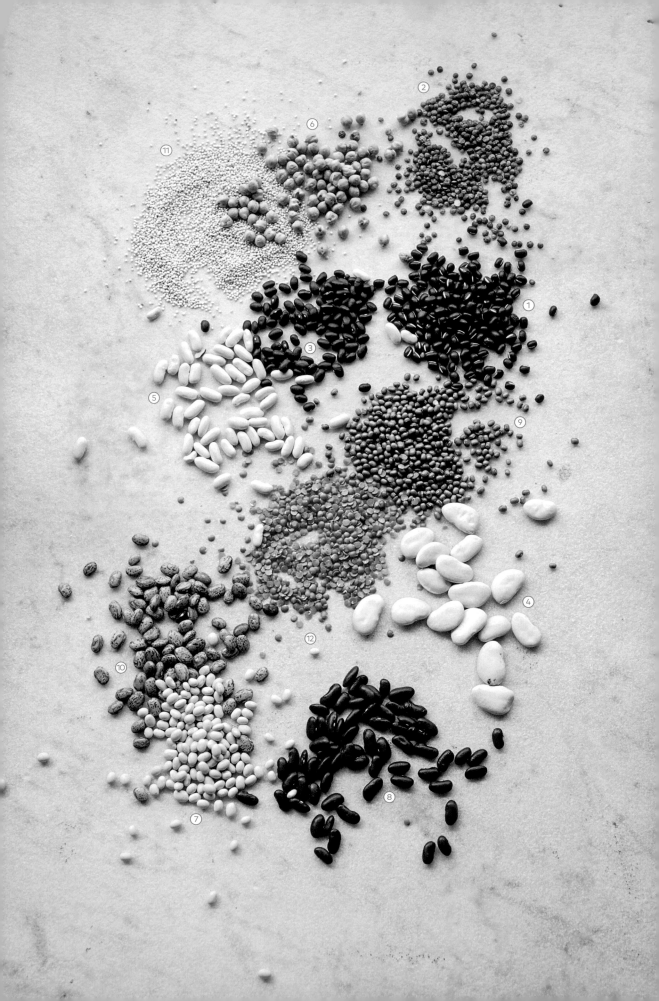

PULSES & QUINOA

Dried beans, peas and lentils form the basis of many of our vegetarian dishes. This is because pulses provide a valuable source of protein, fibre and complex carbohydrates as well as a good source of folate, magnesium, iron and zinc (this is what makes them an essential component of vegetarian and vegan diets). They also add a delicious texture.

Although not a pulse (which is a dried seed from a leguminous crop), quinoa (the seed of a grain) is also a protein source and so we've included it here.

Often people think cooking with dried beans is a long and laborious task, but you only need to soak them in water overnight and allow a little longer for the cooking time. The resulting taste and texture are worth it. If you don't have time for the soaking and cooking, tinned beans can be substituted, but buy a good-quality organic tin – I find organic tinned beans have more flavour than other brands, which can taste very watered-down.

ADUKI BEANS ① These dark red beans are prized for their sweet, nutty flavour and firm texture, which makes them great for soups and stews.

BELUGA & PUY LENTILS ② We cook lentils al dente, not until completely tender, especially when using them as the base of a salad. Black beluga and green Puy lentils hold their shape better than softer red and yellow varieties. Their peppery, rich flavour makes these lentils a staple in our kitchen.

BLACK BEANS ③ Great for adding a statement black colour to any dish, we mainly use these beans in South American-inspired dishes.

BUTTER BEANS ④ Mild and creamy in texture, these are perfect for making a potato-free mash. Adding some tinned butter beans to a salad makes it a little more filling.

CANNELLINI BEANS ⑤ These are buttery, soft and plump, and great for absorbing flavours, which makes them perfect for salads or slow-cooked stews and casseroles.

CHICKPEAS ⑥ Popular in Middle Eastern, Indian and Mediterranean cooking, chickpeas appear often in our recipes. You can use tinned for a quick hummus, or soak dried chickpeas overnight to cook in casseroles for a firmer texture. You can also roast chickpeas to make a crisp snack.

HARICOT BEANS ⑦ Similar to cannellini beans, haricots are lightly sweet and very creamy. We use them for our beans on toast recipe.

KIDNEY BEANS ⑧ So called because of their shape, kidney beans have a thick skin and sweet taste. They are delicious puréed for a creamy side dish or in stews.

MUNG BEANS ⑨ Earthy and nutty, these brilliant green beans are the star of the show in our mung bean curry (see page 167).

PINTO BEANS ⑩ These speckled, light brown Mexican beans are great in stews and salads.

QUINOA ⑪ Packed with protein and fibre plus essential minerals, quinoa has long been considered one of the most nutritious of foods. What makes it unique is that it is a complete protein – it contains all of the essential amino acids. Quinoa has a delicious nutty flavour and crunchy texture. We use it in lots of salads, or overcook it to add to burgers or fishcakes as an alternative to potato.

RED LENTILS ⑫ These are used widely in Indian cooking – red lentil dal is one of my favourite dishes. Soft and earthy in flavour, lentils are so easy to cook.

NUTS & SEEDS

Nuts and seeds are a great way to add crunch and depth of flavour to a dish, but the health benefits are also significant. Rich in good fats, protein and minerals, the following nuts and seeds feature heavily in our recipes.

ALMONDS Rich in vitamin E, almonds are great for your skin. Try mixing them with dried goji berries for a quick mid-morning booster, or toast them and toss into a salad or stew to add a delicious crunch. Ground almonds are ideal for baking.

BRAZIL NUTS Great for snacking on, brazils are also good chopped and sprinkled over a salad or bowl of muesli. These nuts are one of the richest sources of the mineral selenium, an antioxidant that helps protect the body from the damaging effects of free radicals.

CASHEW NUTS The creamiest of all the nuts, we use cashews at every opportunity. Once soaked in water, they are perfect for puréeing to add to sauces or dressings. Cashews are rich in magnesium, which helps maintain healthy bones.

CHIA SEEDS A rich source of healthy omega 3 fats and fibre, these tiny black or white seeds can easily be added to your everyday diet for an extra nutritional boost. We sprinkle them on breakfasts or mix into smoothies.

COCONUT We like to use toasted and desiccated coconut in breakfasts and puddings to sweeten them naturally.

FLAXSEEDS Also known as linseeds, the health benefits of these tiny brown or yellow seeds have been appreciated for centuries. They are a great source of omega 3 fatty acids as well as both soluble and insoluble fibre. Crush them and add to smoothies or sprinkle over your breakfast. Flaxseed oil also has beneficial properties.

HAZELNUTS These nuts are perfect for both sweet and savoury dishes. One of my favourite recipes is salmon with green beans, orange and toasted hazelnuts (see page 235).

PECANS Our granola wouldn't be the same without the pecans. Lightly toasted, they become much sweeter and are a great addition to puddings.

PISTACHIO NUTS It is a labour of love shelling pistachios, but they taste so much better, and somehow more nutty, than those you can buy already shelled. We use pistachios in puddings and salads.

PUMPKIN SEEDS A good source of healthy fats and minerals, including magnesium and zinc, pumpkin seeds are a great nutritious addition to breakfasts and puddings. With their subtle flavour, they are also a good, crunchy garnish for most savoury dishes.

SESAME SEEDS Use black and white sesame seeds to add texture and a smoky flavour to dishes. Black sesame looks good in colourful salads, speckling them for contrast. Toast the seeds to extract maximum flavour.

SUNFLOWER SEEDS These have a similar nutritional content to pumpkin seeds (see above). We use masses of sunflower seeds, often lightly toasted, throwing them into any dish to add some crunch and depth. They are also great in pesto.

WALNUTS These nuts are a good source of omega 3 fats. Lightly roasted with a drizzle of honey, they make an excellent snack. Buy the best quality walnuts you can afford as they will taste much creamier and less bitter than cheaper nuts.

DRIED FRUIT

Dried fruit is a great natural sweetener, although it's best used in small quantities as it is high in calories. Sprinkle a little over your breakfast or throw some into salads to add soft texture and sweetness. Dried fruit also provides a good source of fibre, which helps to support digestion. When buying dried fruit, always make sure that it is unsweetened and unsulphured, which means it doesn't contain additives or preservatives.

APRICOTS Unsulphured apricots are darker in colour and less sweet than the sulphured ones. They are delicious in tagines and stews.

DATES We use dates to sweeten our puddings, cakes and oat bars. Puréed, they work well to bind ingredients together in the same way that refined sugar would.

GOJI BERRIES A 'super berry' rich in antioxidants, gojis have a slightly bitter taste. They are perfect on their own as a healthy snack or make a great addition to oat breakfasts.

GOLDEN BERRIES Also known as cape gooseberries, golden berries are sweet/slightly sour berries native to Brazil. Add them to breakfasts or have as a snack during the day.

GOLDEN RAISINS Slightly sweeter than normal sultanas, these are perfect in breakfasts, salads and puddings.

DAIRY ALTERNATIVES

Even if you choose not to completely eliminate dairy foods from your diet, you may want to opt for dairy alternatives most of the time. It is best to choose fortified, plant-based milks that have a similar nutritional profile to cow's milk to ensure you will still get all the nutrients you need.

ALMOND MILK Try our recipe on page 32. We mainly use almond milk in baking and smoothies.

COCONUT MILK (AND YOGURT) Containing good natural fats, coconut milk is perfect for curries and soups as well as puddings. Note though that it is high in calories, so use in moderation or opt for a reduced-fat variety if you're looking to lose weight.

NUT BUTTER So easy to make (see our recipe on page 63), nut butter is a great protein booster. Creamy nuts such as cashews and almonds work particularly well. It makes a nutritious spread, and we sometimes use it to thicken stews too.

OAT MILK The least expensive of the dairy alternatives, oat milk is great for porridge.

RICE MILK The sweetest of all the non-dairy milks, this works well with muesli and granola and in smoothies.

SOYA YOGURT This is looser than normal yogurt and has a slightly bitter flavour, but is delicious mixed with a little honey and fresh fruit.

NATURAL SWEETENERS

Although sugar features very little in our cooking, sometimes something sweet is needed, and for this we always turn to natural sugars found in fruit (and some vegetables), honey or spices.

FRUIT JUICE Add the juice of an apple or pear to a breakfast or pudding for a natural sweet boost. Puréed and reduced apple or pear sauce is also a great alternative to eggs in pancake, cake or muffin mixtures.

HONEY Rich in antioxidants, good-quality honey is the perfect substitute for refined sugar. Raw honey, which hasn't been heated, pasteurised or processed, is the best choice to retain natural flavours. If you can get fresh honey straight from the producer, do so. The taste will be sublime compared to that of shop-bought honey. For most vegans, honey is not suitable; the best alternative is maple syrup.

RAW CACAO POWDER The raw form of chocolate, cacao powder is rich and intense in flavour with a natural sweetness. It is a good source of iron and magnesium, as well as antioxidants and other unique compounds that may benefit health. Use cacao powder in cakes, mousses, chocolate milk, hot chocolate and smoothies for the perfect healthy chocolate fix.

VANILLA A real treat to use, vanilla adds a fragrant, sweet note that can't be matched by any other ingredient. We like to use vanilla pods: although more expensive than extract, one pod can go a long way. Once the seeds inside the pod have been removed, put the empty pod in almond milk to infuse it with vanilla flavour. Try this over your breakfast to add extra sweetness.

FLOURS

There are so many great non-wheat flour options now, which is good news for us healthy bakers. In most supermarkets you can buy a pack that will simply be labelled 'gluten- and wheat-free flour': this tends to made from a mixture of rice and buckwheat. There will be a much wider variety of flours in healthfood shops.

Baking with gluten- and wheat-free flour can be slightly more difficult than using wheat flours because it is gluten that gives cakes and bread their 'spring'. Without it, they may be more crumbly, with a slightly denser texture. Our recipes take all of this into account, and we use ingredients that help to bind and lighten.

ALMOND FLOUR Simply finely ground almonds, this is perfect for making pastry bases, giving them a lovely nutty flavour.

ARROWROOT This is a starch obtained from the tubers of various tropical plants. It will act as a binder when gluten isn't present, so we often add arrowroot when baking if we know that the ingredients will need help holding together.

BAKING POWDER & BICARBONATE OF SODA Gluten-free baking powder and bicarbonate of soda are available in most supermarkets. They act in the same way as the normal versions.

BUCKWHEAT FLOUR Very versatile buckwheat flour acts similarly to a normal plain wheat flour, although it gives a slightly grainier texture. We mix it with equal quantities of rice flour and use it in pancakes, scones and cakes, or as a binder for fishcakes and burgers.

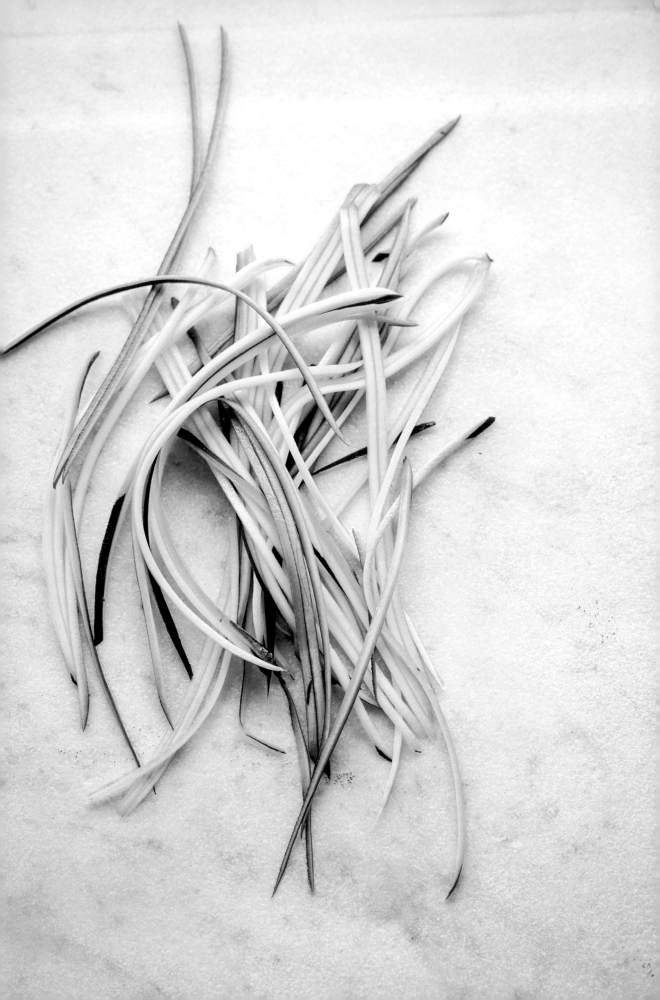

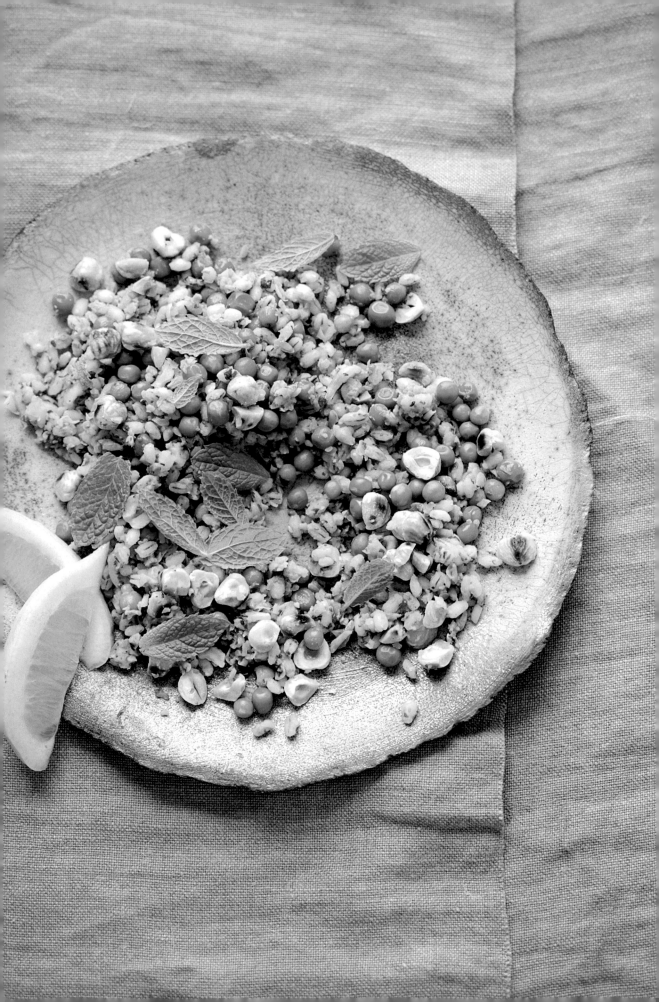

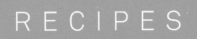

RECIPES

BREAKFASTS

'Breakfast is the most important meal of the day.' It's a familiar phrase, but we all know that it is sometimes hard to put into action. In the morning, every extra minute of sleep seems precious and once you're up, there are always so many things to do. But it's worth making the effort because research shows that those who eat breakfast have a more balanced diet throughout the day and are more likely to maintain a healthy weight.

When we're rushed we often reach for nutrient-poor, sugary cereals or quick fixes made from refined carbohydrates such as white flour. By mid-morning we're starving because these foods are quickly digested, giving a burst of energy that is often swiftly followed by a drop in blood sugar levels. This leaves us grabbing snacks to satisfy our hunger. The key to overcoming this is to eat a breakfast that contains slow-release carbohydrates (to maintain steady energy levels) as well as a little protein, and healthy fats to help keep us feeling fuller for longer.

One great way of ensuring your first meal of the day is a nutrient powerhouse is to supercharge your breakfast with healthy toppings. Try sprinkling some flaxseeds on your cereal; stir nuts and seeds into your fruit and yogurt pot; or add a vegetable-based juice to your morning ritual.

It's a no-brainer to decide to eat a nutrient-rich breakfast each day. The recipes in this section will inspire you to celebrate breakfast-time and ensure that every morning you start the day in the healthiest, most wholesome way.

At the end of most of the recipes, you'll find a list of the main nutrients supplied in a serving as well as a list of health issues that may be benefited by including the recipe in your healthy diet. For more, see page 9.

BEETROOT & APPLE BIRCHER MUESLI

SERVES 2 • 450 CALORIES PER SERVING

Swiss physician Maximilian Bircher-Benner, who created muesli in the 1890s, included more fruit than grains in his recipe. The muesli here is extra fruity too, with a bright pink fruit juice adding a fresh sweetness. Of course, you can serve it instead with your choice of milk – rice milk is a Detox Kitchen favourite – but do give the beetroot and apple juice a go. It has a delicious zing to it that is perfect for a morning boost.

RICH IN Folate • Potassium • Magnesium • Iron • Phytoestrogens • Nitrates • Fibre

USEFUL FOR Heart ①②③ • Bones ① • Digestion ① • Immunity ① • Mind ② • Fatigue ①⑤ • Men ① • Women ①③④

FOR THE MUESLI

160g jumbo oats

1 tbsp rapeseed oil

50ml rice milk

1 tsp desiccated coconut

1 tbsp flaked almonds

20g dried golden berries or sultanas

20g dried goji berries

2 tbsp plain soya yogurt, to serve

FOR THE JUICE

4 large eating apples

1 small raw beetroot

1 Preheat your oven to 200°C/fan 180°C/gas 6. Line a baking tray with greaseproof paper.

2 Put the oats in a large bowl and add the rapeseed oil and rice milk. Use your hands to mix it all thoroughly to ensure the oats are all moistened – unlike granola, you don't want the oats to clump together.

3 Tip on to the lined baking tray and spread out evenly. Bake in the heated oven for 12 minutes until golden. Remove the oats from the oven and allow to cool.

4 Once cold, transfer the oats to a bowl and mix with the desiccated coconut, flaked almonds, golden berries and goji berries. (You can make this muesli in 1kg batches – just multiply the ingredients by five and keep in an airtight container for up to 4 weeks.)

5 Wash the apples and beetroot, then cut them in half and juice them. They should produce around 400ml of juice.

6 Divide the muesli between two bowls. Split the juice between the two portions and add a spoonful of soya yogurt to each, then tuck in.

APPLE, BLUEBERRY & CINNAMON BIRCHER MUESLI

SERVES 2 • 400 CALORIES PER SERVING

Fresh and zingy, this is the perfect summer breakfast to enjoy with a cup of peppermint tea. It is every bit as filling as porridge but with a delicious lightness. Starting your day with an oat-based cereal like muesli or porridge has great benefits because oats contain a type of soluble fibre called beta-glucan that has been shown to help reduce levels of LDL ('bad') cholesterol. In the past, the oats for making muesli were soaked overnight to create a soft creamy texture, but that isn't necessary these days as commercial oats are usually softened through a steaming process.

3 eating apples
140g porridge oats
A handful of flaked coconut
20g blueberries
20g whole blanched (skinned) almonds
1 tbsp plain soya yogurt
A pinch of ground cinnamon
Finely shredded zest of 1 lime

1 Wash two of the apples and juice them, then pour the juice into a large bowl. Grate the other apple – you don't need to peel it, just grate until you get to the core. Add to the juice in the bowl.
2 Now add the porridge oats, flaked coconut, blueberries, whole almonds, yogurt, cinnamon and lime zest. Mix together. Cover with clingfilm, place in the fridge and leave for 15 minutes before serving. (The muesli can be kept in the fridge for 5 days, so you could make enough for the whole week on Sunday night.)

RICH IN Vitamins B1 (thiamin) and E •
Magnesium • Fibre

USEFUL FOR Heart ① ③ • Bones ① • Digestion ① •
Immunity ① • Mind ① • Fatigue ⑤ • Men ① •
Women ① ③

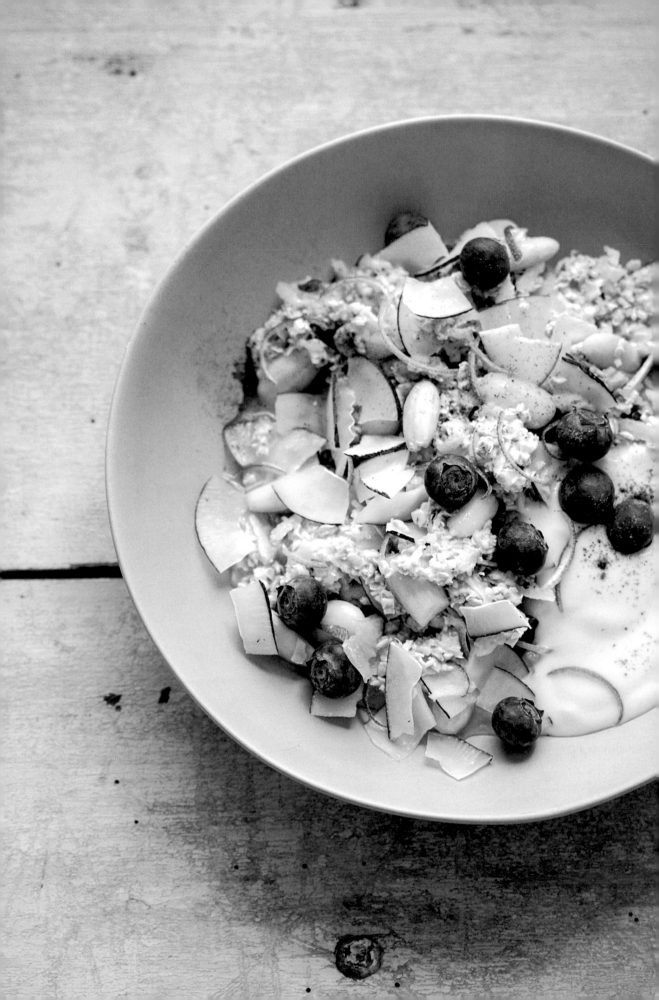

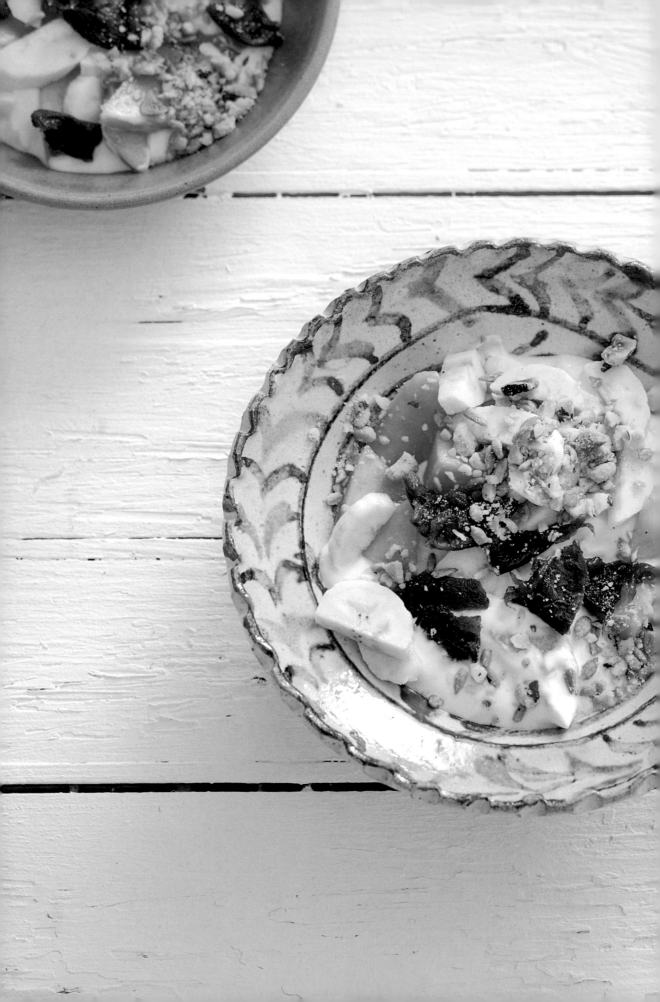

MANGO YOGURT WITH DRIED APRICOTS & BANANA

SERVES 2 • 400 CALORIES PER SERVING

The fruit yogurts you buy are always very sweet. If you make your own, adding fruit and nuts to soya yogurt, the fruit flavours will be fresh and their natural ripe sweetness will make the yogurt taste very indulgent.

1 ripe mango
4 tbsp plain soya yogurt
1 banana, sliced
100g dried apricots, roughly chopped
50g brazil nuts, roughly chopped
A handful of sunflower seeds

1 Cut the mango in half, slicing down on either side of the stone. Score the flesh in each half and scoop it out with a spoon. Then remove the rest of the flesh surrounding the stone. Finely dice all the mango flesh.
2 Put the mango in a bowl with the soya yogurt and fold together. Cover and chill for 20 minutes. This will help the flavours to develop.
3 To serve, simply spoon the yogurt into two bowls, add the sliced banana and top with the dried fruit, nuts and seeds.

RICH IN Vitamins B1 (thiamin), C and E • Selenium • Potassium • Magnesium • Fibre

USEFUL FOR Heart ①② • Bones ① • Digestion ① • Immunity ① • Mind ② • Fatigue ⑤ • Men ① • Women ③

STRAWBERRY SOYA YOGURT

SERVES 4 • 70 CALORIES PER SERVING

This recipe is based on soya yogurt, which contains a group of phytoestrogens (oestrogen-like chemicals found in plants) known as soy isoflavones; these may help to ease the symptoms of PMS. The yogurt also works brilliantly with raspberries, blueberries, blackberries, kiwi, mango or banana – just finely dice the fruit and mix it through. If the fruit you use is sweet and ripe, you won't need to add much honey for sweetening.

4 large strawberries (for drying)
100g strawberries, finely diced
½ vanilla pod, split open lengthways
300ml plain soya yogurt
1 tsp runny honey, or to taste

1 Preheat your oven to 70°C/fan 50°C/gas low. Line a baking tray with baking parchment.
2 Thinly slice the large strawberries, then lay them on the baking tray in one layer. Leave to dry in the oven for 1 hour, then allow to cool – the strawberries will become crisp.
3 Put the diced fresh strawberries in a large mixing bowl. Scrape the seeds from the vanilla pod and add to the bowl along with the yogurt. Sweeten to taste with honey.
4 Serve in little bowls topped with a sprinkle of dried strawberry.

RICH IN Vitamin C • Phytoestrogens • Fibre

USEFUL FOR Heart ①② • Digestion ① • Immunity ① • Men ① • Women ①③④

PECAN & COCONUT GRANOLA

MAKES 500G FOR 10 SERVINGS • 200 CALORIES PER SERVING

Typically, granola is bound together with honey and oil in fairly large quantities, meaning that it can be quite an unhealthy breakfast option. The easy version here uses just a drizzle of honey and a small quantity of coconut oil. This oil contains unique medium-chain fatty acids (MCFAs) that are directed straight to the liver, where they are broken down and used as a quick energy store. The granola is best served with lots of fresh berries and a big dollop of coconut yogurt or plain soya yogurt.

1 tbsp coconut oil
400g porridge oats
150ml rice milk
1 tbsp runny honey
40g pecans
A pinch of ground cinnamon
20g flaked coconut

1 Preheat your oven to 200°C/fan 180°C/gas 6. Line a baking tray with greaseproof paper.
2 Melt the coconut oil, either in a small pan on a low heat or in the microwave. Combine the oats, rice milk, coconut oil and honey in a bowl and mix together using your hands. You want to create little chunks and the mixture will naturally stick together.
3 Spread the oat mixture evenly in the lined baking tray and bake in the heated oven for 20 minutes.
4 Spread the pecans on another baking tray and put into the oven to toast with the oat mixture for the last 10 minutes of the cooking time.
5 Remove the oats and pecans from the oven and leave to cool. Once cold, mix them together and add the cinnamon and flaked coconut. The granola will keep for 2 weeks stored in an airtight jar.

RICH IN Phosphorus • Fibre

USEFUL FOR Heart ① • Bones ① • Digestion ① • Immunity ①

GRANOLA WITH PINEAPPLE & STRAWBERRIES

SERVES 2 • 335 CALORIES PER SERVING

Pineapple and strawberry make a wonderful fruit combination. Both are juicy and succulent, and they complement each other in equal measures of sourness and sweetness. The fruit works deliciously well with granola and slightly tart soya yogurt. Pineapple contains an enzyme called bromelain, which has the ability to break down protein, so may be useful to aid digestion (particularly after a meal rich in protein).

100g strawberries, cut in half or into quarters (depending on size)
100g fresh pineapple chunks
100g Pecan & Coconut Granola (see left)
150ml plain soya yogurt
25g toasted pumpkin seeds
2 sprigs of fresh mint, leaves picked

1 Layer up the strawberries, pineapple, granola and dollops of soya yogurt in two small bowls.
2 Garnish each bowl with toasted pumpkin seeds and mint leaves before serving.

RICH IN Vitamin C • Magnesium • Phytoestrogens • Bromelain • Fibre

USEFUL FOR Heart ①②③ • Bones ① • Immunity ① • Mind ② • Fatigue ⑤

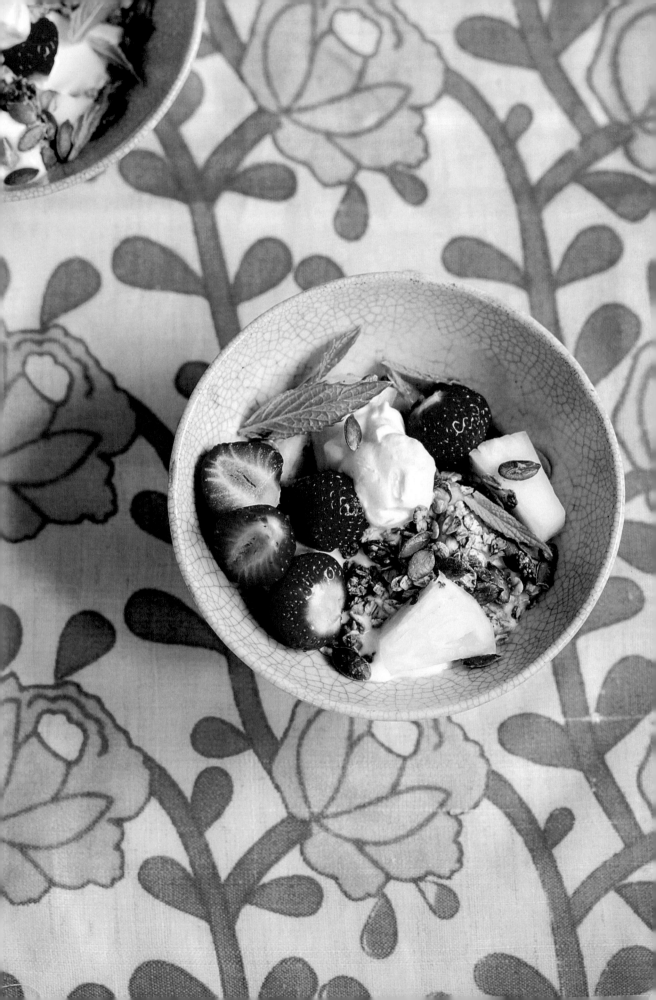

VANILLA ALMOND MILK

SERVES 4 • 155 CALORIES PER SERVING

Although it sounds like it might be a bit time-consuming, creating nut milk is surprisingly simple. All it requires is some good-quality unsalted nuts, a piece of muslin and a bit of elbow grease. This recipe is made with almonds, a rich source of the antioxidant vitamin E, which enhances the body's immune system (this almond milk provides 50 per cent of the RDA in one serving). The milk is flavoured with vanilla, which gives it a natural sweet note.

100g blanched (skinned) almonds
A pinch of salt
½ vanilla pod, split open lengthways

1 Soak the almonds in water overnight.
2 Drain the almonds and place them in a blender with 500ml fresh water and the salt. Scrape the seeds from the vanilla pod and add to the blender. Blend for about 2 minutes until the nuts are finely ground and the liquid is milky.
3 Place a piece of muslin over a large bowl and strain the almond liquid through it. Gather up the ends of the muslin and squeeze tightly to ensure all the liquid has been strained out.
4 Transfer the almond milk to a bottle, seal and chill. This will keep in the fridge for up to 3 days.

RICH IN Vitamin E • Beta-sitosterol

USEFUL FOR Heart ① • Men ① • Women ③

MANGO CUP WITH POMEGRANATE

SERVES 2 • 210 CALORIES PER SERVING

When I was a child, I was shown how to make a mango hedgehog and my love for this fruit was born. The orange flesh is unique in taste and texture – soft, creamy and wonderfully sweet with just a hint of sourness. Like other bright orange fruits and vegetables, mango is a fantastic source of beta-carotene as well as vitamin C, both of which act as antioxidants protecting the body's cells from free radical damage.

1 ripe mango
1 pomegranate
2 sprigs of fresh mint, leaves picked and finely chopped
1 tsp pumpkin seeds
Plain soya yogurt, to serve

1 Using a knife, gently cut into the top of the mango to feel where the long, flat stone is. Once you have found the top of the stone, carefully cut down either side of it to remove two halves of flesh. Score the mango flesh, not cutting through the skin, to create small cubes, then turn each half inside out. (It will look like a little hedgehog.) Slice the cubes off the skin – don't cut through the skin as you will need it for serving. Put the cubes of mango in a bowl.

2 Cut the pomegranate in half and remove the seeds (see Edamame & Seed Salad, page 73). Add to the bowl along with the mint and pumpkin seeds. Mix gently together.

3 Spoon into the mango skins and top each serving with a dollop of soya yogurt.

RICH IN Vitamin C • Phytoestrogens • Beta-carotene • Fibre

USEFUL FOR Heart ①② • Digestion ① • Immunity ① • Skin, hair & nails ①③ • Men ①② • Women ①③④

QUINOA & OAT PORRIDGE WITH BLACKBERRY COMPOTE

SERVES 2 • 425 CALORIES PER SERVING

This is a recipe for a morning when you can linger a little longer at breakfast, particularly in winter when you want something warming and filling. Jumbo oats and quinoa create a slightly coarser texture than normal porridge, which makes this version feel more substantial, yet it is still comfortingly creamy due to the almond milk. It is sustaining, too, as quinoa – a low-carbohydrate grain with a very low glycaemic load – releases energy slowly, helping to maintain steady blood sugar levels. The porridge is topped off with a sharp and sweet blackberry compote.

50g quinoa
250ml Vanilla Almond Milk (see page 32)
100g jumbo oats

FOR THE COMPOTE
1 pear
100g blackberries
1 tsp runny honey
A pinch of freshly grated nutmeg

1 Put the quinoa in a saucepan and cover with the almond milk and 100ml water. Bring to the boil on a medium heat, then turn the heat to low and simmer for 15 minutes, stirring occasionally.

2 While the quinoa is cooking, make the compote. Peel and core the pear, then finely dice. Place in a small saucepan with the blackberries, honey, nutmeg and a splash of water. Bring to the boil on a medium heat, then turn the heat to low and simmer for 10 minutes. Once cooked, remove from the heat and allow to cool slightly. (I like a chunky texture but if you would prefer to have smooth compote, blitz in a food processor and pass through a sieve.)

3 Once the quinoa is soft, add the jumbo oats to the pan and stir for 3 minutes until completely warmed through. Add more almond milk if you prefer a wetter porridge.

4 Spoon the porridge into bowls and top with the warm compote.

RICH IN Folate • Magnesium • Fibre

USEFUL FOR Heart ①③ • Bones ① • Digestion ① • Immunity ① • Mind ② • Fatigue ⑤ • Women ①③

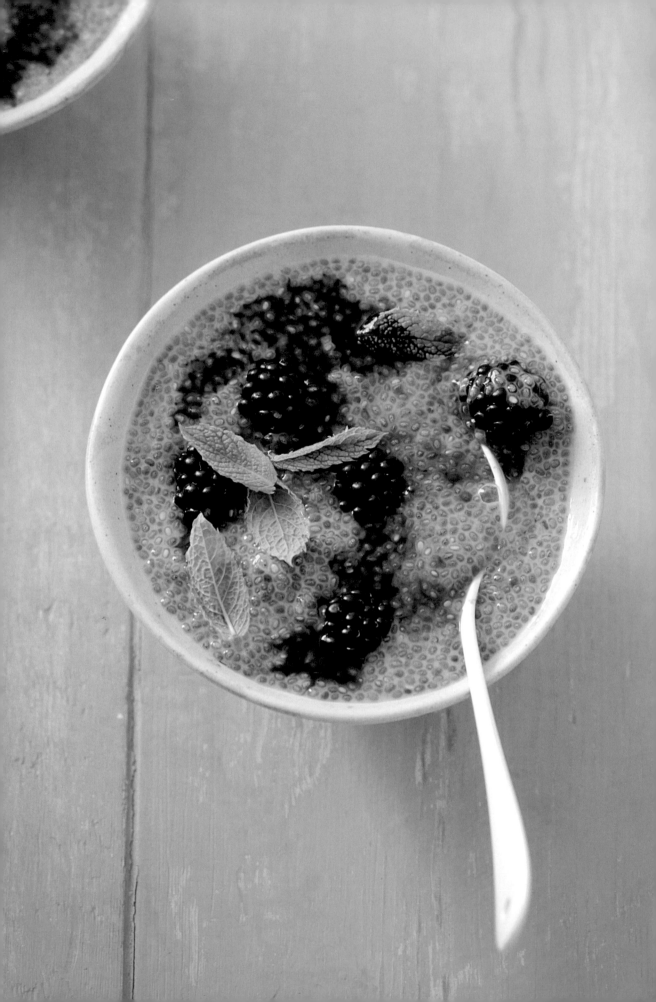

CHIA SEED PUDDING WITH BLACKBERRY & LIME COULIS

SERVES 4 • 270 CALORIES PER SERVING

A great breakfast that you can prepare the night before, this is based on chia seeds, which are a rich source of antioxidants and fibre (with the help of the chia seeds, this pudding provides over a third of your recommended daily fibre intake). When soaked in a liquid they become gelatinous, with a texture very similar to that of tapioca. The blackberry coulis adds a sharpness that is balanced by the addition of honey.

400ml almond milk
3 tbsp runny honey
100g white chia seeds

FOR THE COULIS
Grated zest of ½ lime
150g blackberries
1 tbsp runny honey

TO GARNISH
Blackberries
Fresh mint leaves

1 Put the almond milk, honey and chia seeds in a bowl. Cover with clingfilm and leave in the fridge overnight.

2 For the coulis, combine all the ingredients in a blender or food processor and blitz until smooth. Press through a sieve into a small bowl. Cover with clingfilm and keep in the fridge.

3 In the morning, stir the pudding, then pour it into four small bowls or glasses. Top with the coulis and garnish with a few blackberries and some fresh mint leaves.

RICH IN Vitamins B2 (riboflavin) and E • Magnesium • Calcium • Selenium • Omega 3 • Fibre

USEFUL FOR Heart ①②③ • Bones ①② • Digestion ①②③ • Immunity ① • Mind ① • Fatigue ②③⑤ • Men ①② • Women ①③④

AVOCADO SMASH WITH TOASTED NUTS & SEEDS

SERVES 2 • 460 CALORIES PER SERVING

You may be apprehensive about having a salad for breakfast, but if you try this one with a few slices of toast, you will be converted. The creamy avocado mixed with all of our favourite nuts and seeds and some protein-packed lentil sprouts tastes wonderfully fresh and really will keep you feeling full until lunch. Avocados contain high levels of a plant compound known as beta-sitosterol, which is thought to help balance cholesterol levels.

20g cashew nuts

20g hazelnuts

1 tsp sunflower seeds

1 tsp white sesame seeds

1 tsp black sesame seeds

2 ripe avocados

Juice of 1 lemon

4 fresh chives, finely chopped

50g lentil sprouts

Salt and pepper

TO SERVE

Chopped fresh coriander or micro coriander

Lime wedges

1 Preheat your oven to 200°C/fan 180°C/gas 6.

2 Spread all the nuts and seeds in a small baking tin and toast in the heated oven for 8 minutes until golden. Tip them into a mortar and lightly crush with the pestle. Set aside.

3 Cut the avocados in half and remove the stones, then scoop out the flesh and put it in a large bowl. Add the lemon juice, chives and some salt and pepper and crush with a fork. You want to create a creamy but chunky texture. Add the lentil sprouts and mix through.

4 Add the crushed nuts and seeds to the avocado mix. Serve sprinkled with coriander and with wedges of lime to squeeze over.

RICH IN Vitamins B6 and E • Potassium • Magnesium • Phytoestrogens • Beta-sitosterol • Fibre

USEFUL FOR Heart ①②③ • Bones ① • Digestion ①② • Mind ①② • Fatigue ③⑤ • Men ① • Women ①③④

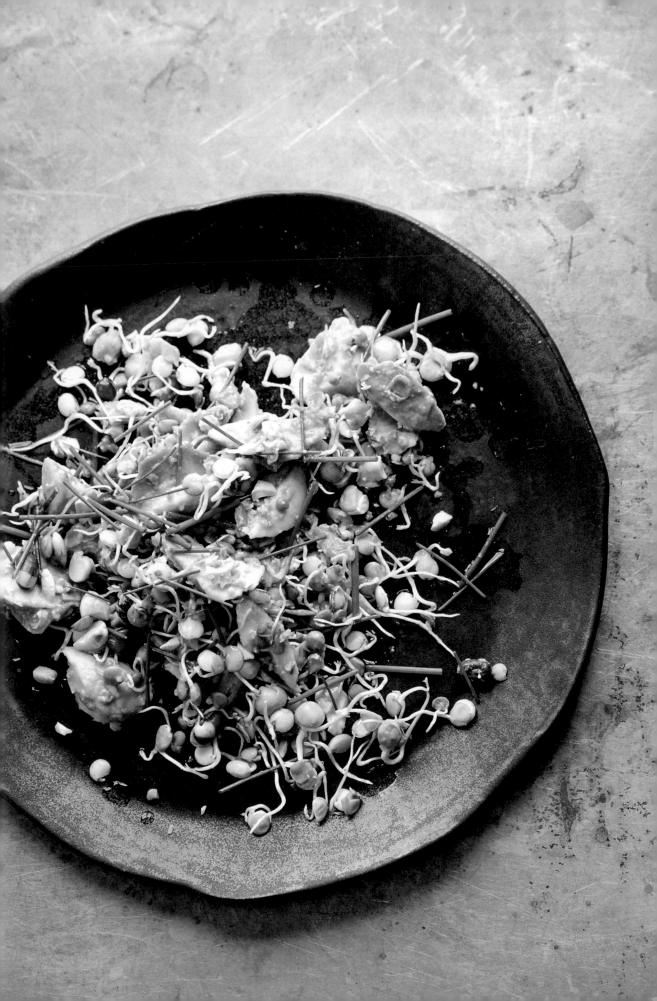

BAKED EGGS WITH SPINACH & TOMATO

SERVES 2 • 265 CALORIES PER SERVING

Eggs baked on a colourful vegetable base make a great sharing breakfast for two. If you multiply the quantities, this is perfect for serving a group of people. Try it with a big pot of fresh mint tea and toasted Quinoa Bread (see page 44). In addition to all their other benefits, eggs are a good source of the mineral iodine, which is needed to make thyroid hormones that control the body's metabolism. A significant number of women in the UK do not get enough iodine in their diets.

1 tsp rapeseed oil
2 shallots, finely diced
1 garlic clove, finely chopped
4 large beef tomatoes, seeded and thinly sliced
10 cherry tomatoes, halved
2 handfuls of fresh coriander leaves, finely chopped
A pinch of paprika
2 handfuls of baby spinach
4 eggs
1 tsp sunflower seeds
Salt and pepper

1 Preheat your oven to 200°C/fan 180°C/gas 6.
2 Heat the oil in a shallow, heavy-based flameproof baking dish or ovenproof frying pan. Add the shallots and garlic and cook on a medium heat for 5 minutes until the shallots start to soften.
3 Now add the beef and cherry tomatoes, half of the coriander, the paprika and a splash of water. Cook, stirring occasionally, for 10 minutes to reduce and thicken.
4 Add the spinach and stir until it has wilted. Make four holes in the mixture and crack an egg into each, making sure not to break the yolk. Sprinkle with the sunflower seeds and season with salt and pepper.
5 Transfer the dish to the heated oven and bake for about 8 minutes until the eggs are cooked (whites firm and yolks soft, or however you like your eggs to be). Sprinkle with the rest of the coriander and serve hot.

RICH IN B vitamins • Vitamins C and D • Potassium • Iron • Tryptophan • Lycopene

USEFUL FOR Heart ②③ • Bones ① • Immunity ① • Mind ① • Fatigue ①③ • Men ①

SOFT-BOILED EGGS WITH AVOCADO SALAD

SERVES 2 • 245 CALORIES PER SERVING

This has become something of a signature dish for the Detox Kitchen – when we cater for breakfast meetings, this salad always features on the menu. It really is a perfectly balanced breakfast: the boiled egg is filling and tasty, and the avocado and lemon combination is tangy and refreshing. Avocados are a good source of the fat-soluble antioxidant vitamin E, which can help to promote healthy skin by protecting skin cell membranes from damage.

2 large eggs, at room temperature
1 avocado
1 lemon, cut in half
1 tbsp pumpkin seeds, toasted
1 tbsp chopped fresh coriander
½ yellow pepper, seeded and finely diced
1 spring onion, finely sliced
Salt and pepper

1 Bring a medium saucepan of water to the boil, then reduce to a simmer. Gently place the eggs in the water, using a tablespoon to ensure the shells don't crack. Cook for 6 minutes. This will give you slightly runny eggs, not completely soft and not completely hard. Cook for a minute more or less, if you prefer. (If the eggs are cold or straight from the fridge, they will take slightly longer to cook.)
2 While the eggs are cooking, peel the avocado and remove the stone. Chop the avocado flesh into small chunks. Place in a bowl and add a squeeze of lemon juice, the pumpkin seeds, coriander, yellow pepper and spring onion. Season to taste, then mix together gently. Divide between two small serving bowls or plates.
3 Once the eggs are cooked, peel them and set on top of the avocado salad. When you cut open the egg, the yolk will mix with the avocado salad to create a rich dressing.

RICH IN Vitamins B6, B12, C and E • Beta-sitosterol • Tryptophan

USEFUL FOR Heart ① • Immunity ① • Mind ① • Fatigue ③ • Men ① • Women ③

POACHED EGGS & SWEET POTATO HASH

SERVES 4 • 275 CALORIES PER SERVING

This is a great recipe for a leisurely weekend breakfast: perfectly poached eggs served on a crisp, spicy potato hash. When you split open the egg, the runny yellow yolk mixes with the orange hash and the fresh red tomato – a feast for the eye! Eggs are one of the few food sources of vitamin D, which is essential for healthy bones.

1 large or 2 small sweet potatoes
2 spring onions, finely sliced
1 tbsp gluten- and wheat-free flour
1 tbsp olive oil
75ml rice milk
A handful of finely chopped fresh coriander
½ fresh red chilli, seeded and finely chopped
Grated zest of 1 lemon
4 or 8 very fresh eggs
Salt and pepper

TO GARNISH
1 beef tomato, seeded and finely chopped
A handful of finely chopped fresh coriander

1 Preheat your oven to 200°C/fan 180°C/gas 6. Line a large baking tray with greaseproof paper.
2 Peel the sweet potato and grate it on to some kitchen paper. Sprinkle with 1 teaspoon of salt and leave for 10 minutes.
3 Transfer the sweet potato to a colander and rinse off the salt, then tip on to a kitchen towel and squeeze out any excess water. Place the potato in a large mixing bowl and add the spring onions, flour, oil, rice milk, coriander, chilli and lemon zest. Mix together using your hands.
4 Divide the mixture into four portions and place, spaced well apart, on the lined baking tray. Flatten each portion roughly to a round cake about 5mm thick: it will be slightly bobbly and misshapen. Bake in the heated oven for about 20 minutes until golden.
5 Meanwhile, poach the eggs. You'll need two wide pans of water (four eggs in each) or you can cook in batches. Bring the water to the boil, then reduce the heat to low so that there are no big bubbles rising.
6 Gently stir the water, then crack the eggs and plop them in – don't try to be gentle, otherwise they will disperse. Turn up the heat to medium so that the water is lightly simmering and poach for 1½ minutes for a runny yolk, or longer if you prefer your yolks firmer. Lift the eggs from the water using a slotted spoon and drain briefly on kitchen paper.
7 Remove the sweet potato hash from the oven and transfer to plates. Set the poached eggs on the hash. To garnish, season the tomato and mix with the coriander, then spoon on top of the eggs. Serve immediately.

RICH IN Vitamins B12 and D • Folate • Selenium • Tryptophan • Beta-carotene

USEFUL FOR Bones ① • Immunity ① • Skin, hair & nails ① • Mind ① • Fatigue ③ • Men ①

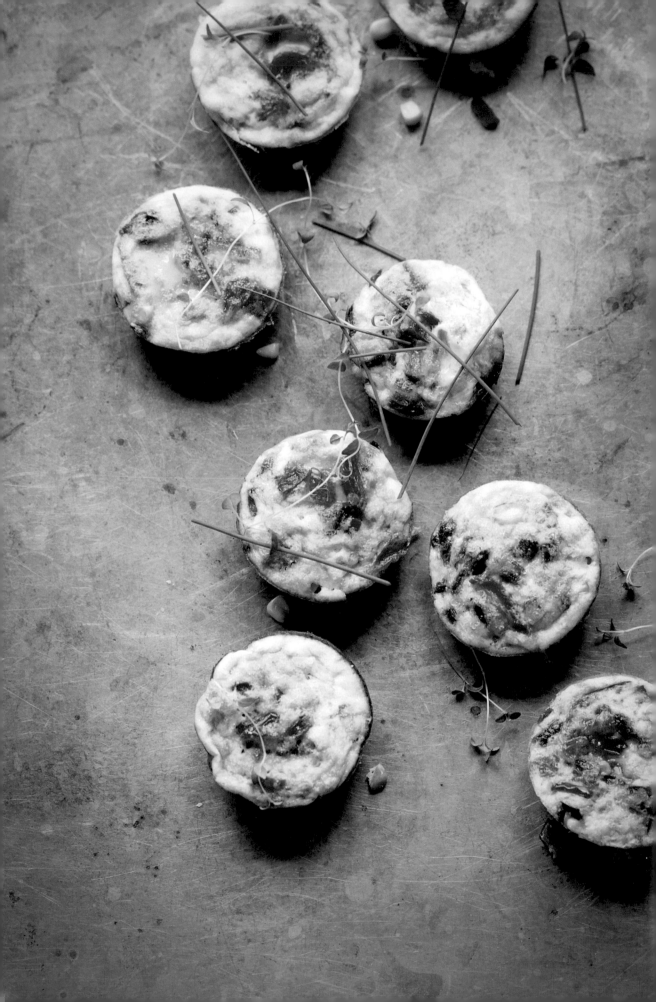

MINI FRITTATAS

MAKES 12 FRITTATAS TO SERVE 4 • 300 CALORIES PER SERVING

These frittatas have a very simple courgette and red pepper filling, but you can vary this. Just keep the egg base the same and add any vegetables you fancy. They are great for a special breakfast and also make a lighter alternative to quiche at a picnic. One serving provides a third of your daily requirement for selenium, which is needed for the proper functioning of the thyroid gland. A significant number of UK adults don't get enough of this essential mineral in their diet.

RICH IN B vitamins • Vitamins C and D • Potassium • Selenium • Beta-carotene

USEFUL FOR Heart ② • Bones ① • Immunity ① • Skin, hair & nails ① • Mind ① • Fatigue ② • Men ① • Women ①③④

1 large red onion
2 garlic cloves
2 red peppers, seeded
1 courgette
1 ear of sweetcorn (corn on the cob), husks and silk removed
1 sprig of fresh thyme, leaves picked
9 eggs
100ml rice milk
Salt and pepper
Snipped fresh chives or micro rocket, to garnish

1 Preheat your oven to 200°C/fan 180°C/gas 6. Lightly oil a non-stick 12-hole muffin tin.
2 Finely dice the onion, garlic, red peppers and courgette and place in a large bowl.
3 Now cut the sweetcorn kernels from the cob. The easiest way to do this is to hold the cob at one end, upright at an angle, with the other end in the centre of a kitchen towel on your work surface, and to run a knife down the cob to remove the kernels. Do this all the way round. Discard the cob and tip the sweetcorn kernels into the bowl.
4 Add the thyme leaves to the vegetables and season with salt and pepper. Spoon the mixture into the holes in the muffin tin, distributing the vegetables equally. Place in the heated oven and cook for 12 minutes.
5 Meanwhile, crack the eggs into a large jug or bowl. Add the rice milk and a pinch of salt and whisk until well mixed.
6 Remove the tin from the oven and set it on a heatproof surface. Pour the egg mixture over the vegetables so that each hole is three-quarters full. Bake for a further 6 minutes until the egg is completely set.
7 The mini frittatas should fall out of the holes easily. Place them on a large plate, garnish with chives or micro rocket and serve.

RASPBERRY PANCAKES

MAKES 8 SMALL PANCAKES TO SERVE 4 •
115 CALORIES PER SERVING

Why not make something a little different and more colourful than the usual big beige griddle cakes – like these pink baby pancakes that look almost too pretty to eat? You can use rice or almond milk instead of the oat milk. Or replace the raspberries with blackberries to create purple versions. Coconut oil makes a great substitute for butter or margarine for frying the pancakes. It contains a type of fat called lauric acid, which holds unique anti-viral properties that may help kill harmful invaders in the body such as bacteria and viruses.

150g raspberries

50ml oat milk

A pinch of ground cinnamon

2 eggs, separated

50g gluten- and wheat-free flour

½ tsp baking powder

1 tsp coconut oil

1 tbsp toasted desiccated coconut

1 Put 100g of the raspberries, the oat milk, cinnamon and egg yolks in a blender or food processor and blitz to make a loose paste. Pour into a bowl.

2 Whisk the egg whites to stiff peaks, then fold gently into the raspberry mixture.

3 Sift the flour and baking powder into another bowl. Add the egg mixture and gently fold into the dry ingredients.

4 Heat the coconut oil in a non-stick frying pan until melted. For each pancake, pour a small ladleful of the batter into the pan, spacing them apart to allow for spreading. Cook the pancakes for 2 minutes on each side.

5 Serve warm, with the remaining raspberries and a sprinkling of toasted coconut.

RICH IN Vitamin B12

USEFUL FOR Mind ①

BANANA MUFFINS

MAKES 12 MUFFINS • 340 CALORIES EACH

These have a slightly denser texture than other muffins due to the high banana content. Everyone who tries them becomes hooked because they are just on the right side of sweet and their oat topping adds a delicious crispness. Bananas are high in potassium, which is essential for maintaining healthy blood pressure. Although our muffins are not a rich source, each one still provides a useful 20 per cent of the RDA.

150g gluten- and wheat-free flour
110g ground almonds
2 tbsp arrowroot powder
1 tsp salt
2 tsp baking powder
2 tsp ground cinnamon
4 ripe bananas, cut into chunks
8 eggs
300g runny honey
3 tbsp rapeseed oil
3 tbsp pumpkin seeds
A handful of porridge oats

1 Preheat your oven to 200°C/fan 180°C/gas 6. Line a 12-hole muffin tin with paper cases.
2 Sift the flour, almonds, arrowroot, salt, baking powder and cinnamon into a large bowl and stir together with a wooden spoon. Set aside.
3 Put the bananas, eggs, honey and oil in a blender and blitz for 1–2 minutes until very smooth.
4 Scatter the pumpkin seeds into a small tin and toast them in the heated oven for 5 minutes. Remove the tin and then turn the oven down to 170°C/fan 150°C/gas 3.
5 Add the pumpkin seeds to the bowl with the dry ingredients, then gradually add the banana mixture, stirring with a wooden spoon. When thoroughly amalgamated, transfer the mixture to a jug.
6 Pour the mixture into the muffin cases until each one is just over half full. Sprinkle the oats on top.
7 Bake for 35 minutes. Transfer the muffins to a wire rack and leave to cool completely. They will keep for 3 days in an airtight container.

RICH IN B vitamins • Vitamins C, D and E

USEFUL FOR Mind ① • Men ① • Women ③

BLUEBERRY & APPLE MUFFINS

MAKES 12 MUFFINS • 260 CALORIES EACH

Ideal for a grab-and-go breakfast, these muffins are perfectly sweet, with little pieces of blueberry and apple running through to add a lovely texture. It was no mean feat creating them – wheat-free, refined sugar-free and dairy-free, but still with the light, fluffy texture that all muffins should have. Ground almonds were the answer. Almonds are one of the richest food sources of vitamin E – you can obtain half of your daily requirement from a 25g serving (12 almonds), so they make a highly nutritious snack. At the Detox Kitchen we often make a batch of these muffins just before people arrive for a meeting, so they're greeted by the delicious sweet aroma of baking.

4 eggs
50ml coconut oil
2 tbsp runny honey
1 large eating apple, cored and cut into 1cm cubes
300g ground almonds
2 tsp baking powder
250g blueberries

1 Preheat your oven to 200°C/fan 180°C/gas 6. Line a 12-hole muffin tin with paper cases.
2 Put the eggs, oil, honey and apple in a blender and blend for 1 minute. Add the ground almonds and baking powder and blend until smoothly combined, with little chunks of apple. Transfer the mixture to a jug.
3 Pour into the muffin cases to fill each one to about 1cm below the rim. Place 7 blueberries in each case and press them into the mixture using a toothpick or the back of a spoon.
4 Bake in the heated oven for 30–35 minutes until risen and golden brown. Leave the muffins to cool before serving.

RICH IN Vitamin E • Beta-sitosterol

USEFUL FOR Heart ① • Men ① • Women ③

QUINOA BREAD

**MAKES 1 SMALL LOAF (CUTS INTO 12 SLICES) •
190 CALORIES PER SLICE**

At the Detox Kitchen we are avid fans of quinoa, so decided to try to create a wheat-free bread based on this powerhouse of a grain (it provides a source of all the essential amino acids). Surprisingly, the first attempt was a success. You will be amazed by how easy this recipe is and how delicious the bread tastes. It is the perfect bread for toasting and serving with some fresh avocado – a great protein-boosting breakfast for vegetarians and vegans in particular.

30g chia seeds

350g quinoa

70ml olive oil

½ tsp bicarbonate of soda

A pinch of flaked sea salt

Juice of ½ lemon

A handful of sunflower seeds

15g nigella seeds

1 Put the chia seeds in a bowl with 100ml water, stir well and leave for 30 minutes. This should form into a gel.

2 Preheat your oven to 200°C/fan 180°C/gas 6. Line a small loaf tin (25.5 x 13.5 x 6cm) with baking parchment.

3 Place the weighed quinoa in a measuring jug, then tip it into a saucepan. Cover with three times its volume of cold water. Bring to the boil and simmer for 3 minutes – the quinoa will only be part-cooked, which is what you want. Drain in a sieve and rinse under running cold water until completely cooled. Leave to drain for a few minutes. This is important because if it is too wet, your bread will be stodgy.

4 Combine the chia gel and quinoa in a food processor and blitz to combine. Add 150ml water together with the olive oil, bicarbonate of soda, salt and lemon juice. Run the food processor for 5 minutes – you want the consistency of the mixture to be quite wet, similar to a muffin batter.

5 Pour the mixture into the loaf tin and cover the top with the sunflower and nigella seeds. Bake in the heated oven for 1 hour until the bread is firm and slightly golden on top.

6 Remove from the oven and allow to cool in the tin for 15 minutes, then transfer to a wire rack and leave to cool completely. Wrap in clingfilm and keep in the fridge, ready to slice when wanted.

RICH IN Folate • Omega 3

USEFUL FOR Heart ①② • Bones ② •
Digestion ③④ • Skin, hair & nails ①③ •
Mind ① • Fatigue ② • Men ② •
Women ①③④

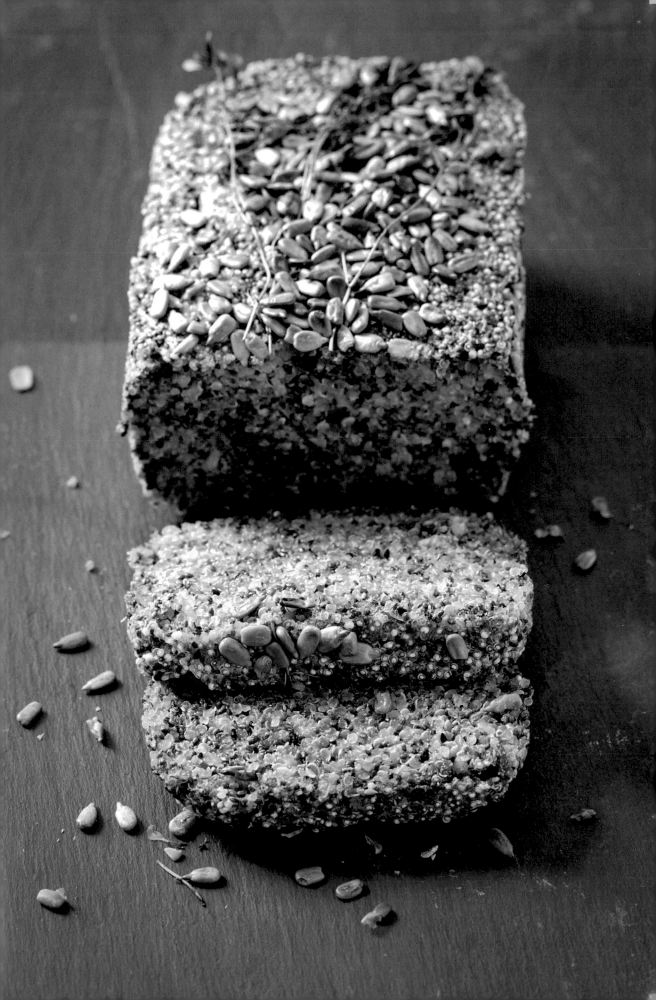

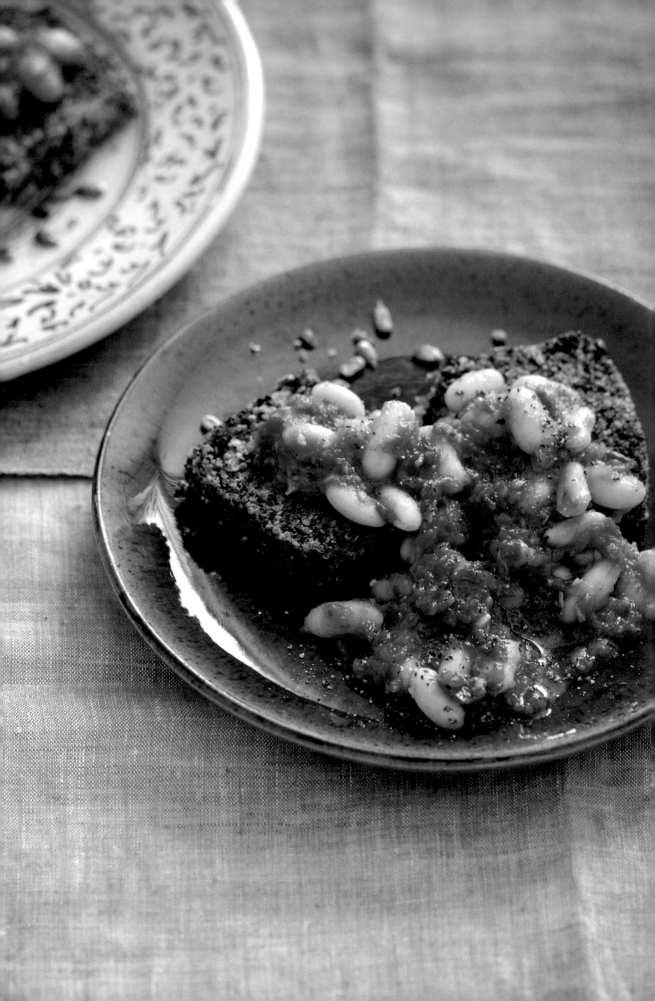

BEANS ON TOAST

SERVES 2 • 220 CALORIES PER SERVING
(WITHOUT TOAST)

Most children seem to have been brought up on beans on toast, and as an adult I feel rather nostalgic about them. But tinned baked beans are packed with hidden sugars. This re-creation of the classic is healthier and, we think, much better. One of the flavourings we've used is dried oregano. Dried herbs provide a concentrated source of iron, making them useful additions to dishes if you're trying to increase this nutrient in your diet (low levels can cause tiredness and fatigue).

300g large vine tomatoes, roughly chopped
1 shallot, roughly chopped
1 garlic clove
1 tsp ground ginger
1 tsp dried oregano
1 tsp runny honey
400g tin cannellini beans or haricot beans, drained and rinsed
Slices of Quinoa Bread (see page 44), toasted, to serve

1 Put the vine tomatoes, shallot, garlic, ginger and oregano in a blender or food processor and blitz to a fairly loose, smooth texture.
2 Pour into a saucepan and add the honey and 4 tablespoons water. Set on a medium heat and bring to the boil, then reduce to a simmer and cook for 30 minutes, stirring occasionally. If the mixture starts sticking to the pan, just add a splash more water.
3 Now add the beans, stir and heat through for a few minutes. Serve on warm slices of toast.

RICH IN Vitamin B6 • Folate • Potassium • Iron • Lycopene • Fibre

USEFUL FOR Heart ② • Digestion ① • Mind ① • Fatigue ① • Men ① • Women ①

JUICES & SMOOTHIES

Over the last few years, it's as if a day hasn't gone by without a celebrity being flashed across the web with a green juice in tow. Freshly pressed fruit and vegetable juices have become all the rage now and cooks across the world are investing in high-tech juice machines. With this has come a lot of information in the press about the health benefits – or lack of them – of juices and smoothies. So the question is: are they actually good for us?

When you juice a piece of fruit or a vegetable you are separating the fibre from the juice. This makes it slightly less nutritious, but it still retains a significant amount of goodness from other nutrients and antioxidants. The fibre is what helps to regulate your blood sugar levels after you eat a whole piece of fruit or vegetable, which is why juices should really be drunk alongside your breakfast or other meal. Although juices add nutritional value to the diet, they don't provide everything you need, so are certainly not a substitute for food.

Instead, a juice or a smoothie should form a welcome addition to your diet. Making a quick green smoothie or juice will give you an extra lift if you are going to be rushing around all day. They should be seen as a nutrient booster rather than a meal replacement. As the sugar and calories are comparable to any other type of soft drink, stick to one glass of juice or smoothie a day.

Always drink a juice as soon as it has been pressed to ensure that you benefit from the nutrients: the longer you leave a juice, the less its nutritional impact will be, because water-soluble vitamins soon start to become depleted (this applies to pressed juices you buy on the go, too).

We like to add little extra boosters to our juices and smoothies, such as stirring a few tablespoons of oats into smoothies. To make a more filling snack, try adding a spoonful of wheatgrass powder (made from the sprouted part of the wheat plant) or spirulina (powdered blue/green freshwater algae) for a small dose of additional nutrients, including certain B vitamins, iron, magnesium and copper. If you're a vegetarian, you could add chia seed oil or crushed flaxseeds for an omega 3 boost.

At the end of most of the recipes, you'll find a list of the main nutrients supplied in a serving as well as a list of health issues that may be benefited by including the recipe in your healthy diet. For more, see page 9.

RASPBERRY, BLUEBERRY & COCONUT WATER SMOOTHIE

SERVES 2 • 110 CALORIES PER SERVING

This is a real treat, very rich and creamy. The coconut water and yogurt create a silky texture and it's packed full of zingy berries. Blueberries and other purple/blue-coloured fruits contain anthocyanins from a group of compounds called flavonoids, which have both antioxidant and anti-inflammatory properties that benefit health. If you keep the smoothie in the freezer, you'll have a quick frozen yogurt – perfect for summer.

100g raspberries

100g blueberries

350ml coconut water

2 tbsp plain soya yogurt

1 tsp runny honey

2 ice cubes

1 Place all the ingredients in a blender and blitz until smooth.

2 Pour into glasses and serve.

RICH IN Vitamin C • Potassium

USEFUL FOR Heart ② • Immunity ①

FRESH GINGER LEMONADE

SERVES 2 • 15 CALORIES PER SERVING

This is a lovely summer drink, delicious served chilled at a barbecue. It's the perfect alternative to sugary fizzy drinks and will have you feeling instantly refreshed.

1 tsp finely grated fresh ginger

Juice of 2 lemons

1 tsp runny honey

Ice cubes, to serve

Edible flowers, to garnish (optional)

1 Put the grated ginger in a jug and add the lemon juice and honey. Stir well, then gradually stir in 400ml water. Leave to chill in the fridge until you are ready to serve.

2 Strain the lemonade over ice cubes in glasses and garnish with small edible flowers, if you like.

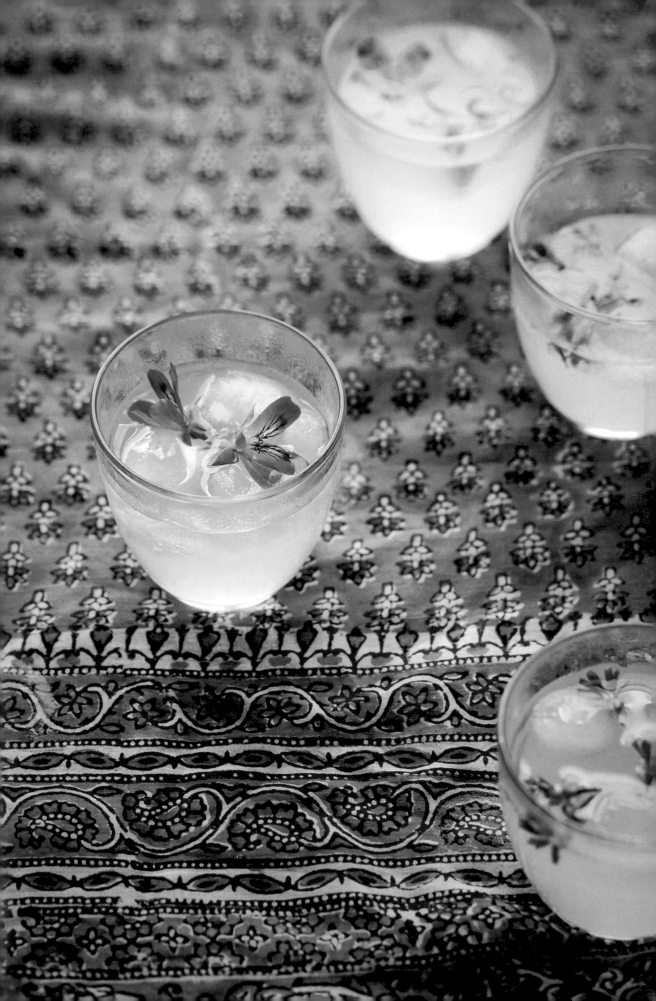

CHIA SEED, COCONUT & PINEAPPLE SMOOTHIE

SERVES 2 • 120 CALORIES PER SERVING

This tropical-tasting juice will whisk you off to a far-away island. The addition of chia seeds adds a delicate crunchy texture. If the core of the pineapple is soft enough, include it in the juice for a supply of the enzyme bromelain, which assists the body in the breakdown of protein, so aiding digestion.

2 pears
1 ripe pineapple, peeled, cored and diced
300ml coconut water
1 tsp chia seeds
1 tbsp plain soya yogurt

1 Wash the pears, then juice them.
2 Place the pineapple in a blender and blitz for 5 minutes. Add the coconut water, pear juice, chia seeds and soya yogurt and blitz for a further 1–2 minutes until smooth. Serve immediately.

RICH IN Vitamin C • Potassium • Bromelain

USEFUL FOR Heart ② • Digestion ④ • Immunity ① • Men ②

GINGER, LEMONGRASS & CLOVE TEA

SERVES 2 • 20 CALORIES PER SERVING

When I was pregnant I completely went off tea. I also suffered from terrible morning sickness, so discovering this genius tea was wonderful. It helped me feel less nauseous – ginger is known to be useful for quelling mild nausea. (And even if you are not pregnant, you'll find this a delicious and refreshing drink!)

A thumb-sized piece of fresh ginger
1 stick of lemongrass, roughly chopped
Grated zest and juice of 1 lemon
1 tbsp runny honey
1 clove

1 Put the ginger, lemongrass, and lemon zest and juice in a blender and blitz to a rough paste.
2 Transfer the paste to a medium-sized saucepan and add the honey, clove and 400ml water. Bring to the boil and leave to simmer for 5 minutes.
3 Strain through a sieve or tea strainer into heatproof glasses and serve hot.

CACAO MILK

SERVES 2 • 270 CALORIES PER SERVING

Raw cacao is a source of the plant chemical theobromine, which acts as a mild stimulant. That's why this drink is the favourite pick-me-up for our Detox Kitchen chefs. It's so delicious and chocolaty, it seems a bit naughty. Best when served chilled.

70g pitted dates
400ml Vanilla Almond Milk (see page 32), or use shop-bought almond milk
1 tbsp raw cacao powder
A pinch of ground cinnamon

1 Put the dates in a bowl and cover with boiling water. Leave to soak for 10 minutes.
2 Drain off the water and place the dates in a blender with 300ml of the almond milk, the cacao powder and cinnamon. Blitz for at least 5 minutes until completely smooth.
3 Add the rest of the almond milk and blitz for a further minute, then serve.

RICH IN Vitamin E • Magnesium • Potassium • Theobromine • Phenylethylamine

USEFUL FOR Heart ②③ • Bones ① • Mind ①② • Fatigue ③⑤ • Women ①③

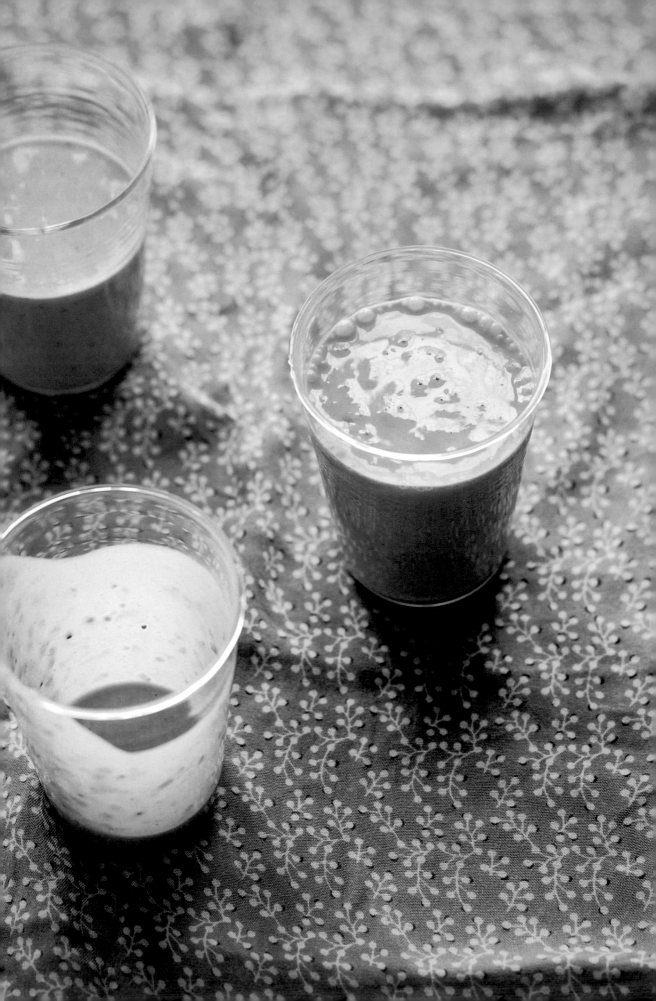

STRAWBERRY & MANGO LASSI

SERVES 2 • 140 CALORIES PER SERVING

This Indian drink is normally made with cow's milk yogurt. We use soya yogurt, which creates a very similar texture. Perfectly ripe fruit will give you a luscious sweet, smooth finish. The drink is rich in vitamin C due to the strawberries; studies have suggested these berries may also hold properties that help to reduce inflammation within the body. Serve the lassi chilled – perfect on a summer's day.

1 ripe mango, peeled and stone removed
100g ripe strawberries, hulled and cut in half
2 tbsp plain soya yogurt
Juice of ½ lime
250ml rice milk
2 ice cubes

1 Place all the ingredients in a blender and blitz until smooth.
2 Serve immediately, over ice. (If you don't have any ice cubes, put the lassi in the fridge to chill a bit before serving.)

RICH IN Vitamin C • Beta-carotene • Phytoestrogens

USEFUL FOR Heart ①② • Bones ② •
Skin, hair & nails ①③ • Men ①② •
Women ①③④

AVOCADO, APPLE, KIWI & SPINACH SMOOTHIE

SERVES 2 • 200 CALORIES PER SERVING

Adding a highly nutritious avocado to your morning juice is a great way to get healthy fats as well as key nutrients, such as beta-carotene (which converts to vitamin A in the body) and vitamin E, into your diet. It's just like adding banana to a smoothie to give it the classic texture, except that the avocado offers an earthy, less sweet flavour. It actually creates a much creamier result than banana.

4 eating apples
6 celery sticks
2 kiwi fruits
1 avocado
2 handfuls of spinach
2 ice cubes
A squeeze of lemon

1 Wash the apples and celery, and peel the kiwi fruits, then put them all through the juicer.
2 Pour the juice into a blender and add the avocado flesh, spinach, ice and lemon juice. Blitz for 1–2 minutes until completely smooth. Serve immediately.

RICH IN Vitamins C and E • Potassium •
Beta-carotene • Beta-sitosterol

USEFUL FOR Heart ①② • Immunity ① •
Men ①② • Women ③

HOT APPLE SMOOTHIE

SERVES 2 • 110 CALORIES PER SERVING

At the Detox Kitchen, we like to have a fresh juice every day, even in winter. On cold days, though, something warm is called for. This hot smoothie, which is one of our favourites, is comforting and delicious. It's spiced with cinnamon, which research suggests may help to reduce blood glucose levels and so could be useful for people trying to manage their blood sugar.

4 eating apples
2 celery sticks
A pinch of freshly grated nutmeg
1 cinnamon stick
1 star anise

1 Wash the apples and celery, then put them through the juicer.
2 Pour the juice into a medium-sized saucepan and add the nutmeg, cinnamon stick and star anise. Bring to the boil, then leave to simmer for 5 minutes.
3 Strain through a sieve or tea strainer into heatproof glasses and serve hot.

USEFUL FOR Heart ② • Immunity ①

CARROT, BEETROOT, APPLE & CELERY JUICE

SERVES 2 • 105 CALORIES PER SERVING

Consisting of three vegetables and a fruit, this juice has a deep, earthy flavour with a little sweetness. The squeeze of lime at the end is essential to give a little sour kick. Beetroot juice is rich in nitrates, which widen blood vessels and may help to reduce high blood pressure.

1 raw beetroot
3 carrots
4 eating apples
5 celery sticks
2 ice cubes
A squeeze of lime

1 Wash the beetroot, carrots, apples and celery, then put them all through the juicer.
2 Pour the juice into a blender. Add the ice and lime juice and blitz until the ice has melted. Serve immediately.

RICH IN Vitamin C • Folate • Potassium • Nitrates

USEFUL FOR Heart ② • Immunity ① • Men ②

CUCUMBER, PEAR, MINT & WHEATGRASS JUICE

SERVES 2 • 115 CALORIES PER SERVING

Fresh cucumber juice mixed with nutrient-dense wheatgrass powder makes a great pick-me-up during the day. Mint adds a light, clean taste. The kale is blended to a purée rather than juiced, which preserves more of its nutrients as well as giving the finished juice a thicker texture and brighter green colour.

2 cucumbers
4 pears
200g kale
1 tsp wheatgrass powder
A handful of fresh mint leaves
2 ice cubes
A squeeze of lemon

1 Wash the cucumbers and pears, then put them through the juicer.
2 Pour the juice into a blender and add the kale, wheatgrass powder, mint, ice and lemon juice. Blitz until smooth, then serve.

RICH IN B vitamins • Vitamin C • Potassium • Calcium • Magnesium • Iron

USEFUL FOR Heart ② • Bones ① • Immunity ① • Mind ①② • Fatigue ①③⑤ • Men ② • Women ①③

SNACKS & DIPS

Whilst snacking on unhealthy foods can lead to weight gain, we are big believers in the benefits of healthy snacking, because busy lives can leave you hungry between meals. In the detox plans at the back of this book – and for our Detox Kitchen delivery service – your day's meals will generally look like this: breakfast, snack, lunch, snack, dinner.

It's a good idea to have simple snack foods such as nuts or dried berries within reach – a couple of handfuls of these will tide you over until the next meal and quash that craving for sugary foods. They will also help regulate blood sugar levels.

In this chapter you'll find recipes for a variety of snacks to satisfy your level of hunger. Many of our main dishes are light, so opting for a nutritious dip in between meals, or as a starter, may be just the ticket to make you feel satiated.

At the end of most of the recipes, you'll find a list of the main nutrients supplied in a serving as well as a list of health issues that may be benefited by including the recipe in your healthy diet. For more, see page 9.

GUACAMOLE

SERVES 4–6 • 140–200 CALORIES PER SERVING

This classic Mexican dip is so quick and easy to put together. The key is to always make it fresh so that it has vibrant colour and tastes zingy. Guacamole is one of the most popular ways to use avocado, which provides oleic acid, shown to lower LDL ('bad') cholesterol. Try this with Mixed Seed Crackers (see page 77).

4 ripe avocados

Juice of 1 lime

3 ripe vine tomatoes, seeded and finely diced

½ red onion, finely diced

A handful of fresh coriander, finely chopped

½ fresh red chilli, seeded and finely chopped

Salt and pepper

1 Scoop the flesh from two of the avocados into a blender or food processor. Add half of the lime juice and blitz to a smooth paste.

2 Scoop out the flesh from the remaining avocados and place in a mixing bowl with the rest of the ingredients. Add the blitzed avocado and combine well to a lumpy texture. Season to taste with salt and pepper.

RICH IN Vitamins B6 and E • Potassium • Lycopene • Beta-sitosterol

USEFUL FOR Heart ①② • Mind ① • Men ① • Women ①③

AVOCADO & BROAD BEAN SMASH ON BROWN RICE CAKES

SERVES 2 • 335 CALORIES PER SERVING

Here, brown rice cakes make a light, crisp backdrop for a vibrantly green and fresh-tasting avocado and broad bean smash. This is a great snack, but just double the portion and you can have a delicious breakfast or lunch. Beans and pulses provide a valuable source of protein for vegetarians and vegans.

2 avocados
1 tsp lemon juice
A handful of spinach
50g cooked broad beans (podded but unskinned)
½ cucumber, diced
1 tsp lime juice
A pinch of crushed dried chilli
1 tbsp chopped fresh coriander, plus extra leaves
4 fresh mint leaves, finely chopped, plus extra leaves
Salt and pepper

TO SERVE
4 brown rice cakes
Lime wedges

1 Peel the avocados and remove the stone. Place the flesh from one avocado in a blender with the lemon juice, spinach and broad beans, and blitz to a rough paste.
2 Dice the remaining avocado and place in a bowl with the cucumber, lime juice, chilli, and chopped coriander and mint. Mix through the avocado paste with salt and pepper to taste.
3 Pile on top of the brown rice cakes, add the whole herb leaves and serve, with lime wedges for squeezing over.

RICH IN Vitamins B6, C and E • Folate • Potassium • Beta-sitosterol • Fibre

USEFUL FOR Heart ①② • Digestion ① • Immunity ① • Mind ① • Men ①② • Women ①③

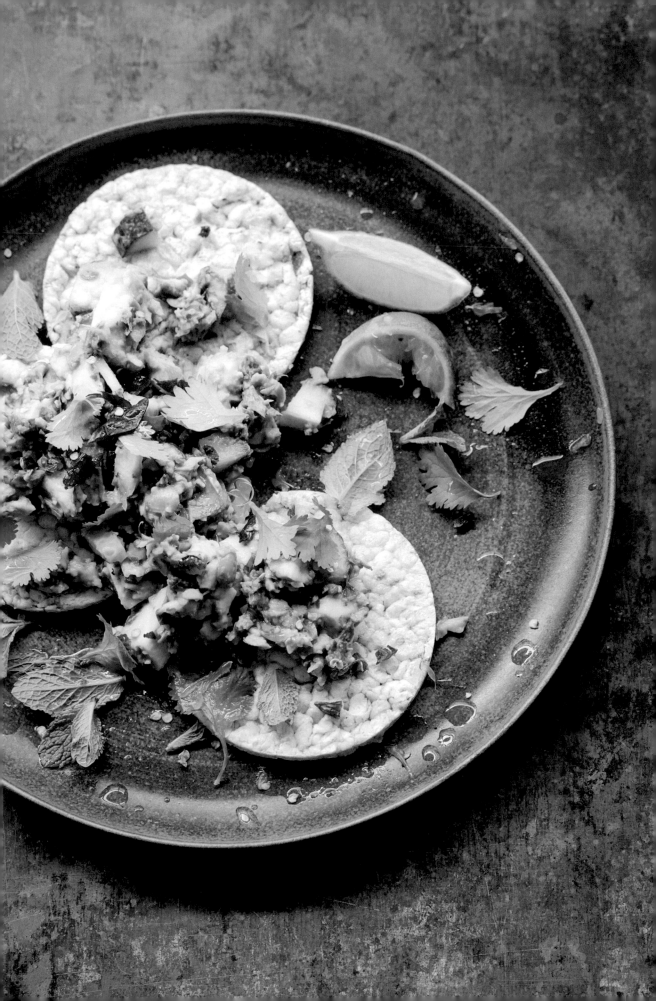

TOMATO & CASHEW CREAM

SERVES 6 • 155 CALORIES PER SERVING

Sun-dried tomatoes have a very concentrated sweet, slightly smoky tomato taste. You only need a few to add deep, rich flavour to a dish. All types of tomatoes offer a rich source of potassium, which can help reduce the chances of cramping after an intense workout. Try teaming this creamy dip with a few oatcakes for a nourishing post-training snack.

2 ripe vine tomatoes
100g sun-dried tomatoes
150g cashew nuts
Juice of ½ lemon
1 tbsp rapeseed oil
A pinch of flaked sea salt
A pinch of pepper

1 Score a cross on the base of each tomato, then place them in a pan of boiling water. Blanch for 20–30 seconds. Remove with a slotted spoon and place straight into a bowl of cold water. Drain and peel off the skin, then cut the tomatoes in half and remove the seeds.

2 Put the peeled tomatoes in a blender with the rest of the ingredients and blitz until smooth.

RICH IN Potassium • Lycopene

USEFUL FOR Heart ①② • Men ①

BROCCOLI STALK & CASHEW SPREAD

SERVES 6 • 165 CALORIES PER SERVING

Here's a great way to use up broccoli stalks when you've taken the florets for another recipe. It's a very savoury mix that can be used as a dip or as an alternative to nut butter – delicious on brown rice crackers.

4 broccoli stalks
Juice of 1 lemon
150g cashew nuts
1 tbsp rapeseed oil
A pinch of flaked sea salt
A pinch of white pepper

1 Bring a medium-sized saucepan of water to the boil. Add the broccoli stalks and boil for 15 minutes until very soft. Drain and rinse under cold water to cool.
2 Put the stalks in a blender, add the remaining ingredients and blitz for 5 minutes until completely smooth.

RICH IN Vitamin C • Chromium

USEFUL FOR Immunity ① • Women ④

CASHEW NUT BUTTER

SERVES 4 • 135 CALORIES PER SERVING

A rich, nutty cream, this makes a perfect alternative to dairy butter. Spread it on toast, add to smoothies, or stir into curries for extra thickness and depth of flavour. Thanks to the cashews, a serving of this butter provides 20 per cent of your recommended daily intake of magnesium. It is important to soak the nuts beforehand to ensure a smooth, creamy texture.

200g cashew nuts
2 tbsp rapeseed oil
A pinch of flaked sea salt

1 Soak the nuts in warm water for 20 minutes.
2 Drain and transfer to a blender. Add the oil and salt and blitz for 5 minutes until completely smooth.
3 Transfer the nut butter to a small container, cover and keep in the fridge for up to 2 weeks.

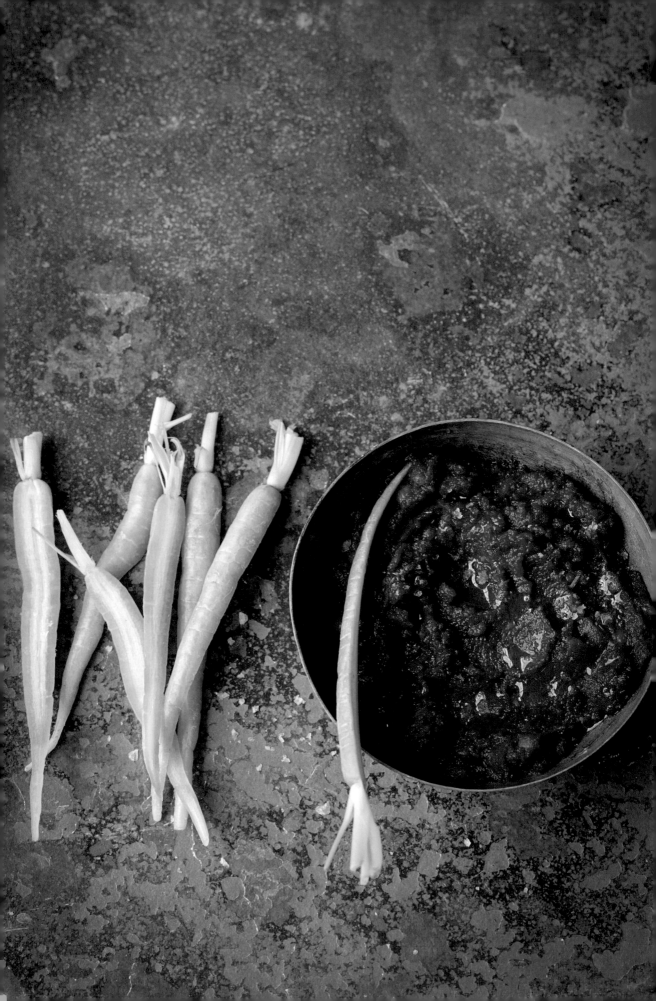

BEETROOT HUMMUS

SERVES 4–6 • 80–120 CALORIES PER SERVING

An unusual alternative to classic hummus, this gorgeous red dip tastes earthy and sweet, and looks brilliantly inviting. Its creamy texture makes it the perfect dip for crudités.

4 large raw beetroots
400g tin chickpeas
Grated zest of 1 orange
Juice of 1 lime
A pinch of ground cumin
1 tsp rapeseed oil
A pinch of flaked sea salt
A pinch of white pepper
Shredded orange zest or chopped fresh coriander, to garnish (optional)
Lime wedges, to serve

1 Preheat your oven to 200°C/fan 180°C/gas 6.
2 Lay out a sheet of foil twice the size of the baking tray you will use, and place the beetroots in the middle of it. Gather up the corners of the foil to create a sealed parcel and place it on the baking tray. Roast in the heated oven for about 40 minutes.
3 Remove from the oven. When the beetroots are cool enough to handle, peel them and put the flesh in a blender.
4 Drain the chickpeas, rinse them with cold water and pat dry with kitchen paper. Add them to the blender along with the orange zest, lime juice, cumin, oil, sea salt and pepper. Blitz until smooth.
5 Transfer to a serving bowl and garnish with the shredded orange zest or coriander, if you like. Serve with lime wedges for squeezing over.

RICH IN Folate • Phytoestrogens • Nitrates • Fibre

USEFUL FOR Heart ①② • Digestion ① •
Women ①③④

RADISHES & CAULIFLOWER WITH HUMMUS

SERVES 4 • 215 CALORIES PER SERVING

Two of the prettiest crudités, cauliflower and radishes both have a slightly peppery flavour and wonderful crunchy texture. They're delicious with this hummus, which is so easy to whizz up that once you've made it fresh, you won't go back to shop-bought ever again. The snack is simple, but it still offers one of your five-a-day!

1 cauliflower
20 radishes
Salt and cracked black pepper

FOR THE HUMMUS
400g tin chickpeas, drained and rinsed
2 tbsp rapeseed oil
1 tsp tahini
Juice of 1 large lemon
A pinch of salt
A pinch of paprika, to garnish

1. To make the hummus, put all the ingredients in a blender and blitz for 2–3 minutes until completely smooth. Remove from the blender and place in a small bowl. Add a dusting of paprika before serving.
2. To prepare the cauliflower, take off all the florets. You want them to be bite-sized, so cut them in half if you need to. Place them in a colander and rinse well.
3. For the radishes, cut off the stringy part of the root and trim the leaves – or keep the leaves on if you wish; they look so pretty and taste great too. Give the radishes a good wash and soak them in cold water for a minute or so to help them to plump up.
4. Add the radishes to the colander with the cauliflower and give everything a final rinse and shake together. Sprinkle the vegetables with salt and cracked pepper and place them in a bowl. Serve with the hummus.

RICH IN Vitamins B6 and C • Potassium • Phytoestrogens • Fibre

USEFUL FOR Heart ①② • Digestion ① • Immunity ① • Mind ① • Men ① • Women ①③④

TENDERSTEM & TAHINI

SERVES 2 • 240 CALORIES PER SERVING

Tenderstem has a slightly sweeter flavour than regular broccoli, and the stem has a texture similar to asparagus. The spears are perfect for dipping into a tahini and avocado mixture as a delicious alternative to classic crudités. Tahini is a great ingredient to include in a vegan diet as it contains a rich source of both iron and calcium, which can be depleted in the absence of meat and dairy foods.

200g Tenderstem broccoli
1 tsp rapeseed oil
1 tbsp sesame seeds
1 tbsp tahini
½ avocado, peeled and diced
Juice of 1 lemon
A pinch of ground cumin
Salt

1. Bring a medium-sized pan of water to the boil and add a pinch of salt. Drop in the Tenderstem and boil for 30 seconds. Drain in a colander and cool quickly under cold running water.
2. Place the Tenderstem on a serving plate. Drizzle the rapeseed oil over the spears and sprinkle with the sesame seeds.
3. Put the remaining ingredients in a blender or small food processor and blitz until smooth. Serve in a little bowl alongside the Tenderstem.

RICH IN Vitamins B6, C and E • Potassium • Iron • Calcium • Chromium • Beta-sitosterol • Fibre

USEFUL FOR Heart ①②③ • Digestion ① • Immunity ① • Mind ① • Fatigue ① • Men ① • Women ①④

TAPENADE

SERVES 2 • 200 CALORIES PER SERVING

A classic Mediterranean dip made with olives and capers, tapenade can have a rough or smooth texture. We prefer it fairly coarse and slather it on Quinoa Bread (see page 44) or Mixed Seed Crackers (page 77).

4 tbsp black olives, pitted

1 tbsp capers

Grated zest and juice of 1 lemon

1 sprig of fresh mint, leaves picked

A handful of fresh coriander

A handful of fresh flat-leaf parsley leaves

1 garlic clove

1 tbsp olive oil

A pinch of flaked sea salt

1 Place all the ingredients in a blender and blitz for 20–30 seconds. This will result in a fairly coarse texture, so if you would prefer it to be smoother, blitz a little longer.

2 Transfer to a bowl for serving.

RICH IN Beta-sitosterol

USEFUL FOR Heart ① • Men ①

RED PEPPER & BUTTER BEAN MASH

SERVES 4–6 • 65–100 CALORIES PER SERVING

Charring red peppers gives them a rich, smoky flavour that blends beautifully with smooth, buttery beans. This is a quick dip to knock up for your friends and is very easy to double if you are expecting more people. Serve it with crudités, in particular raw cauliflower florets or celery sticks.

2 red peppers
400g tin butter beans, rinsed, drained and dried on kitchen paper
A pinch of paprika
A pinch of crushed dried chilli
A pinch of flaked sea salt
Juice of ½ lemon
1 tsp rapeseed oil

1 If you have a gas hob, turn on a burner to medium heat. Place each pepper directly on the flame (or hold the pepper over the flame on a long-handled metal fork). Once one side has blackened, turn the pepper using long-handled metal tongs. Continue doing this until the whole pepper is charred black. Alternatively, you can char the peppers under a hot grill, turning to blacken all sides.
2 Remove the charred peppers from the heat and place in a glass bowl. Cover with clingfilm and leave to sweat for 10 minutes. The peel should now come away easily.
3 Cut the peeled peppers in half and remove the stalk and seeds. Place the flesh in a blender with the rest of the ingredients and blitz until smooth. Transfer to a bowl for serving.

RICH IN Vitamin C • Beta-carotene • Fibre

USEFUL FOR Heart ① • Digestion ① •
Skin, hair & nails ①③ • Men ②

BUTTER BEAN & SPINACH MASH WITH CRUDITÉS

SERVES 2 • 240 CALORIES PER SERVING

This is a quick, pretty dish. Butter beans, which are packed with fibre, make a nutty-tasting, creamy mash. Adding spinach turns it a delightful pale green, which looks beautiful next to the bright crudités. You could also serve the mash in place of mashed potato as part of a main meal.

FOR THE BUTTER BEAN MASH
2 handfuls of spinach
400g tin butter beans, drained and rinsed
Grated zest and juice of ½ lemon
4 fresh chives, roughly chopped
1 tsp rapeseed oil

FOR THE CRUDITÉS
1 carrot, cut into batons, or a handful of baby carrots, halved lengthways
2 celery sticks, cut into batons
1 red pepper, seeded and cut into strips
1 baby cucumber, cut into strips

1 Put all the ingredients for the butter bean mash in a blender and blitz to a chunky consistency. You can blitz it for longer to create a smooth texture, if you prefer.
2 Place the mash in a bright bowl and serve with the crudités.

RICH IN Vitamins B6 and C • Folate • Potassium • Beta-carotene • Fibre

USEFUL FOR Heart ② • Digestion ① •
Immunity ① • Skin, hair & nails ①③ •
Mind ① • Women ①

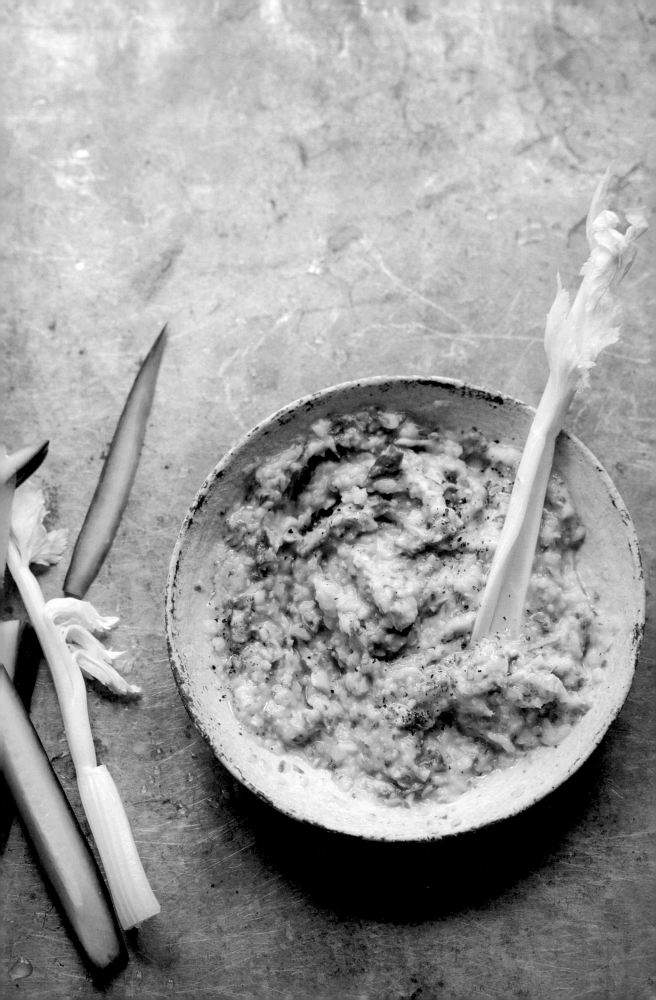

BROAD BEAN & MINT DIP

SERVES 4–6 • 60–90 CALORIES PER SERVING

This is a vibrant green dip to make in springtime when broad beans are in season. These sweet beans are a good source of prebiotics (non-digestible fibres) to help maintain a healthy digestive system. Used raw in this dip, the beans are perfectly complemented by fresh mint. This is particularly refreshing with cucumber crudités.

300g podded young broad beans
A handful of fresh mint leaves
1 spring onion, chopped
2 handfuls of baby spinach
2 tbsp rapeseed oil
Juice of 1 lemon

1 Place all the ingredients in a blender and blitz for 30 seconds to make a fairly coarse texture but one that is smooth enough for dipping.
2 Transfer to a bowl for serving.

RICH IN Vitamin C • Folate • Prebiotics • Fibre

USEFUL FOR Heart ① • Digestion ①② • Immunity ①

CUCUMBER, MINT & YOGURT DIP

SERVES 4–6 • 25–35 CALORIES PER SERVING

A classic in Indian cooking, where it is known as raita, this refreshing yogurt dip is typically served with hot, spicy curries to act as a cooling agent, but it's also great for a quick snack with some cucumber batons. It's very easy to make.

1 large cucumber
2 sprigs of fresh mint, leaves picked and finely chopped
½ onion, very finely chopped
4 tbsp plain soya yogurt
A pinch of paprika
Salt

1 Peel the cucumber, then cut it in half lengthways and remove the seeds with a teaspoon. Place the cucumber halves on kitchen paper and sprinkle with salt. Leave for 10 minutes.
2 Pat off the excess water with more kitchen paper, then cut the cucumber into small cubes. Place in a mixing bowl.
3 Add the mint to the cucumber along with the onion and yogurt. Mix together. Transfer to a serving bowl and sprinkle with paprika.

RICH IN Phytoestrogens

USEFUL FOR Heart ①② • Bones ① • Men ① • Women ①③④

APRICOT & GINGER JAM

**MAKES ABOUT 230G • 20 CALORIES PER 45G
(ABOUT 1 HEAPED TBSP)**

This is a recipe inspired by my travels in India –
it seems to be a popular jam in Rajasthan as well
as Goa and Kerala. It is sweet from the apricots
and fiery from the ginger, making it a great
morning jam to awaken your tastebuds. Ginger
has anticoagulant properties, so is particularly
good for heart health.

5 cardamom pods

2 cloves

1 cinnamon stick

10 fresh apricots

A thumb-sized piece of fresh ginger, peeled
and grated

1 Put the cardamom, cloves and cinnamon in
  a saucepan and cover with 600ml of water.
  Bring to the boil and simmer for 20 minutes.
2 Meanwhile, cut the apricots in half and remove
  the stones. Roughly slice the apricots.
3 Strain the spiced liquid into another pan and
  add the apricots and ginger. Bring to the boil,
  then simmer for about 40 minutes, stirring
  occasionally. To check if the jam is ready, dip
  in a teaspoon, then lift it out: the jam should
  slowly drizzle off the spoon.
4 Remove from the heat and leave to cool. Store
  in a sterilised airtight jar in the fridge.

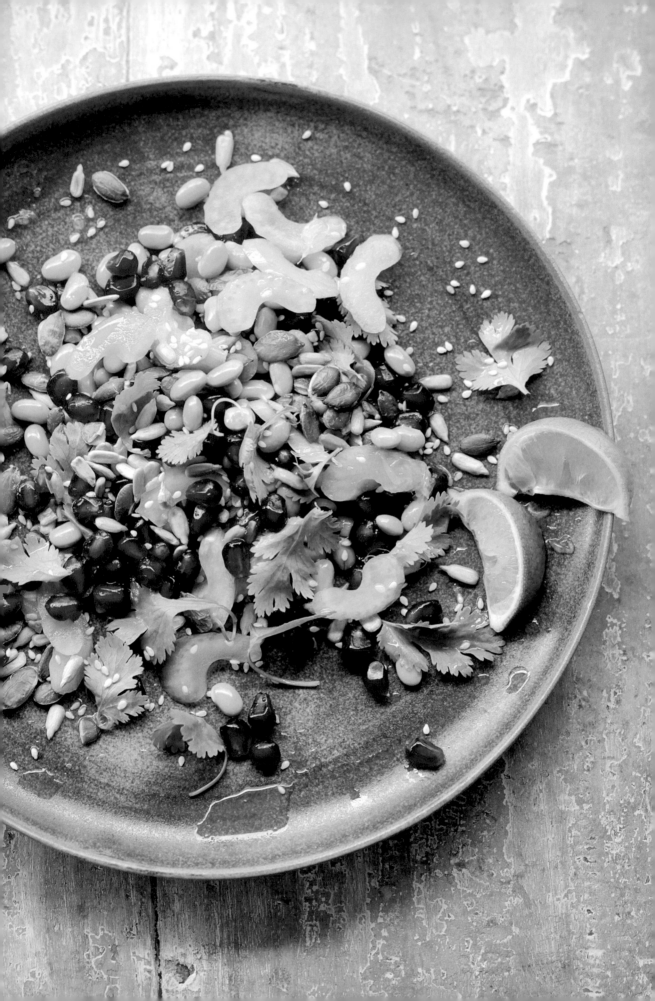

EDAMAME & SEED SALAD

SERVES 2 • 230 CALORIES PER SERVING

Edamame beans are high in protein and low in fat. Keep some in the freezer so that when you are in a rush and need to get some goodness down you, you can knock up this snack. Not only does it taste delicious, nutty and fresh, it is also surprisingly filling. It's a great post-training snack too.

10g sesame seeds
20g sunflower seeds
20g pumpkin seeds
1 pomegranate
100g edamame beans, thawed if frozen
1 celery stick, thinly sliced
1 tsp chopped fresh coriander, plus extra leaves
Juice of 1 lime, plus wedges to serve
Salt and pepper

1 Preheat your oven to 180°C/fan 160°C/gas 4.
2 Spread out the sesame, sunflower and pumpkin seeds on a baking tray and toast in the heated oven for 8 minutes.
3 Meanwhile, cut the pomegranate in half and place the halves cut side down on some kitchen paper. Gently tap them with a wooden spoon until all the seeds have fallen out. You will have to remove some of the skin that has fallen out too, but it's worth it for these little jewels!
4 Combine the pomegranate seeds, edamame, celery, coriander (both chopped and leaves) and lime juice in a bowl. Add the toasted seeds, season with salt and pepper, and mix together. Serve immediately, with lime wedges for squeezing over.

RICH IN Vitamin E • Folate • Magnesium • Beta-sitosterol • Phytoestrogens • Fibre

USEFUL FOR Heart ①②③ • Bones ① • Digestion ① • Mind ② • Fatigue ③⑤ • Men ①② • Women ①③④

QUAIL'S EGGS, CELERY SALT & CHERRY TOMATOES

SERVES 2 • 285 CALORIES PER SERVING

It's a myth that eating too many eggs will result in high cholesterol levels, meaning there's no limit on the number you can have each week. So when you want a savoury, substantial snack between meals, you can happily enjoy quail's eggs. Although delicate in size, they fill you up instantly. They're delicious sprinkled with the classic celery salt.

12 quail's eggs
A pinch of celery salt
100g cherry tomatoes, cut in half
A pinch of cracked black pepper

1 Bring a medium-sized pan of water to the boil. Reduce to a simmer and add the quail's eggs. Cook on a medium heat for 5 minutes.
2 Drain and cool under cold running water to stop the cooking process. Now gently peel the eggs.
3 Sprinkle the quail's eggs with celery salt and mix with the tomatoes and pepper.

RICH IN Vitamin B2 (riboflavin) • Iron • Lycopene • Tryptophan

USEFUL FOR Mind ① • Fatigue ①③ • Men ①

BUTTERNUT & BEETROOT CRISPS

MAKES 400G TO SERVE 8 | 45 CALORIES PER SERVING

These colourful vegetable crisps are a much lower calorie alternative to the usual potato crisp. To ensure the crispiest texture, they need time to dry out – if you try to cook them for a shorter period and at a higher temperature than specified, they will tend to go soggy fairly quickly. Believe me, they are worth the wait.

2 raw beetroots
1 butternut squash
1 tbsp flaked sea salt
1 tsp olive oil
A pinch of paprika
A pinch of chilli powder

1 Preheat your oven to 70°C/fan 50°C/gas low.
2 Peel the beetroots and butternut squash, then use a potato peeler to take very thin slices – the longer and wider the better – from the beetroot and squash flesh (discard the squash seeds and fibres). Place the slices on a baking tray, sprinkle with the salt and drizzle the oil over them, then dust them with the paprika and chilli powder.
3 Place in the oven and leave to dehydrate for about 1 hour 10 minutes until crisp – check every now and then towards the end of the time to be sure they don't burn. Allow to cool before eating. Store in an airtight container.

KALE CRISPS WITH CASHEW NUTS & PAPRIKA

MAKES 200G TO SERVE 8 • 50 CALORIES PER SERVING

We are always looking for new and interesting ways to use kale, and created these crisps when we wanted a healthy vegetable snack that felt a little bit naughty. To make them, you need to dehydrate the kale in the oven rather than bake it, which means a little patience is required for your crispy treats.

30g cashew nuts
1 tsp rapeseed oil
500g kale
1 tsp paprika
A pinch of flaked sea salt

1 Preheat your oven to 70°C/fan 50°C/gas low. Soak the cashew nuts in water for 20 minutes.
2 Drain the nuts and place them in a blender with the rapeseed oil and 50ml water. Blitz for about 5 minutes until completely smooth. Add more water if necessary: the consistency should be similar to single cream.
3 Take the kale leaves off the stalk and tear them into bite-sized pieces. Place in a large bowl and pour over the cashew cream. Toss with your hands to ensure that every piece is coated.
4 Spread out the kale on a baking tray and sprinkle with the paprika and sea salt. Dry out in the heated oven for about 1 hour until crispy. Leave to cool. The crisps can be kept in an airtight container for up to 2 days.

RICH IN Vitamin C • Folate

USEFUL FOR Immunity ① • Men ②

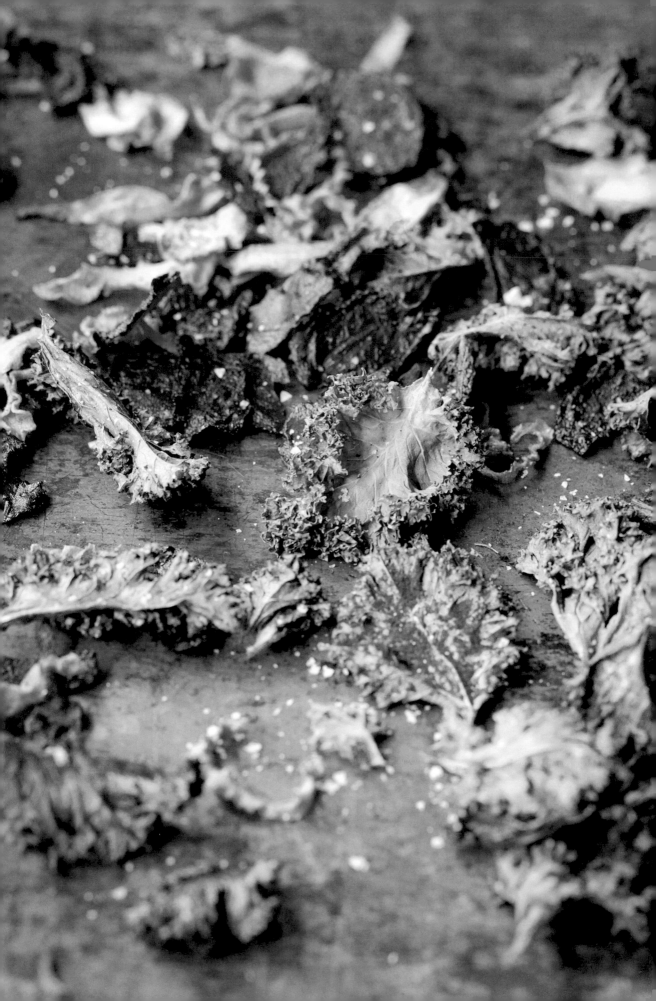

SPICY NUTS

SERVES 2 • 260 CALORIES PER SERVING

Although high in calories, nuts make a good snack because they contain monounsaturated fat that can benefit heart health by lowering levels of blood cholesterol. The spices used for these nuts give them a real kick, with honey providing a welcome sweetness. You can substitute any nuts and seeds you have in your cupboard.

50g whole almonds
50g cashew nuts
50g home-shelled pistachios
50g brazil nuts, cut in half
1 tsp paprika
1 tsp chilli powder
1 tsp ground cinnamon
A pinch of ground cumin
A pinch of ground turmeric
1 tsp runny honey

1 Preheat your oven to 180°C/fan 160°c/gas 4. Line a baking tray with greaseproof paper.
2 Put all the nuts in a mixing bowl and add the spices and honey. Mix together well.
3 Spread out on the baking tray and toast in the heated oven for 8 minutes. Leave to cool completely. The nuts can be kept in an airtight container for a few weeks.

RICH IN Vitamin E • Selenium • Magnesium • Beta-sitosterol • Phytoestrogens

USEFUL FOR Heart ①②③ • Bones ① • Immunity ① • Fatigue ③⑤ • Men ① • Women ①③④

ROASTED CURRIED CHICKPEAS

MAKES 250G TO SERVE 2 • 210 CALORIES PER SERVING

Spicy, crunchy, healthy and delicious, this is our favourite kind of snack. It is quick and easy to knock up, and then is left to crisp up in the oven. The chickpeas, which also make a punchy addition to salads, provide a great source of iron for vegans, who are particularly at risk of low stores of this important mineral.

½ tsp ground cumin
½ tsp ground coriander
½ tsp paprika
½ tsp garam masala
A pinch of flaked sea salt
1 tbsp rapeseed oil
250g tinned chickpeas (drained weight), rinsed

1 Preheat your oven to 180°C/fan 160°C/gas 4.
2 Mix together the cumin, coriander, paprika, garam masala, salt and oil in a bowl to create a paste.
3 Pat the chickpeas dry with kitchen paper. Add to the bowl and mix to coat them with the spice paste. Spread the chickpeas on a baking tray.
4 Bake in the heated oven for 1 hour until crisp. Leave to cool completely. Eat within 2–3 days.

RICH IN Iron • Phytoestrogens • Fibre

USEFUL FOR Digestion ① • Fatigue ① • Women ①③④

MIXED SEED CRACKERS

MAKES 20 CRACKERS • 60 CALORIES EACH

These crackers are packed full of deep nutty flavours, and potent onion seeds give them a wonderful savoury edge. They are fantastic topped with hummus (see a recipe on page 66). Pumpkin, flax and sunflower seeds contain plant hormones that may be helpful in relieving a number of female health conditions.

50g pumpkin seeds

20g flaxseeds

30g sunflower seeds

40g brown rice flour

1 tbsp olive oil

1 tbsp runny honey

10g white sesame seeds

30g black sesame seeds

10g onion seeds

1 Preheat your oven to 180°C/fan 160°C/gas 4. Line a 20cm square baking tin with greaseproof paper.

2 Put the pumpkin seeds and flaxseeds in a blender and grind to a powder. Transfer this to a bowl and add the sunflower seeds, rice flour, olive oil, honey and 150ml water. Mix well. The mixture should be runny enough to pour.

3 Spread the mixture evenly on the baking tray using a wooden spoon, then sprinkle with the sesame and onion seeds.

4 Bake in the heated oven for 40 minutes. Cut into 20 small squares and leave to cool. These can be kept in an airtight container for 2 weeks.

RICH IN Beta-sitosterol • Phytoestrogens

USEFUL FOR Heart ① • Men ① • Women ①③④

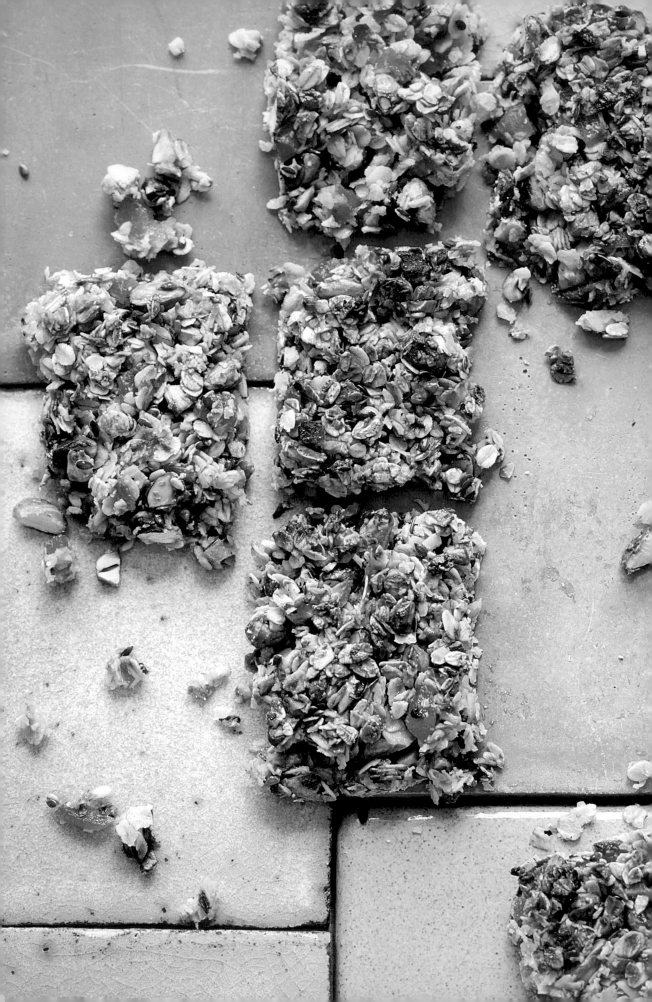

PISTACHIO OAT BARS

MAKES 12 BARS • 280 CALORIES EACH

Our reduced-sugar version of the flapjack was created by happy accident when we were trying to make a pistachio brittle with honey. It didn't set properly so we mixed in some porridge oats, flaxseeds, psyllium husks and dried apricots. The result was a filling crunchy, delicately sweet oat bar that offers a great source of fibre.

300g runny honey

200g porridge oats

200g home-shelled pistachios, roughly chopped

2 tbsp rapeseed oil

1 tbsp flaxseeds

1 tsp psyllium husks (don't worry if you don't have any; just use extra flaxseeds)

100g dried apricots, roughly chopped

1 Preheat your oven to 190°C/fan 170°C/gas 5. Line a 20cm square shallow baking tray with greaseproof paper.

2 Combine all the ingredients in a large bowl and mix well together.

3 Tip the mixture into the tray and flatten with a wooden spoon. Cover with some greaseproof paper and set another baking tray of the same size and shape on top, then gently push down to flatten the mixture evenly (don't apply too much pressure or the bars will come out very hard). Remove the extra baking tray and paper.

4 Bake in the heated oven for about 20 minutes until golden.

5 Remove from the oven and allow to cool before cutting into 12 small bars. These will keep in an airtight jar or tin for 10 days.

RICH IN Phytoestrogens • Fibre

USEFUL FOR Heart ① • Digestion ① • Immunity ① • Women ①③④

CASHEW & GOJI BERRY FLAPJACKS

MAKES 9 FLAPJACKS • 275 CALORIES EACH

There is nothing better than healthy fast food. These squares are energising and wholesome, and will keep you going for hours. Not too sweet and with just the right balance of crunchy and chewy, they include goji berries, which are rich in the antioxidants lutein and zeaxanthin – these help to protect the eyes from free radical damage and may help protect eyesight as you age. (The subtle taste of the berries also makes a great tea – just add a handful to hot water.)

300g porridge oats
30g flaked almonds
80g cashew nuts
200g runny honey
1 tsp ground cinnamon
A pinch of salt
2 rice cakes, broken into 2.5cm pieces
A handful of dried goji berries

1 Preheat your oven to 200°C/fan 180°C/gas 6. Line a 20cm square baking tin with baking parchment.
2 Spread out the oats and nuts on a large baking tray and toast in the oven for 10 minutes until slightly golden. Remove from the oven and allow to cool. Keep the oven on for later.
3 In a large bowl, mix together the honey, cinnamon, salt and 2 tablespoons water. Add the oats, nuts, rice cakes and goji berries and mix thoroughly.
4 Transfer the mixture to the lined baking tin and press down lightly (don't push down too hard as this will make the bars very dense). Bake in the heated oven for about 25 minutes until slightly golden on top. Leave to cool in the tin before cutting into nine squares. Keep in an airtight container and enjoy for 2 weeks.

RICH IN Magnesium • Fibre

USEFUL FOR Heart ①②③ • Bones ① • Digestion ① • Immunity ① • Mind ② • Fatigue ⑤ • Women ①③

SESAME SEED COOKIES

MAKES 12 COOKIES | 100 CALORIES EACH

These sweet and savoury cookies will satisfy the pickiest of palates even though they are much lower in sugar than typical recipes. Tahini, made from ground sesame seeds, gives a pleasantly earthy depth to the flavour, and honey provides a subtle sweetness.

200g gluten- and wheat-free flour
A pinch of salt
¼ tsp baking powder
2 tbsp runny honey
2 tbsp tahini
1 tbsp coconut oil
2 tbsp sesame seeds

1 Preheat your oven to 180°C/fan 160°C/gas 4. Line a baking tray with greaseproof paper.
2 Sift the flour, salt and baking powder into a large mixing bowl. In a separate bowl combine the honey, tahini and oil. Add to the dry ingredients and mix together with a wooden spoon until you have an even consistency.
3 Form the mixture into small balls, about the diameter of a 10p coin. Roll the balls in sesame seeds to coat all over, then place them on the baking tray, spacing them well apart. Flatten each ball to a disc about 1cm thick.
4 Bake in the heated oven for about 8 minutes until golden. Remove from the oven and allow to cool on the baking tray for 1–2 minutes, then transfer to a wire rack to finish cooling. These can be kept in an airtight container for 10 days.

CANDIED WALNUTS

SERVES 2 • 380 CALORIES PER SERVING

Not only are these sweet walnuts great to snack on but they are also delicious in salads or puddings, adding extra crunch and nourishing sweetness. Walnuts are a great vegetarian source of omega 3 fatty acids.

300g walnut halves
2 tbsp runny honey
1 tbsp groundnut oil
1 tsp ground cinnamon
1 tsp freshly grated nutmeg

1 Preheat your oven to 180°C/fan 160°C/gas 4. Line a baking tray with greaseproof paper.
2 Mix together all the ingredients in a bowl, then spread out on the baking tray. Bake in the heated oven for 15 minutes. Leave to cool completely. Store in an airtight jar for up to a month.

RICH IN Vitamin B6 • Omega 3 • Phytoestrogens

USEFUL FOR Heart ① • Bones ② • Digestion ③④ • Skin, hair & nails ①③ • Mind ① • Fatigue ② • Men ② • Women ①③④

SOUPS

A warming soup will nourish your soul and your body – soup can provide a surprisingly good source of many nutrients, making it the perfect meal when you're not overly hungry or if you're feeling unwell. Most of our soups offer you more than two servings of your minimum five-a-day. Those that include pulses can make a meal, whilst some of our lighter soups can be a handy nutritious snack.

The key to a good soup is to use a flavourful stock. Keep all your vegetable trimmings (in the fridge), then add them to water with some onions and a bay leaf, and voilà! You have already given your soup a tasty head start (see our vegetable stock recipe on page 283).

For the best taste, make soups using ingredients in season. In order to retain as much of the goodness from the vegetables as possible, don't over-cook them. If you're making a puréed soup, it may take longer to blitz in a blender until velvety smooth, but your soup will be richer in colour, taste and nutrients. You can get even more flavour by adding a garnish of chopped herbs or flavoured oils.

Soups also offer a brilliant opportunity to fortify your diet. You could increase your fibre intake by adding pulses, or chia seed oil for omega 3, or lentils for iron. Throwing another veggie into the mix is another easy way to boost goodness.

At the end of most of the recipes, you'll find a list of the main nutrients supplied in a serving as well as a list of health issues that may be benefited by including the recipe in your healthy diet. For more, see page 9.

BROWN RICE, PAK CHOI & GINGER BROTH

SERVES 2 • 350 CALORIES PER SERVING

This broth is bursting with heart-healthy foods (brown rice, chillies, onion, garlic and ginger), all of which can help with high cholesterol, inflammation and circulation. The lightness of the flavoursome broth bulked out with rice and vegetables makes the soup feel cleansing yet filling.

RICH IN Vitamins B1 (thiamin), B6 and C • Folate • Potassium • Magnesium • Iron • Fibre

USEFUL FOR Heart ①②③ • Bones ① • Digestion ① • Mind ① • Fatigue ①③⑤ • Women ①

150g brown rice
1 tsp olive oil
1 red onion, finely sliced
2 garlic cloves, finely sliced
2 large thumb-sized pieces of fresh ginger, grated with the skin on
1 stick of lemongrass, gently bashed with a rolling pin to break up the fibres, then finely chopped
½ fresh red chilli, seeded and finely chopped
Juice of 1 lime
1 celery stick, finely diced
1 tsp salt
2 bunches of pak choi
1 spring onion, finely sliced on the diagonal
½ iceberg lettuce, finely shredded
A handful of fresh coriander leaves, finely chopped

1 Bring a medium-sized pan of water to the boil. Add the rice and cook for 20 minutes until just tender – it should still have a little bite. Drain and set aside.

2 While the rice is cooking, prepare the broth. Set a large saucepan on a high heat. Add the olive oil, then add the onion and turn the heat to medium. Cook for 10 minutes until translucent. Add the garlic, ginger, lemongrass, chilli and lime juice, and cook for a further 3 minutes. Add the celery, salt and 600ml water. Bring to the boil, then simmer for 20 minutes.

3 Trim the base of the pak choi, then cut lengthways into 1cm slices, through the base. Add the pak choi to the broth along with the cooked rice and spring onion. Simmer for 2 more minutes. Remove from the heat and stir in the lettuce and coriander. Serve immediately in large bowls.

BROCCOLI & GINGER SOUP
SERVES 2 • 220 CALORIES PER SERVING

This hearty soup makes a deliciously satisfying supper. The heat of fresh ginger, which is considered to be a powerful anti-inflammatory, works really well with the earthy flavour of broccoli, but you could also use pak choi, mange tout or shredded white cabbage.

1 tsp rapeseed oil
1 onion, diced
A thumb-sized piece of fresh ginger, grated with the skin on
2 broccoli heads, about 400g in total
500ml vegetable stock (see page 283)
4 celery sticks, diced
1 tsp salt
A pinch of pepper
A handful of toasted pumpkin seeds

1 Set a large saucepan on a high heat, add the oil and then add the onion. Reduce the heat and cook for 5 minutes. Add the ginger and cook for another 5 minutes.
2 Meanwhile, cut the stalk from the broccoli and dice it. Break the rest of the heads into florets.
3 Pour the stock into the pan and add the broccoli, celery, salt and pepper. Bring to the boil, then simmer for 10 minutes until the pieces of broccoli stalk are soft.
4 Use a hand blender to blitz the soup in the pan until smooth (or do this in a blender). Serve sprinkled with the toasted pumpkin seeds.

RICH IN Vitamins B1 (thiamin), B6, C and E • Folate • Potassium • Iron • Calcium • Chromium • Beta-carotene • Fibre

USEFUL FOR Heart ①② • Bones ① • Digestion ① • Immunity ① • Skin, hair & nails ①③ • Mind ① • Fatigue ① • Women ①③④

KING PRAWN, NOODLE & LEMONGRASS BROTH
SERVES 2 • 340 CALORIES PER SERVING

This version of the classic noodle soup uses Thai flavours – ginger, coriander and lemongrass – to create a really fresh, fragrant, cleansing broth. If you can't find brown rice noodles, any wheat-free noodles will work well. You could also add some courgette spaghetti (see page 127). Lemongrass, which is thought to enhance circulation, can be used to make a refreshing alternative to tea or coffee. Just put a crushed stick in a cup of hot water with some fresh mint.

1 red onion, finely sliced
A thumb-sized piece of fresh ginger, peeled and cut into very thin matchsticks
1 garlic clove, finely diced
1 stick of lemongrass, gently bashed with a rolling pin to break up the fibres but kept whole
1 tsp rapeseed oil
600ml chicken or vegetable stock (see page 283)
200g peeled raw king prawns
100g brown rice noodles
Juice of 1 lime
1 tbsp tamari
2 spring onions, sliced on the diagonal
A handful of fresh coriander leaves, finely chopped, plus extra to garnish
A pinch of salt
½ red chilli, thinly sliced

1 Combine the onion, ginger, garlic, lemongrass, rapeseed oil and a splash of water in a large pan and cook on a low heat for 5 minutes. Add the stock and bring to the boil. Boil for 10 minutes, then turn down the heat to low.
2 Add the prawns and cook for 5 minutes. Next add the noodles along with the lime juice, tamari, spring onions, coriander and salt. Turn the heat back up and bring to the boil, then boil for 1 minute.
3 Remove from the heat, take out the lemongrass and serve, garnished with the chilli and extra coriander.

RICH IN Vitamins B12 and C • Potassium • Zinc • Selenium • Iron • Tryptophan

USEFUL FOR Heart ② • Immunity ① • Skin, hair & nails ①④ • Mind ① • Fatigue ①③ • Men ①②

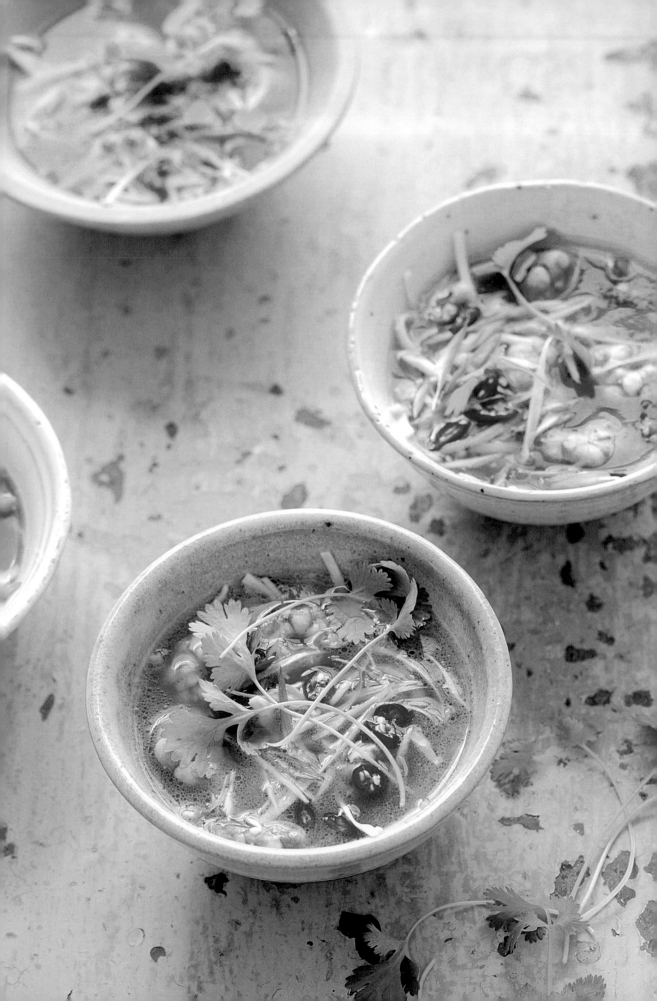

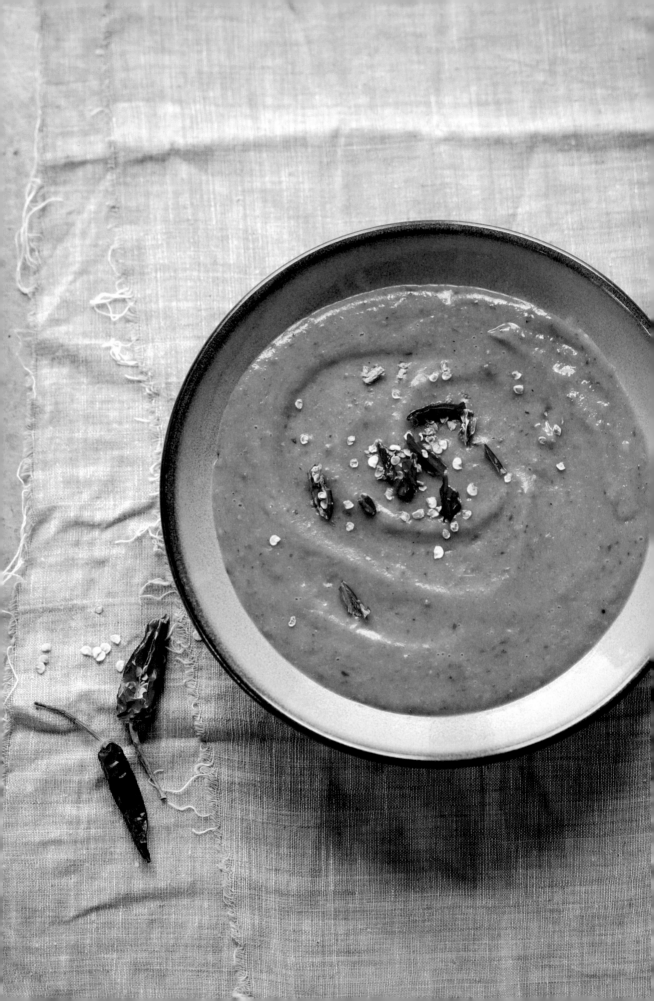

BUTTERNUT, COCONUT & CHILLI SOUP

SERVES 2 • 190 CALORIES PER SERVING

This is a delightfully smooth, spicy, creamy soup. The coconut and butternut squash happily melt into one another, with the coconut mellowing the sweetness of the butternut. The chilli gives this soup the fiery kick it needs. It's worth the effort to make your own stock as the fresh vegetables used give any dish an additional nutrient boost.

1 butternut squash
1 tsp crushed dried chilli
1 red onion, finely sliced
600ml vegetable stock (see page 283)
200ml coconut milk
Salt and pepper

1 Preheat your oven to 180°C/fan 160°C/gas 4. Line a baking tray with greaseproof paper.
2 Peel the butternut squash and cut it lengthways in half. Scoop out the seeds and fibres, then cut the flesh into 2.5cm pieces. Spread the pieces on the baking tray and roast for 15 minutes.
3 Remove the tray from the oven and scatter the chilli and onion over the pieces of squash. Roast for a further 10 minutes. Remove from the oven and allow to cool for a few minutes.
4 Pour the stock into a medium saucepan and bring to the boil, then turn the heat to low. Stir in the coconut milk and warm for 2 minutes. Remove from the heat.
5 Put the squash, onions and chilli in a blender and add the coconut milk/stock. Blitz until smooth, then season to taste. Serve hot.

RICH IN Vitamins B6, C and E • Folate • Potassium • Magnesium • Beta-carotene • Fibre

USEFUL FOR Heart ① ② ③ • Bones ① • Digestion ① • Immunity ① • Skin, hair & nails ① ③ • Mind ① ② • Fatigue ③ ⑤ • Women ① ③

FRESH SWEETCORN SOUP

SERVES 2 • 205 CALORIES PER SERVING

This bright yellow soup is the complete opposite of what you might imagine a sweetcorn soup to be (gloopy and grey). Using fresh corn on the cob is the key – it makes a well-flavoured soup with a vibrant colour.

3 ears of sweetcorn (corn on the cob)
3 spring onions, finely sliced
2 garlic cloves, finely sliced
2 celery sticks, finely diced
½ fresh red chilli, seeded and finely chopped
500ml vegetable stock (see page 283)

1 Remove the husks and 'silk' from the sweetcorn, if necessary, then shave the kernels off the cob. The easiest way to do this is to hold the sweetcorn at an angle in a shallow bowl and to cut down the cob with a sharp knife.
2 Put the sweetcorn kernels in a large saucepan with the spring onions and garlic and cook gently for 5 minutes, stirring occasionally. Add the celery, chilli and stock. Bring to the boil, then simmer for 20 minutes.
3 Blitz in a blender until smooth. Serve hot.

RICH IN Vitamins B1 (thiamin), B6 and C • Folate • Potassium • Beta-carotene • Fibre

USEFUL FOR Heart ② • Digestion ① • Immunity ① • Skin, hair & nails ① ③ • Mind ① • Women ①

MEXICAN BEAN SOUP

SERVES 4 • 300 CALORIES PER SERVING

The big, bold flavours of Mexican spices and herbs come together in this hearty soup. It's packed with beans – cannellini, borlotti and red kidney – which provide a useful source of phytoestrogens that may help with hormone imbalances in women. If you don't have time to soak and cook dried beans, you can use 400g tinned beans, although they won't have the same texture.

100g dried red kidney beans
100g dried borlotti beans
100g dried cannellini beans
1 tbsp rapeseed oil
1 large red onion, finely sliced
2 garlic cloves, finely sliced
A thumb-sized piece of fresh ginger, finely grated with the skin on
1 tbsp paprika
1 tsp chilli powder
1 tsp ground coriander
1 bay leaf
1 tsp dried thyme
1 carrot, finely diced
6 ripe vine tomatoes, finely chopped
700ml chicken or vegetable stock (see page 283)
1 courgette, diced
A handful of fresh coriander leaves, finely chopped
Salt and pepper

1 Soak the beans in two to three times their volume of water overnight, or for at least 8 hours. Drain and tip them into a saucepan. Cover with fresh water, bring to the boil and boil for 10 minutes. Drain again.

2 Set a large saucepan on a high heat, add the oil and then add the onion. Cook for 10 minutes until slightly browned. Add the garlic, ginger, paprika, chilli powder, ground coriander, bay leaf and dried thyme. Add a splash of water so that the spices don't stick, then cook for 2 minutes, stirring frequently.

3 Add the beans along with the carrot, tomatoes and stock. Bring to the boil, then reduce the heat and simmer for 1½ hours until the beans are soft but still intact.

4 Add the courgette, stir and cook for a further 10 minutes. Remove from the heat. Season the soup and discard the bay leaf. Leave to stand for 10 minutes before serving with a sprinkle of chopped coriander on each bowlful.

RICH IN Vitamins B1 (thiamin), B6 and C • Potassium • Magnesium • Iron • Beta-carotene • Lycopene • Phytoestrogens • Fibre

USEFUL FOR Heart ①②③ • Bones ① • Digestion ① • Immunity ① • Skin, hair & nails ①③ • Mind ①② • Fatigue ①③⑤ • Men ① • Women ①③④

RED LENTIL SOUP

SERVES 2 • 315 CALORIES PER SERVING

Soup is just the thing you need when you're feeling under the weather, and this one is soothing and surprisingly refreshing. It's also easy to make and totally delicious. The lentils in the recipe provide a healthy dose of zinc and iron, both of which are associated with a healthy immune system. Try topping the soup with some shredded chicken and serve with a bowl of brown rice for a wholesome and filling dinner.

1 tbsp rapeseed oil

1 large onion, diced

A thumb-sized piece of fresh ginger, grated with the skin on

2 garlic cloves, finely chopped

100g red lentils

1 cardamom pod

2 cloves

1 bay leaf

2 carrots, diced

750ml vegetable stock (see page 283)

Juice of ½ lemon

A handful of fresh coriander

Salt and pepper

1 Set a large saucepan on a medium heat and add the oil. Add the onion and cook for 10 minutes until translucent. Add the ginger and garlic and cook for a further 3 minutes.

2 Add the red lentils, cardamom pod, cloves and bay leaf and mix well. Cook for 1–2 minutes before adding the carrots and stock. Bring to the boil, then simmer for 20 minutes until the lentils are soft. From time to time during cooking, you will need to skim off the foam from the surface with a slotted spoon.

3 Fish out the cardamom pod, cloves and bay leaf and discard them. Add the lemon juice and fresh coriander to the pan, then pour the soup into a blender and blitz until smooth. Season with salt and pepper before serving hot.

RICH IN Vitamins B6 and C • Folate • Potassium • Iron • Zinc • Beta-carotene • Fibre

USEFUL FOR Heart ①② • Digestion ① • Immunity ① • Skin, hair & nails ①④ • Fatigue ① • Men ①② • Women ①

BEETROOT & CUMIN SOUP

SERVES 2 • 270 CALORIES PER SERVING

This recipe comes from my older brother Hayden, who has a restaurant in the Isles of Scilly. It's a rich and creamy soup, heavily spiced but perfectly balanced, and a beautiful colour due to the red and yellow spices, carrots and beetroot. It's heart-healthy too because beetroot is rich in phytochemicals (found in plants) that may help to lower the risk of heart disease.

5 large raw beetroots

1 tbsp rapeseed oil

1 large onion, finely diced

2 garlic cloves, finely chopped

A thumb-sized piece of fresh ginger, peeled and finely grated

1 tsp ground cumin

1 tsp paprika

A pinch of ground turmeric

1 tsp dried thyme

2 carrots, finely diced

2 celery sticks, finely diced

500ml vegetable stock (see page 283)

2 tbsp plain soya yogurt, to serve

1 Preheat your oven to 200°C/fan 180°C/gas 6.

2 Wrap up the beetroots in foil to create a sealed parcel and place it on a baking tray. Roast for 40 minutes. Remove from the oven. When the beetroots are cool enough to handle, peel them, then dice and set aside.

3 Set a large saucepan on a medium heat and add the oil, then fry the onion for 10 minutes until translucent. Add the garlic, ginger, cumin, paprika, turmeric and dried thyme. Cook for 3 minutes, stirring, then add the carrots and celery. Cook for a further 2 minutes.

4 Pour in the vegetable stock. Bring to the boil, then simmer for 15 minutes until all the vegetables are soft. Add the beetroot and cook for 5 more minutes.

5 Transfer the soup to a blender and blitz until completely smooth. Serve each bowlful topped with a dollop of soya yogurt.

RICH IN Vitamins B6 and C • Folate • Potassium • Iron • Beta-carotene • Nitrates • Fibre

USEFUL FOR Heart ①② • Digestion ① • Immunity ① • Skin, hair & nails ①③ • Mind ① • Fatigue ① • Women ①

CREAMY CAULIFLOWER & ROASTED GARLIC SOUP

SERVES 2 • 160 CALORIES PER SERVING

Roasting garlic makes it sweeter and creamier, perfect with cauliflower in this spicy, aromatic soup. Garlic has anticoagulant properties that can help to prevent blood clotting, so it's a useful food to include in a heart-healthy diet.

1 bulb of garlic
1 cauliflower
A pinch of ground cumin
A pinch of freshly grated nutmeg
1 tbsp rapeseed oil
1 large onion, chopped
500ml vegetable stock (see page 283)
Salt and white pepper
Smoked paprika, to serve

1 Preheat your oven to 180°C/fan 160°C/gas 4. Line a baking tray with greaseproof paper.
2 Place the garlic bulb on the baking tray and roast for 20 minutes. Remove from the oven, wrap the garlic in foil and set it back on the tray. Roast for a further 30 minutes. Remove the garlic from the oven, keep it wrapped in the foil and set aside to cool. Leave the oven on.
3 Separate the cauliflower florets from the core. Dice the core and set aside. Spread the florets on the baking tray and sprinkle with the cumin and nutmeg. Roast for 10 minutes. Set aside.
4 Break the garlic bulb into cloves and peel them. You only need half of them (the rest can be kept in the fridge for 5 days covered with olive oil in an airtight container; you'll then have the bonus of some subtly flavoured garlic oil).
5 Heat the oil in a large pan, add the onion and cook on a medium heat for 10 minutes until translucent. Add the diced cauliflower core with the roasted garlic cloves and stock. Bring to the boil, then simmer for 10 minutes until softened.
6 Add the spiced florets, then season and simmer for a further 5 minutes. Remove from the heat and leave to sit for 5 minutes.
7 Pour everything into a blender and blitz until smooth. Serve with a dusting of paprika.

RICH IN Vitamins B6 and C • Folate • Potassium • Iron • Phytoestrogens • Tryptophan • Fibre

USEFUL FOR Heart ①② • Digestion ① • Immunity ① • Mind ① • Fatigue ①③ • Women ①③④

CAULIFLOWER, CELERIAC & PAPRIKA SOUP

SERVES 2 • 215 CALORIES PER SERVING

This is a silky classic: the queen of the smooth soups. Sweet celeriac provides a good background flavour for earthy cauliflower, and paprika adds depth and spice. Roasting the cauliflower first gives it a more complex flavour. Like other cruciferous vegetables, it contains substances known as glucosinolates, which are broken down into active compounds that may help to protect against disease, including cancer.

1 cauliflower
½ celeriac, finely diced
½ tsp smoked paprika, plus extra for dusting
A pinch of salt
1 tbsp rapeseed oil
1 large onion, finely diced
2 garlic cloves, finely diced
1 celery stick, diced
500ml vegetable stock (see page 283)

1 Preheat your oven to 200°C/fan 180°C/gas 6.
2 Cut the core out of the cauliflower and finely chop it. Roughly chop the florets. Spread all of the cauliflower and the celeriac in a roasting tin and sprinkle with the paprika and salt. Roast for 20 minutes.
3 Meanwhile, heat the oil in a large saucepan, add the onion and cook for 10 minutes until it is translucent. Add the garlic and cook for a further 3 minutes. Add the celery and stock. Bring to the boil, then simmer for 5 minutes.
4 Tip the cauliflower and celeriac into the pan and stir to mix, then simmer for a further 15 minutes.
5 Transfer everything to a blender and blitz for about 3 minutes until completely smooth. Serve hot, with a light dusting of paprika.

RICH IN Vitamins B1 (thiamin), B6 and C • Folate • Potassium • Fibre

USEFUL FOR Heart ①② • Digestion ① • Immunity ① • Mind ①

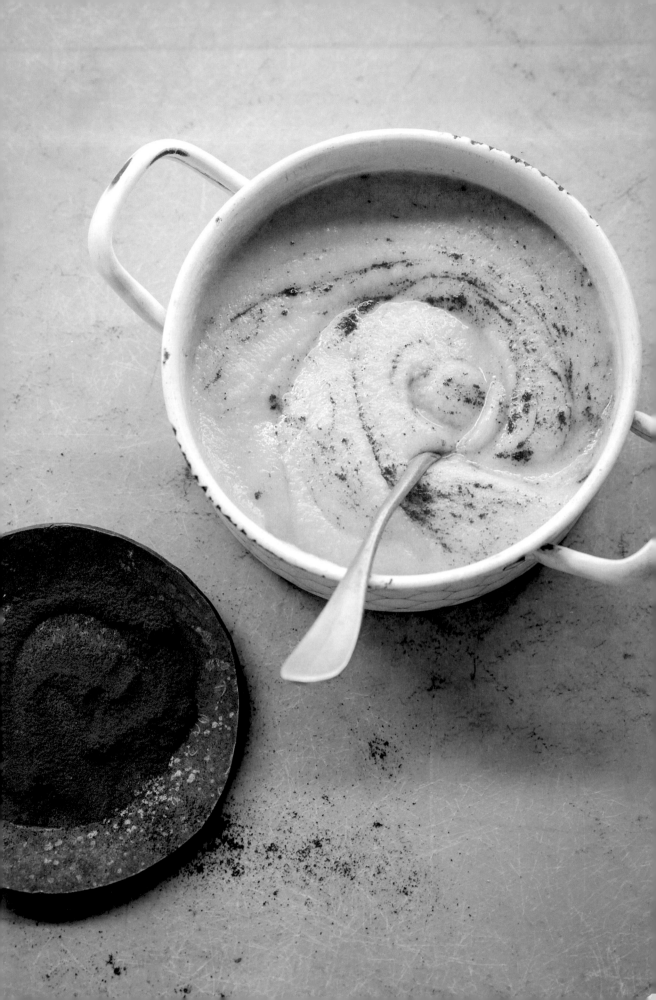

SCOTCH BROTH

SERVES 2 • 355 CALORIES PER SERVING

When our Scottish head chef, Sarah, started at the Detox Kitchen, this was one of the first things we asked her to make. It is her detox version of the traditional Scottish soup, made without lamb. A well-flavoured stock is essential, though. Thanks to the barley, this hearty soup is high in fibre, which is vital for good digestive health.

1 tbsp rapeseed oil

1 onion, finely diced

1 leek, finely diced

600ml chicken or vegetable stock (see page 283)

100g pearl barley

2 celery sticks, finely diced

1 swede, finely diced

1 turnip, finely diced

2 carrots, finely diced

A handful of fresh flat-leaf parsley, finely chopped

Salt and pepper

1 Heat the oil in a large saucepan and cook the onion and leek for 5 minutes. Pour in the stock and add the pearl barley. Bring to the boil, then simmer for 20 minutes.

2 Add the rest of the vegetables and cook for a further 25 minutes until they are tender. Stir in the parsley and season to taste, then serve hot.

RICH IN B vitamins • Vitamin C • Potassium • Iron • Beta-carotene • Fibre

USEFUL FOR Heart ①②③ • Digestion ① • Immunity ① • Skin, hair & nails ①③ • Mind ① • Fatigue ① • Women ①

NETTLE & KALE BROTH

SERVES 2 • 165 CALORIES PER SERVING

It may seem strange to eat a plant that is notorious for causing a horribly itchy rash. Fear not, though, because as soon as nettles hit boiling water, their sting dissipates. At their best in March and April, nettles contain more than twice the amount of calcium found in kale, which provides a great source of this mineral. A serving of this bone-friendly soup will supply nearly half your recommended daily intake of calcium.

1 tbsp rapeseed oil

1 leek, finely diced

2 garlic cloves, finely sliced

2 celery sticks, finely diced

1 carrot, finely diced

500ml vegetable stock (see page 283)

100g kale, finely shredded

100g nettles, finely shredded

Salt and pepper

1 Set a medium-sized saucepan on a medium heat and add the oil, then add the leek and garlic and cook for 2 minutes.

2 Add the celery, carrot and vegetable stock. Bring to the boil, then turn the heat down and simmer for 15 minutes until the carrot is cooked.

3 Add the kale and nettles and cook for 2 more minutes until the kale wilts. Season to taste. Serve immediately.

RICH IN Vitamins B6 and C • Folate • Potassium • Calcium • Iron • Fibre

USEFUL FOR Heart ①② • Bones ① • Immunity ① • Mind ①② • Fatigue ① • Men ② • Women ①

WATERCRESS & TURKEY SOUP

SERVES 2 • 255 CALORIES PER SERVING

The pepperiness of watercress not only gives a kick to a salad, but it also lends a delicious depth of flavour to soups. Adding it at the last minute will ensure your soup is a beautiful bright green. This soup offers 60 per cent of the RDA for potassium, which is essential for maintaining healthy blood pressure.

1 tbsp rapeseed oil
1 large onion, finely diced
2 garlic cloves, finely chopped
4 celery sticks, finely chopped
500ml vegetable stock (see page 283)
200g watercress, roughly chopped
100g spinach
200g skinless boneless turkey breast, thinly sliced
Salt and pepper

1 Set a large saucepan on a medium heat. Add 1 teaspoon of the oil and then the onion. Cook for 10 minutes until translucent. Add the garlic and cook for a further 3 minutes.
2 Stir in the celery, stock and 1 teaspoon salt and bring to the boil. Reduce the heat slightly and simmer for 10 minutes.
3 Add the watercress and spinach and cook for 2 more minutes. Remove from the heat and leave for a few minutes until the leaves have wilted, then blitz the soup in the pan using a hand blender until smooth (or blitz in a blender). Set aside.
4 Place a frying pan on a high heat and add the remaining oil, then add the turkey. Cook for about 8 minutes, turning frequently, until the slices are golden. Remove from the heat. Season the turkey and leave it to cool slightly, then shred it very finely with your fingers.
5 Add the turkey to the soup and heat through before serving.

RICH IN B vitamins • Vitamin C • Potassium • Beta-carotene • Tryptophan • Fibre

USEFUL FOR Heart ①②③ • Digestion ① • Immunity ① • Skin, hair & nails ①③ • Mind ① • Fatigue ①③ • Women ①

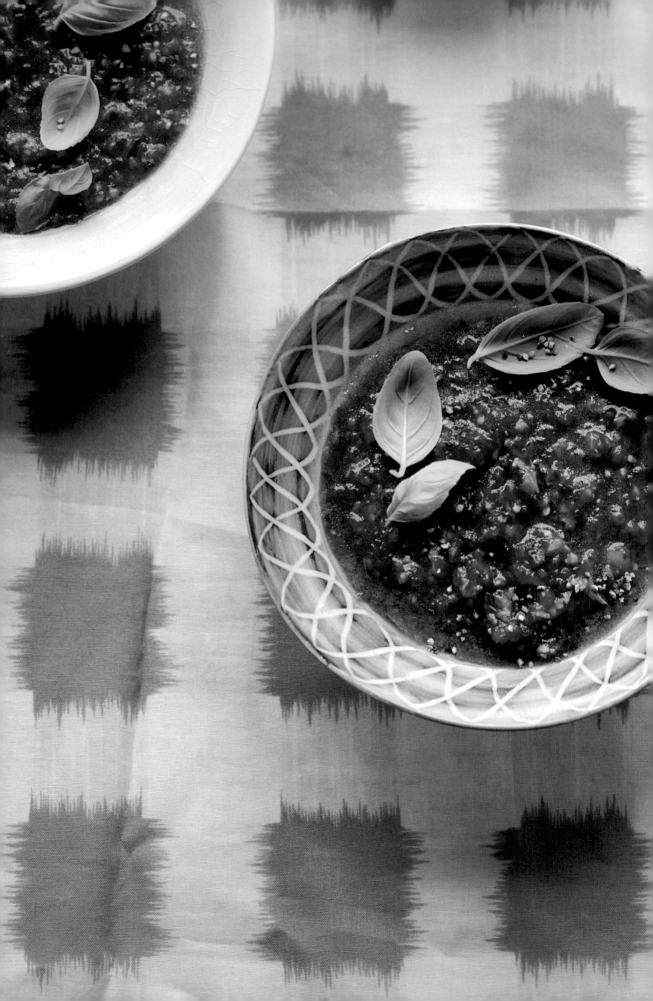

GAZPACHO

SERVES 2–4 • 80–160 CALORIES PER SERVING

No two gazpachos ever taste the same. It's like a Bloody Mary – everyone has their own way of concocting it. We think that this sweet and tangy Spanish classic should be chunky yet smooth enough to slip down without too much chewing, and contain an abundance of vegetables. Sweet peppers are one of the richest sources of vitamin C, which is essential for maintaining a strong immune system. They are partnered with tomatoes in our gazpacho, which offers three times the RDA for this vitamin in a single serving. On a hot summer's day in the garden, sun blazing down, there is nothing better than chilled gazpacho.

2 beef tomatoes (the riper the better)
8 vine tomatoes (the riper the better)
10 cherry tomatoes
1 cucumber, peeled, seeded and roughly chopped
1 red pepper, peeled (see Red Pepper & Butter Bean Mash, page 68) and seeded
1 celery stick, diced
1 tbsp olive oil
½ fresh red chilli, seeded and chopped
2 garlic cloves, diced
A pinch of flaked sea salt
A pinch of cracked black pepper
Juice of ½ lemon
A handful of fresh chives, finely chopped
A handful of fresh basil leaves, chopped, plus extra leaves to garnish

1 Roughly chop all of the tomatoes and place them in a blender. Add the cucumber, red pepper, celery, olive oil, chilli, garlic, sea salt and pepper. Pulse to a fairly chunky consistency.
2 Add the lemon juice, chives and basil and blitz for a few more seconds.
3 Pour into a jug or bowl, cover and leave to chill in the fridge for a few hours.
4 Before serving, taste and add more salt and pepper if needed, then garnish with basil leaves.

RICH IN Vitamins B6, C and E • Potassium • Lycopene • Beta-carotene • Fibre

USEFUL FOR Heart ①② • Digestion ① • Immunity ① • Skin, hair & nails ①③ • Mind ① • Men ① • Women ①

PEA & ROCKET SOUP

SERVES 2 • 115 CALORIES PER SERVING

Rocket gives an extra little peppery kick and adds to the brilliant colour of this pea soup – to create the greenest soup possible, the rocket isn't cooked. Rocket is in the top five richest vegetable sources of iron, and just a single serving of this soup can boost your intake by 30 per cent of the RDA, which can help tackle the tiredness and fatigue associated with low levels of this mineral. The soup is light and fresh in flavour, and is also delicious chilled.

1 tbsp olive oil
2 spring onions, finely sliced
1 garlic clove, finely diced
4 celery sticks, finely diced
600ml vegetable stock (see page 283)
100g frozen peas
100g rocket
A pinch of flaked sea salt
A pinch of white pepper
Fresh mint leaves, to garnish

1 Set a large saucepan on a medium heat and add the olive oil. Add the spring onions and garlic and cook for 2 minutes until softened. Then add the celery and stock, bring to the boil and simmer for 5 minutes until the celery is soft.
2 Add the peas and bring back to the boil. Take the pan off the heat.
3 Add the rocket to the pan and use a hand blender to blitz the soup until smooth. Season with the sea salt and pepper before serving garnished with fresh mint leaves.

RICH IN Vitamins B6 and C • Folate • Potassium • Iron • Calcium • Beta-carotene • Fibre

USEFUL FOR Heart ①② • Digestion ① • Skin, hair & nails ①③ • Mind ① • Fatigue ① • Men ② • Women ①③

SALADS & VEGETABLES

I hope you will forgive me for stating the obvious: all vegetables are good for you. Each one contains vitamins and minerals (some are richer in certain vitamins and minerals than others) as well as a variety of antioxidants that help to protect us from disease. So it makes sense that vegetables form the biggest part of a healthy diet, and have a part to play in all meals and most snacks. This needn't be a hardship: you can weave vegetables into your diet in the most delicious ways. Celebrate and enjoy them in all their diversity.

In the UK, the average daily intake of vegetables and fruit is four portions. New research suggests the more we eat, the greater the benefit, and that we should be aiming for ten, not five, servings each day. Sound daunting? It shouldn't. Have a portion at breakfast (usually fruit), a couple of vegetables for lunch and two or three portions for dinner. Then throw in a few more portions for snacks and a juice for an additional boost. Hey presto!

Try to eat vegetables in the most colourful way possible. Greens are very nutritious but including a variety of colours will ensure you glean a complete range of key nutrients to support your good health. There are some vegetables that feature particularly high on our superstar list: kale, broccoli, squash, beetroot, avocado, garlic, edamame beans, cabbage and tomatoes. You'll see these colourful favourites appearing prominently in the recipes that follow.

At the end of most of the recipes, you'll find a list of the main nutrients supplied in a serving as well as a list of health issues that may be benefited by including the recipe in your healthy diet. For more, see page 9.

AVOCADO SALAD

SERVES 4 • 215 CALORIES PER SERVING
(WITHOUT RICE OR BREAD)

This salad is a best-seller in our deli. Smooth avocado with lots of finely diced vegetables, it's a bit like a chunky guacamole but it's definitely enough to have on its own. Remember that the riper the avocados, the more delicious your salad will be. Avocados are a good source of vitamin B6, a lack of which has been associated with PMS-related depression.

A handful of pumpkin seeds
3 ripe avocados
Juice of 1 lemon
½ iceberg lettuce, very finely sliced
2 celery sticks, diced
½ red onion, finely diced
A pinch of crushed dried chilli
1 yellow pepper, seeded and finely diced
Brown rice or Quinoa Bread (see page 44), to serve

1 Set a small non-stick pan on a medium heat, add the pumpkin seeds and gently toast them for 3–4 minutes. Set aside.
2 Peel each avocado and remove the stone. Place the flesh of two of the avocados in a blender with half the lemon juice and blitz until smooth. Remove with a spatula and place in a large mixing bowl.
3 Dice the remaining avocado and add to the bowl along with the rest of the ingredients, including the pumpkin seeds and remaining lemon juice. Mix well so that all the ingredients are coated with the avocado cream. Serve immediately with brown rice or quinoa bread.

RICH IN Vitamins B1 (thiamin), B6, C and E • Potassium • Beta-sitosterol • Fibre

USEFUL FOR Heart ①②③ • Digestion ① • Immunity ① • Mind ① • Fatigue ① • Men ① • Women ①③

FRESH PEA & RAW COURGETTE SALAD

SERVES 2 • 280 CALORIES PER SERVING

Sweet, tender, freshly picked peas are a real treat during the summer months, which is the time to make this salad. Peas are a useful non-meat source of iron, which is good to keep in mind if you're thinking of going meat-free – this dish provides more than half your daily requirement. It also contains a rich source of vitamin C to help your body to absorb more of the iron. If you are not lucky enough to grow your own peas, or to get fresh peas from your grocer, use podded and blanched broad beans instead.

400g podded fresh peas
Grated zest of 1 lemon
2 courgettes, very finely diced
A handful of fresh flat-leaf parsley, finely chopped
A few fresh mint leaves, finely chopped
4 fresh chives, finely chopped
1 tbsp olive oil
A pinch of flaked sea salt
A pinch of cracked black pepper

1 Bring a pan of water to the boil and blanch the peas for 1 minute. Drain in a colander and rinse under cold water to cool and retain the bright green colour.

2 Tip the peas into a blender, add the lemon zest and pulse for a second or two. You just want to lightly break up the peas, not make them mushy. The texture is very important in this dish.

3 Transfer the peas to a bowl and add the courgettes, parsley, mint, chives and olive oil. Mix gently together. Season with the salt and pepper and serve.

RICH IN Vitamins B1 (thiamin), B3 (niacin) and C • Folate • Potassium • Iron • Magnesium • Beta-carotene • Fibre

USEFUL FOR Heart ①②③ • Bones ① • Digestion ① • Immunity ① • Skin, hair & nails ①③ • Mind ①② • Fatigue ①③⑤ • Women ①

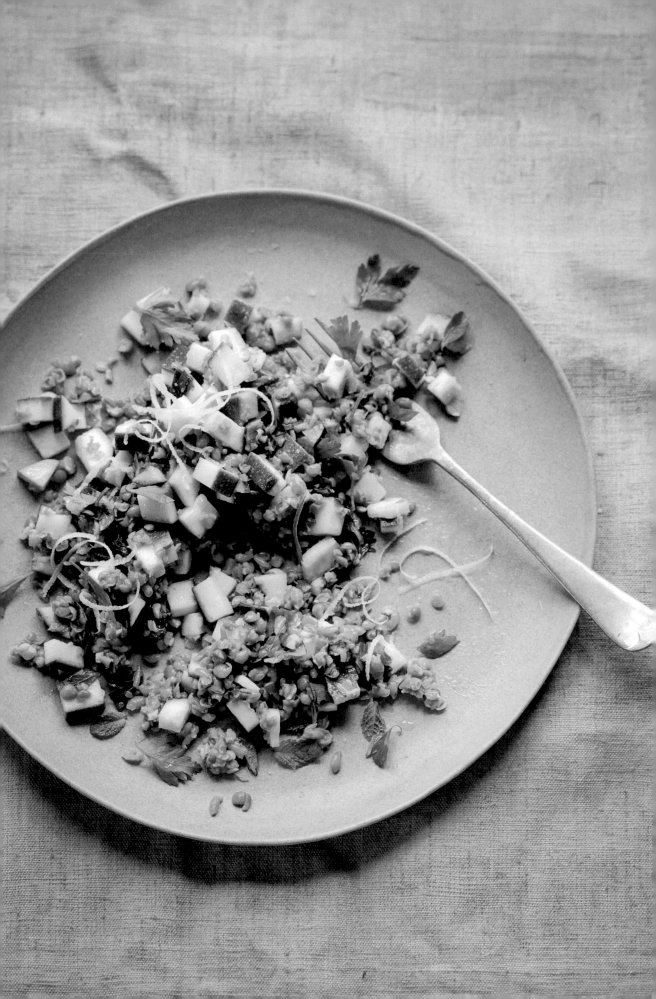

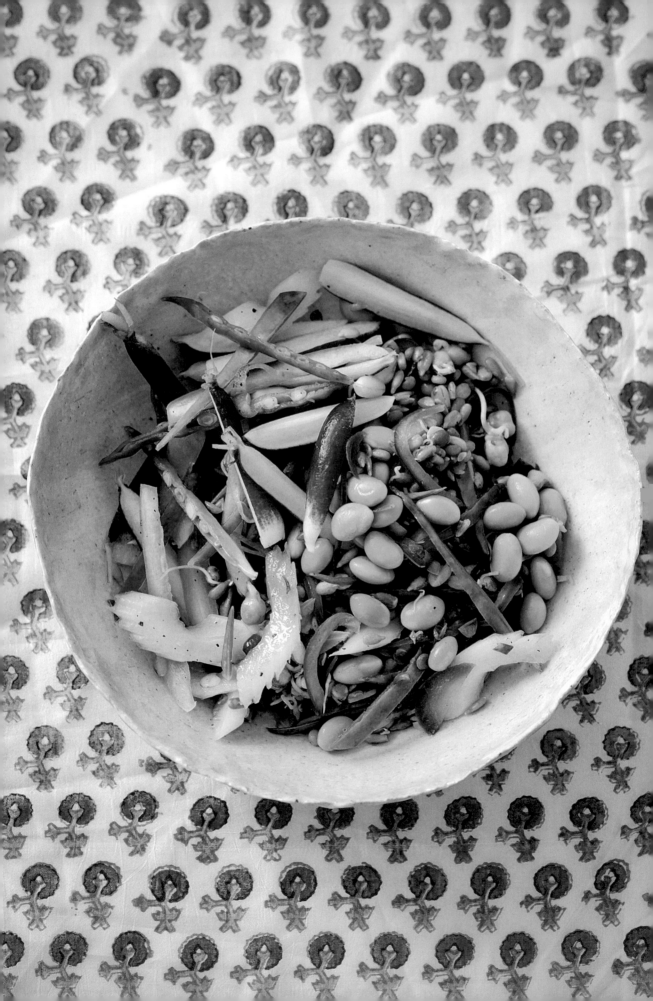

RADISH, EDAMAME & LENTIL SPROUT SALAD

SERVES 2 • 250 CALORIES PER SERVING

This salad has a wonderful texture – everything is crunchy and fresh tasting. It is perfect during summer months when you want something that is refreshing but also fills you up and keeps you going. The art of this salad is all in the chopping, keeping everything long, then adding the small sprouts and edamame. Opting for rapeseed oil in salad dressings is a useful way for vegetarians and vegans who don't eat fish to obtain omega 3 and help balance their fatty acid intake.

1 tsp rapeseed oil, plus extra for drizzling
½ red onion, finely sliced
150g lentil sprouts
1 tbsp sunflower seeds
Grated zest and juice of 1 lemon
100g edamame beans, thawed if frozen
100g mange tout, sliced lengthways
100g 'breakfast' radishes, sliced lengthways
2 celery sticks, sliced
½ yellow pepper, seeded and sliced
Salt and pepper

1 Heat the oil in a frying pan over a medium heat, then add the onion and sauté for 3 minutes until softened. Add the lentil sprouts and sunflower seeds and cook until the seeds are lightly golden. Stir in the lemon zest and a pinch each of salt and pepper, then remove from the heat.
2 Transfer the sprout and seed mixture to a large mixing bowl and add the edamame, mange tout, radishes, celery and yellow pepper. Add the lemon juice, a drizzle of rapeseed oil and some salt and pepper. Toss together, then serve.

RICH IN Vitamins B1 (thiamin), B6, C and E • Folate • Potassium • Iron • Phytoestrogens • Fibre

USEFUL FOR Heart ①② • Digestion ① • Immunity ① • Mind ①② • Fatigue ① • Women ①③④

GREEN PAPAYA SALAD

SERVES 2 • 170 CALORIES PER SERVING

This Thai-inspired salad is incredibly more-ish. The sweetness of tomatoes and orange juice mixed with the sharpness of lime and crunch of green papaya and green beans creates a brilliantly fresh, zingy salad that's great with grilled salmon or king prawns. Both green beans and sesame seeds provide a useful source of phytoestrogens. A diet rich in these plant chemicals may help with hot flushes during the menopause. Look for green papaya in your local ethnic store.

150g green beans, finely chopped
1 green papaya
100g cherry tomatoes, cut in half
1 spring onion, finely diced
1 garlic clove, finely chopped
A handful of fresh coriander, finely chopped
Juice of 2 limes
Juice of 1 orange
1 tbsp rapeseed oil
1 tbsp toasted sesame seeds
1 tsp flaked sea salt
A pinch of cracked black pepper

1 Bring a pan of water to the boil. Drop in the green beans and blanch for 1 minute. Drain in a colander and rinse under cold water until completely cool. Drain and set aside.
2 Peel the papaya and cut it lengthways in half. Remove the white seeds and discard. Grate the flesh and put into a large mixing bowl.
3 Add the tomatoes and, using your hands, squeeze them so that all the juice comes out and is combined with the papaya. Add the green beans along with the remaining ingredients and mix together well. Serve straight away or chill for 10 minutes before serving.

RICH IN Vitamin C • Folate • Potassium • Papain • Phytoestrogens

USEFUL FOR Heart ②③ • Digestion ④ • Immunity ①

RADISH, CUCUMBER & DILL SALAD

SERVES 2 • 60 CALORIES PER SERVING

Radishes are the prettiest vegetable, with their bright pink skin and contrasting white flesh (round Cherry Belle is my favourite variety). They make a colourful salad mixed with cucumber and fresh herbs – the perfect accompaniment for grilled or barbecued fish. If your radishes are really fresh, you can use the green leaves too. Their peppery flavour contrasts well with the chives.

2 cucumbers

100g radishes

Juice of 1 lemon

1 tsp runny honey

A handful of fresh dill, finely chopped

A handful of fresh chives, finely chopped

Salt and pepper

1 Peel the cucumbers, then slice very finely. (Use a mandoline if you have one as you want the slices to be as thin as possible.) Alternatively, you can cut the cucumber lengthways in half and scoop out the seeds before slicing into thin half-moons. Place in a bowl.

2 Trim off the long root from each radish, then thinly slice them (again, use a mandoline if you have one). Add these to the cucumber.

3 Mix together the lemon juice, honey, dill, chives and some salt and pepper in a small bowl. Add this dressing to the cucumber and radishes and mix well.

4 Cover the salad with clingfilm and leave in the fridge for 30 minutes. Drain off the excess liquid before serving.

RICH IN Vitamin C • Potassium

USEFUL FOR Heart ② • Immunity ①

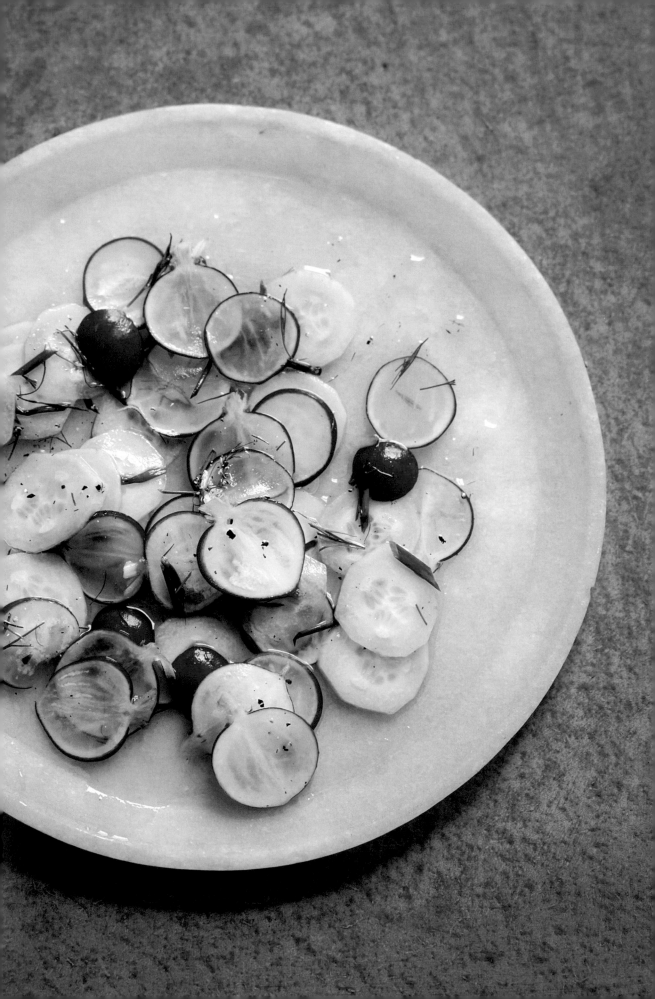

CABBAGE, APPLE & TARRAGON SALAD

SERVES 2 • 120 CALORIES PER SERVING

This is a sharp, crunchy, brightly coloured salad. The pigment in red cabbage that gives it its rich purple colour contains a group of antioxidants which hold anti-inflammatory properties that may help to protect against heart disease. Red cabbages are at their most delicious in January and February, so try this salad with a piece of grilled chicken for a fresh winter lunch. The aniseed flavour of tarragon gives the salad a real taste boost.

1 small red cabbage
1 eating apple
2 sprigs of fresh tarragon, finely chopped
1 garlic clove, finely sliced
Juice of 1 lemon
1 tbsp rapeseed oil
A pinch of salt
A pinch of black pepper

1 Cut the cabbage into four wedges and cut out the core. Using a sharp knife or mandoline, slice the cabbage into very fine strips.
2 Core the apple and cut into very thin slices. (If you can keep them as complete rounds that will look great, but it may be easier to cut them in half and then thinly slice.)
3 Mix the cabbage and apple in a large mixing bowl with the tarragon, garlic, lemon juice, oil, salt and pepper. Serve immediately.

RICH IN Vitamin C • Folate • Fibre

USEFUL FOR Heart ① • Digestion ① • Immunity ①

SAMPHIRE, ROCKET & PEA SALAD

SERVES 2 • 295 CALORIES PER SERVING

Affectionately known as the asparagus of the sea, samphire grows on mud flats on the coast. It is best eaten during May when it is most tender. Along with other sea vegetables, it is high in zinc, which is great for male reproductive health and a no-brainer for any man trying to increase fertility.

300g samphire
300g podded fresh peas
1 tsp olive oil
1 garlic clove, finely sliced
A handful of pumpkin seeds
200g rocket
Juice of ½ lemon
A pinch of cracked black pepper

1 Give the samphire a good wash – it can be very salty, so do this thoroughly. Bring a large pan of water to the boil, then drop in the samphire and cook for 7 minutes. Add the peas and cook for a further 2 minutes. Drain in a colander and rinse under cold water.
2 Heat the olive oil in a non-stick frying pan and fry the garlic and pumpkin seeds until lightly golden. Add the samphire and peas and gently sauté for 2 minutes.
3 Tip into a large salad bowl. Mix through the rocket, lemon juice and pepper, then serve.

RICH IN Vitamins B3 (niacin), B6 and C • Folate • Potassium • Iron • Zinc • Calcium • Beta-sitosterol • Beta-carotene • Fibre

USEFUL FOR Heart ①②③ • Bones ② • Digestion ① • Immunity ① • Skin, hair & nails ①③ • Mind ① • Fatigue ① • Men ①② • Women ①

CARROT & CUCUMBER RIBBONS

SERVES 2 • 180 CALORIES PER SERVING

Fresh and crunchy, this salad is perfect for lunch in the summer. The long slender ribbons of orange and green look wonderfully appetising, and as cucumbers are more than 90 per cent water, they will help keep you well hydrated in warm weather. The salad is delicious served with grilled fish or chicken too.

1 tbsp sesame seeds

2 carrots

2 cucumbers

2 spring onions, finely chopped

FOR THE DRESSING

½ fresh red chilli, seeded and finely chopped

2 garlic cloves, peeled

Juice of 2 limes

1 tbsp toasted sesame oil

1 Preheat your oven to 200°C/fan 180°C/gas 6.

2 Spread the sesame seeds on a small baking tray and toast in the oven for 6 minutes until golden. Set aside.

3 To make the dressing, put the chilli, garlic, lime juice and sesame oil in a small blender and blitz to a paste. If you don't have a small blender you can just finely chop everything and mix together in a bowl, then leave for a few hours to infuse.

4 Peel the carrots. Using a vegetable peeler and working from root end to tip, shave off long ribbons. Keep turning the carrot to take ribbons from all sides.

5 Peel long strips from the cucumber, shaving them from one end to the other. Stop taking ribbons when you get to the seedy centre.

6 Combine the carrots, cucumber and spring onions in a large bowl. Mix through the dressing and toasted sesame seeds, then serve.

RICH IN Vitamin C • Potassium • Beta-carotene • Fibre

USEFUL FOR Heart ①②③ • Bones ① • Digestion ① • Immunity ① • Skin, hair & nails ①③

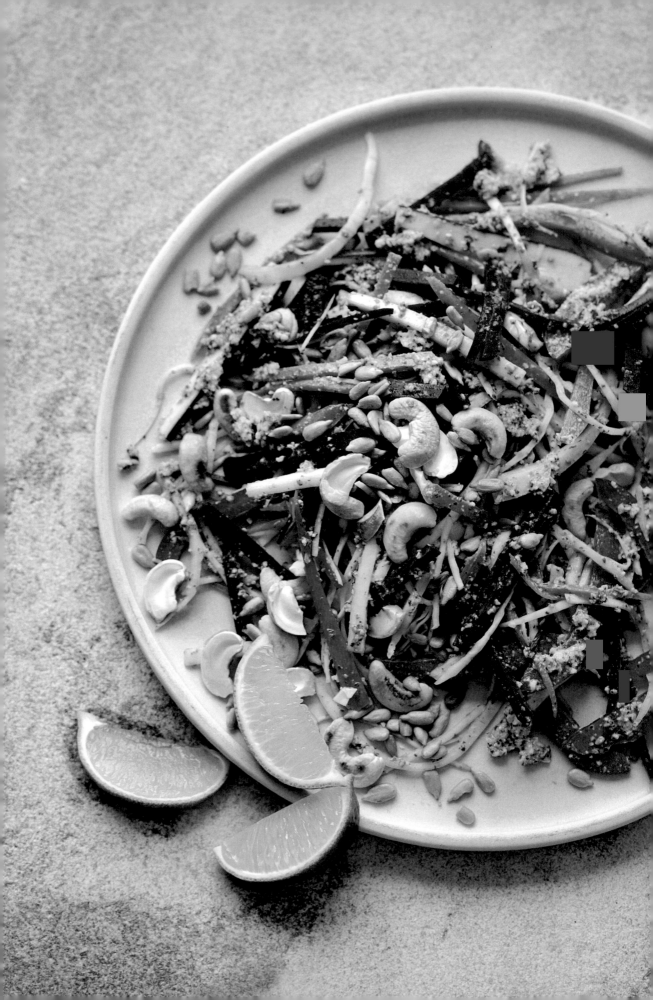

RAW VEGETABLE & GINGER SALAD

SERVES 4 • 215 CALORIES PER SERVING

Crunchy, fragrant and zingy, this salad is a rainbow of vegetables topped with a coarse-textured gingery dressing. Fresh ginger is a powerful anti-inflammatory, so don't be shy about adding a little more to the recipe if you can take the heat. The salad is perfect on its own or served with some grilled chicken or fish.

RICH IN Vitamins B6, C and E • Folate • Potassium • Beta-carotene • Nitrates • Fibre

USEFUL FOR Heart ①②③ • Bones ① • Digestion ① • Immunity ① • Skin, hair & nails ①③ • Mind ① • Women ①③

50g cashew nuts

30g sunflower seeds

2 carrots

1 raw beetroot

1 courgette

1 red pepper, seeded and thinly sliced

½ small white cabbage, cored and very finely sliced

2 spring onions, finely sliced on the diagonal

Lime wedges, to serve

FOR THE GINGER DRESSING

A large thumb-sized piece of fresh ginger, peeled and roughly chopped

1 tbsp rapeseed oil

Juice of 1 lemon

Juice of 1 lime

A handful of fresh mint leaves

2 handfuls of fresh coriander

1 Preheat your oven to 200°C/fan 180°C/gas 6.

2 Spread the cashew nuts and sunflower seeds on a baking tray and toast in the oven for about 8 minutes until golden. Leave to cool.

3 To make the ginger dressing, put half of the toasted nuts and seeds in a blender with all the dressing ingredients and blitz for 1 minute to create a coarse-textured mixture.

4 Peel the carrots, beetroot and courgette, then cut them into long, very thin matchsticks. If you are pressed for time, you can just grate the vegetables.

5 Place all the prepared vegetables in a large mixing bowl and mix through the ginger dressing. Top with the remaining toasted sunflower seeds and cashew nuts and serve with wedges of lime for squeezing over.

FENNEL, APPLE & BUTTERNUT SALAD

SERVES 4 • 145 CALORIES PER SERVING

This is a colourful, tastebud-stimulating salad. It's perfect for a light lunch or served alongside roasted chicken. Apples contain pectin, which is a type of soluble fibre that may help to reduce cholesterol levels in the blood.

1 butternut squash
4 tsp rapeseed oil
1 tsp coriander seeds
1 fennel bulb
2 tbsp lemon juice
1 eating apple, such as Braeburn
½ red onion, thinly sliced
Grated zest and juice of 1 orange
1 tbsp finely chopped fresh coriander
1 tbsp finely chopped fresh chives
Salt and cracked black pepper

1 Preheat your oven to 200°C/fan 180°C/gas 6. Line a baking tray with greaseproof paper.
2 First prepare the butternut squash. You can leave the skin on, if you prefer. Cut lengthways in half and scoop out the seeds and fibres, then cut across in half. Cut the pieces into 1cm wedges. Place them on the lined baking tray, drizzle 1 teaspoon of the oil over them and sprinkle with the coriander seeds, salt and cracked black pepper. Roast for 20–25 minutes until tender.
3 Meanwhile, prepare the fennel and apple. Trim the fennel (keep the delicate leaves for the garnish), then thinly slice lengthways. Place the fennel in a bowl with the lemon juice and remaining oil and toss together with your hands. Peel the apple and slice thinly. Place in the bowl with the fennel.
4 Add the red onion, orange zest and juice, fresh coriander and chives, and some salt and pepper. Toss to mix.
5 Once the butternut is ready, place it on a large plate and leave to cool a bit. Serve it warm, covered with the fennel, apple and onion mixture and garnished with the fennel leaves.

RICH IN Vitamins C and E • Folate • Potassium • Beta-carotene • Fibre

USEFUL FOR Heart ①② • Digestion ① • Immunity ① • Skin, hair & nails ①③

PURPLE KALE, BROCCOLI, SHALLOT & CHILLI SALAD

SERVES 2 • 420 CALORIES PER SERVING

Kale seems to be winning the vegetable popularity contest at the moment – you see it being used everywhere. For this warm salad, don't buy the kale that you find in sealed bags in supermarkets because it can be tasteless and will go mushy when stir-fried. Instead, get a big head of kale, ideally purple kale as it adds wonderful colour to the dish. This is the perfect recipe for healthy bones: calcium from the kale and the broccoli (33 per cent of the RDA) partnered with magnesium from the cashew nuts (60 per cent of the RDA).

1 head of purple kale
1 tsp rapeseed oil
3 shallots, finely sliced
1 garlic clove, finely chopped
100g cashew nuts
1 head of broccoli, separated into small florets (with as much of the stalk as possible)
A pinch of crushed dried chilli

1 Pull the kale leaves from the thick central stalks. Tear the leaves into pieces.
2 Set a large non-stick frying pan or wok on a medium heat and add the oil, then add the shallots and cook for 5 minutes until slightly golden. Add the garlic and cook for a further 3 minutes.
3 Add the cashew nuts and broccoli and stir-fry for 3–5 minutes until the broccoli is starting to get tender. Add a splash of water if the ingredients start to stick.
4 Add the chilli and kale and stir-fry for 4 more minutes until the kale is slightly wilted but still crunchy. Remove from the heat and serve immediately.

RICH IN Vitamins B1 (thiamin), B6 and C • Folate • Potassium • Magnesium • Zinc • Calcium • Chromium • Fibre

USEFUL FOR Heart ①②③ • Bones ① • Digestion ① • Immunity ① • Skin, hair & nails ①④ • Mind ①② • Fatigue ③⑤ • Men ①② • Women ①④

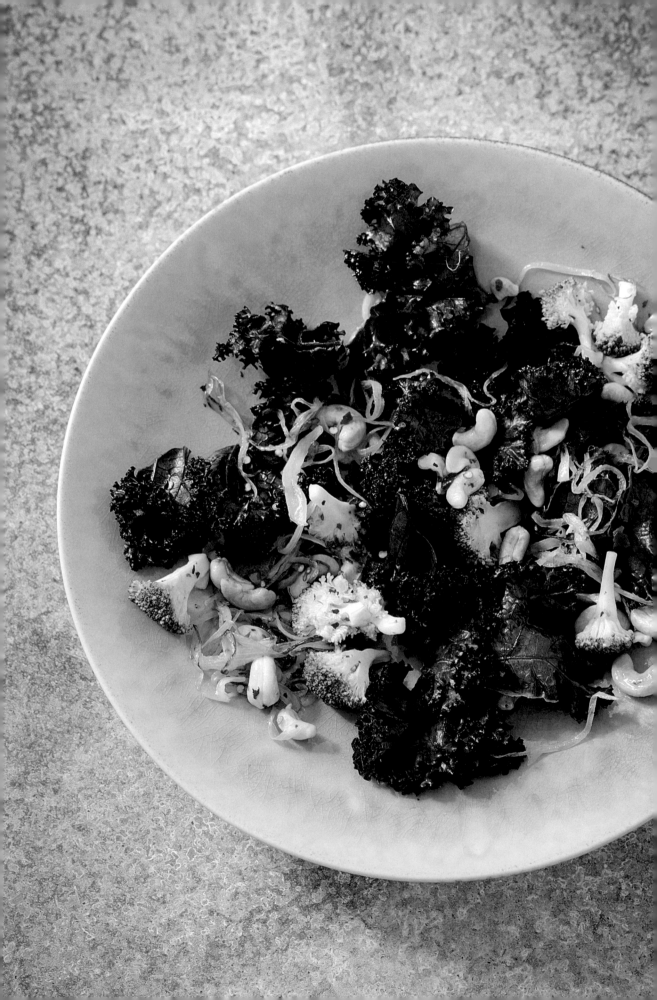

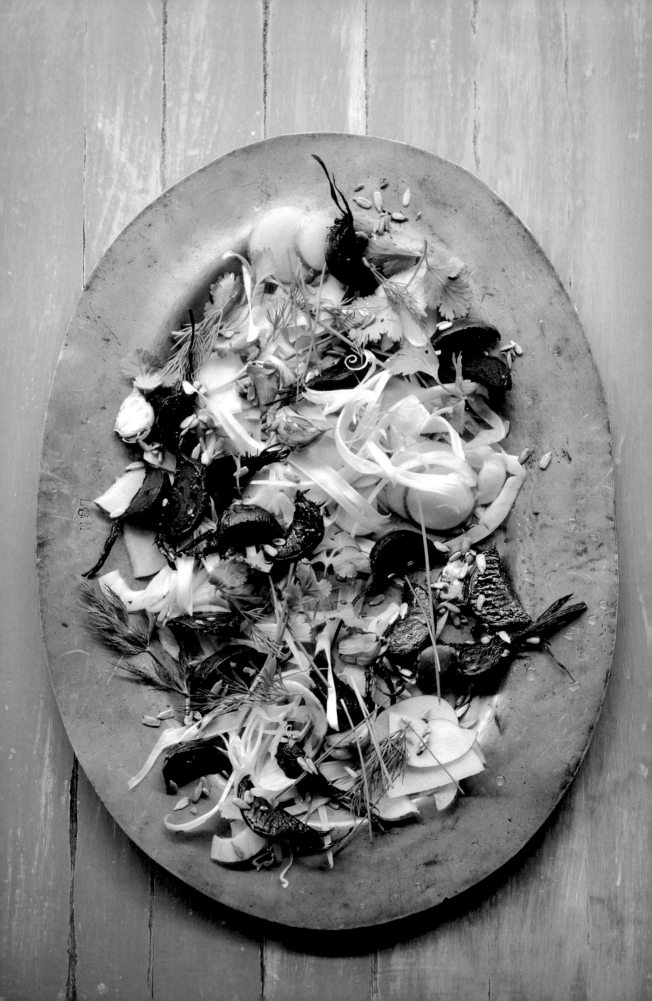

ROASTED BEETROOT, FENNEL & APPLE SALAD

SERVES 2 • 220 CALORIES PER SERVING

This salad is beautiful and colourful, and the flavour combination is complex – sometimes sweet, sometimes earthy, sometimes bitter. Both fennel bulb and seeds, with their distinctive aniseed flavour, are included. Fennel has traditionally been used as a tonic, and a 'tummy tea' can be made by adding fennel seeds and mint to hot water.

4 large raw beetroots
4 garlic cloves, crushed with the skin on
1 tsp fennel seeds
Grated zest and juice of 1 lemon
1 tsp olive oil
A handful of sunflower seeds
1 fennel bulb
3 eating apples, such as Braeburn
2 spring onions, finely sliced
A handful of fresh chives, chopped
A handful of fresh coriander, chopped
Salt and pepper
Fennel leaves or fennel flowers, to garnish

1 Preheat your oven to 200°C/fan 180°C/gas 6.
2 Wash the unpeeled beetroots thoroughly, then cut each into eight wedges. Place them on a baking tray with the garlic, fennel seeds, lemon zest, oil and a pinch each of salt and pepper. Cover with foil and roast in the heated oven for 20 minutes. Remove the foil and cook for a further 15 minutes.
3 Remove the tray from the oven and sprinkle the sunflower seeds over the beetroot. Roast for 5 more minutes.
4 Meanwhile, finely slice the fennel bulb, either using a mandoline or by hand, and place in a large mixing bowl. Wash two of the apples and juice them, then pour the juice over the fennel. Peel, core and finely slice the third apple, then add to the fennel with the spring onions, lemon juice, chives and coriander. Season to taste. Toss together, then transfer to a serving bowl.
5 Place the beetroot mixture on top of the fennel salad and garnish with fennel flowers.

RICH IN Vitamin C • Folate • Potassium • Iron • Nitrates • Fibre

USEFUL FOR Heart ①② • Digestion ① • Immunity ① • Fatigue ①

GRIDDLED COURGETTE & ASPARAGUS WITH ROCKET PESTO

SERVES 2 • 310 CALORIES PER SERVING

Courgettes are the easiest vegetables to grow. As a result, gardeners often have a glut and are always looking for new ways to cook them. Griddling on a ridged griddle/grill pan is perfect because it keeps the crunchy texture whilst adding a light smoky flavour. It's a great method for asparagus too, so this is a dish to make in spring when asparagus is in season. Asparagus contains high levels of an amino acid called asparagine, which acts as a natural diuretic.

12 asparagus spears
12 baby courgettes, cut lengthways in half
2 tbsp rapeseed oil
A pinch of flaked sea salt
A pinch of cracked black pepper
1 tbsp sunflower seeds
1 tsp pine nuts
Grated zest and juice of 1 lemon
200g rocket
Salt

RICH IN Vitamins B1 (thiamin), B6, C and E • Folate • Potassium • Iron • Calcium • Magnesium • Beta-carotene • Asparagine • Fibre

USEFUL FOR Heart ①②③ • Bones ① • Digestion ① • Immunity ① • Skin, hair & nails ①③ • Mind ①② • Fatigue ①⑤ • Women ①③

1 Set a ridged cast-iron griddle/grill pan on a high heat. When the pan is smoking hot, turn the heat down to medium.
2 Meanwhile, snap the tough end of the stalk from each asparagus spear, then cut the spears lengthways in half. Place the asparagus and courgettes, flesh side up, on a chopping board, drizzle over a little of the oil and sprinkle with the sea salt and cracked black pepper.
3 Place the vegetables flesh side down in the griddle/grill pan and cook for 3 minutes until marked with charred lines. Turn over and cook the other side for 2 minutes. Remove from the pan and keep hot.
4 Put the seeds and nuts in a small pan and toast gently for 3 minutes until golden, swirling them in the pan from time to time. Tip them into a blender and add the lemon zest and juice, remaining oil, half the rocket and a pinch of salt. Blitz until smooth.
5 To serve, spread out the rest of the rocket on a plate, top with the griddled vegetables and drizzle the pesto over them.

SWEET POTATO CAKES WITH KALE & GREEN BEANS

SERVES 4 • 355 CALORIES PER SERVING

Choose small/medium-sized sweet potatoes for this recipe because these will be smoother and more tender when cooked, perfect for mashing. Sweet potatoes have a low glycaemic load (GL), meaning they have less of an effect on blood sugar levels after eating. A low GL diet can be a useful approach to losing weight.

4 tbsp rock salt (not to eat)

4 small/medium sweet potatoes

1 egg yolk

2 tbsp gluten- and wheat-free flour

½ red onion, finely diced

2 sprigs of fresh thyme, leaves picked

A pinch of cracked black pepper

200g kale, shredded

150g green beans

40g hazelnuts

40g pumpkin seeds

Grated zest of 1 orange

150g cherry tomatoes

Salt

RICH IN Vitamins B1 (thiamin), B6, C and E • Folate • Potassium • Iron • Beta-carotene • Fibre

USEFUL FOR Heart ①② • Digestion ① • Skin, hair & nails ①③ • Mind ① • Fatigue ① • Women ①

1 Preheat your oven to 200°C/fan 180°C/gas 6. Line a baking tray with greaseproof paper.

2 Make four mounds of rock salt on the baking tray and set a sweet potato on top of each mound. Bake for 35 minutes until soft.

3 Remove from the oven and leave to cool for 15 minutes, then peel off the skin (you could roast the skin a bit longer to enjoy as a sweet, crisp little snack). Place the sweet potato flesh in a bowl. (Discard the salt.)

4 Add the egg yolk, flour, red onion, thyme leaves, cracked black pepper and a pinch of salt. Mix well – the mixture will be quite wet. Form into eight 2cm-thick cakes and place on the baking tray. Bake for 25 minutes until crisp.

5 Meanwhile, bring a large pan of water to the boil. Add the kale and green beans and cook for 1 minute. Drain and refresh under cold running water, then place in a large mixing bowl.

6 Set a small frying pan on a medium heat and toast the hazelnuts and pumpkins seeds for 4 minutes until lightly browned. Tip them into the mixing bowl along with the orange zest, cherry tomatoes and a pinch of salt. Toss to mix.

7 Serve the sweet potato cakes on a bed of kale and green bean salad.

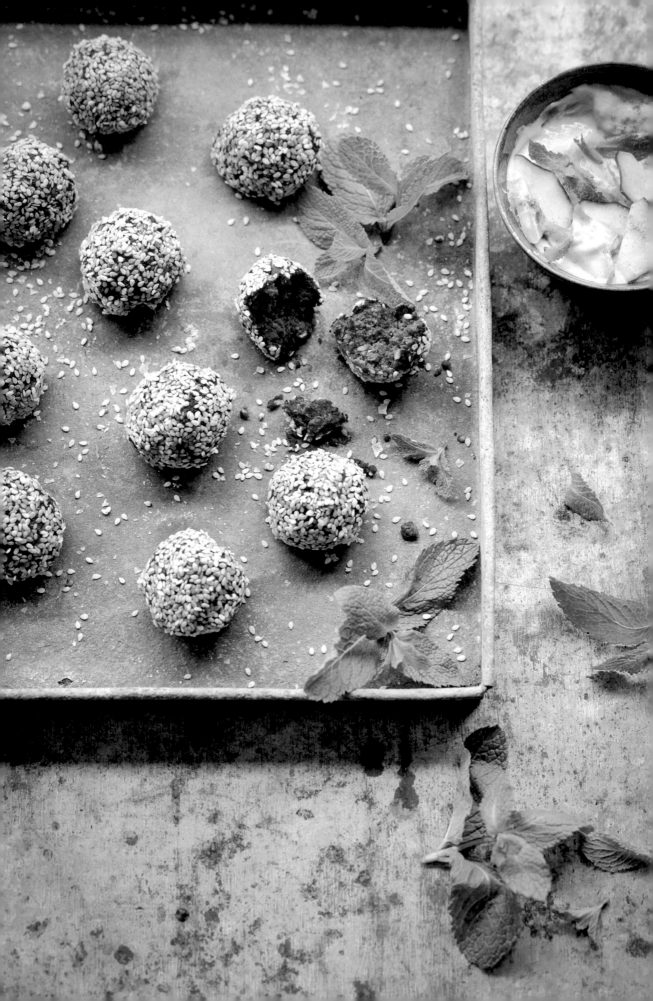

BEETROOT FALAFEL

SERVES 4 • 385 CALORIES PER SERVING

This recipe is the result of a heroic number of falafel trials. The main reason falafels go wrong is taking a short cut and using tinned chickpeas. This always results in wet, mushy, sad-looking falafels. But if you start with dried chickpeas, you will end up with wonderfully crisp, round, textured falafels. We've added beetroot to these for its bright red colour. Beetroot is a rich source of folate, which is used in the production of red blood cells and helps ward off anaemia.

200g dried chickpeas
2 raw beetroots, peeled and finely diced
1 carrot, finely diced
50g cashew nuts
30g home-shelled pistachio nuts
1 tsp olive oil
½ red onion, finely diced
2 garlic cloves, finely chopped
1 egg, lightly beaten with a fork
Grated zest of 1 lemon
2 tsp ground cumin
1 tsp smoked paprika
1 tbsp sesame seeds

FOR THE YOGURT DIP
3 tbsp plain soya yogurt
Grated zest and juice of 1 lemon
1 tsp tahini
1 cucumber, peeled, seeded and finely sliced
A pinch of ground cumin
A pinch of salt

TO SERVE
Iceberg lettuce, separated into leaves
Fresh mint leaves

1 Soak the chickpeas in cold water overnight. The next day, drain and place them in a fresh pan of cold water. Bring to the boil and simmer for about 50 minutes until soft. Drain and pat dry with kitchen paper.

2 Preheat your oven to 180°C/fan 160°C/gas 4. Line a baking tray with greaseproof paper.

3 Place the chickpeas, beetroot, carrot, cashew nuts and pistachios in a blender and pulse until finely chopped. Transfer to a large mixing bowl. Set aside.

4 Heat the olive oil in a non-stick frying pan and cook the onion and garlic until soft. Add them to the bowl along with the rest of the ingredients (except the sesame seeds). Mix together well.

5 Shape the mixture into small balls and roll them in the sesame seeds to coat. Place the balls on the baking tray and bake in the heated oven for 50 minutes.

6 Meanwhile, make the dip by mixing together all the ingredients for it.

7 Serve the falafels with the dip, lettuce leaves and mint. To eat, place three mint leaves on a lettuce leaf, set a falafel on this, add a dollop of yogurt dip and wrap up.

RICH IN Vitamins B1 (thiamin) and B6 • Folate • Potassium • Iron • Magnesium • Beta-carotene • Phytoestrogens • Beta-sitosterol • Nitrates

USEFUL FOR Heart ①②③ • Bones ① • Skin, hair & nails ①③④ • Mind ①② • Fatigue ①③⑤ • Men ① • Women ①③④

BUTTERNUT STEAKS & ROASTED SHALLOTS

SERVES 2 • 155 CALORIES PER SERVING

When you serve these butternut steaks you might be met with a puzzled frown. Where's the meat? But after two mouthfuls there will be silence, followed by a smile, because this rich, savoury dish will satisfy any meat-eater (even my carnivorous brother likes it). Butternut squash is a good source of vitamin B6, which is essential for the proper functioning of both the immune and nervous systems.

1 butternut squash

1 tbsp olive oil

1 tsp flaked sea salt

1 tsp cracked black pepper

4 sprigs of fresh rosemary

4 sprigs of fresh thyme

1 tbsp rapeseed oil

1 tsp runny honey

3 banana shallots, cut in half with the skin on

FOR THE SPINACH AND ROCKET SALAD

2 handfuls of spinach, roughly chopped

2 handfuls of rocket

A handful of basil leaves, roughly chopped

1 tsp olive oil

Juice of ½ lemon

1 tbsp sunflower seeds, toasted

Salt and pepper

1 Preheat your oven to 200°C/fan 180°C/gas 6. Line two baking trays with greaseproof paper.

2 Starting at the stalk end, cut across the squash, on the diagonal, to create four 2.5cm-thick oval slices. When you reach the bulbous bottom part, cut this off (you can keep it for soup).

3 Lay the squash 'steaks' on one of the baking trays. Score a diamond pattern in the squash flesh, then add a drizzle of olive oil and the sea salt and pepper. Place a sprig of rosemary and a sprig of thyme on each steak. Set aside.

4 Heat the rapeseed oil with the honey in a non-stick frying pan over a medium heat. Place the shallots cut side down in the pan and cook for 10 minutes until golden. Transfer them to the other baking tray, keeping the cut side down (this will prevent them from overcooking and drying out).

5 Place both of the baking trays in the oven and roast for 30–40 minutes until the butternut steaks and shallots are tender.

6 Meanwhile, make the salad by tossing the spinach, rocket and basil with the olive oil, lemon juice, salt and pepper. Sprinkle with the sunflower seeds.

7 Remove the skin from the shallots. Set the shallots on top of the butternut steaks and serve with the salad.

RICH IN Vitamins B6, C and E • Folate • Potassium • Magnesium • Calcium • Iron • Beta-carotene • Fibre

USEFUL FOR Heart ①②③ • Bones ① • Digestion ① • Immunity ① • Skin, hair & nails ①③ • Mind ①② • Fatigue ①③⑤ • Women ①③

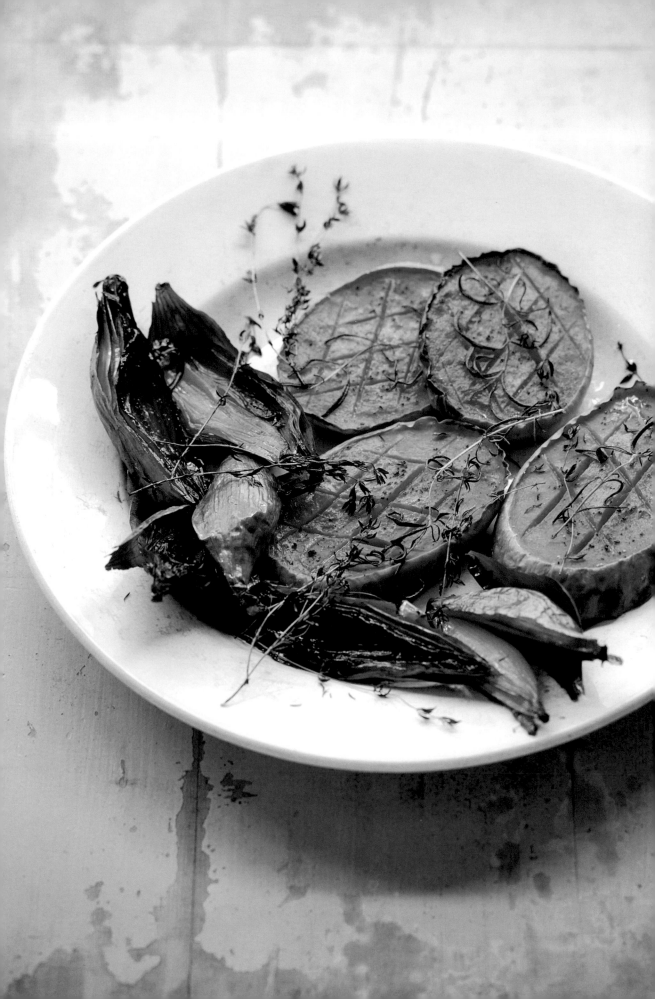

COURGETTE STUFFED WITH BEETROOT & SHALLOT

SERVES 2 • 380 CALORIES PER SERVING

Similar to a dish we had in India, I created this version from taste memory. The key is to buy thick courgettes so that you can fill the pieces with lots of sweet potato and beetroot. The dish is garnished with shallots, which bring all the elements of the dish together and give it a really savoury, more-ish taste. All onions and garlic contain non-digestible fibres that act as prebiotics (more so if eaten raw) and feed friendly bacteria in the gut, which helps to maintain good digestion. The courgettes are great as a main dish, with two each, or a lovely starter for four.

1 tbsp rock salt (not to eat)

1 sweet potato

4 courgettes

1 tsp rapeseed oil

5 shallots, finely chopped

A 2.5cm piece of fresh ginger, grated with the skin on

2 garlic cloves, finely chopped

2 celery sticks, finely diced

2 raw beetroots, peeled and grated

150ml coconut milk

1 tbsp sesame seeds

1 Preheat your oven to 200°C/fan 180°C/gas 6. Line a small baking tray with greaseproof paper.

2 Create a mound of rock salt on the baking tray and set the sweet potato on the mound. Roast for 35 minutes until soft. Remove from the oven (leave it on) and allow to cool, then peel the sweet potato and set it aside. (Discard the rock salt.)

3 While the sweet potato is roasting, cut the courgettes lengthways in half, then scoop out the soft centre with a teaspoon – make sure not to scoop out all the flesh to break through to the skin because the courgette 'boats' need to be thick enough to hold a little liquid in the filling. Set aside.

4 Heat a saucepan, then add the oil and cook the shallots for 5 minutes until soft. Remove half of the shallots and set aside. Add the ginger, garlic, celery and beetroot to the saucepan and cook for 5 minutes, then turn the heat to low. Add the coconut milk and stir to mix. Simmer for 5 minutes to reduce, stirring occasionally. Remove from the heat. Add the cooked sweet potato and mix well.

5 Place the courgette halves on the baking tray. Spoon the sweet potato and beetroot mixture into the courgettes to fill them and top with the reserved cooked shallots and the sesame seeds. Place in the oven and bake for 15 minutes. Serve warm with a spinach and sunflower seed salad.

RICH IN Vitamins B1 (thiamin), B6 and C • Folate • Potassium • Iron • Calcium • Magnesium • Beta-carotene • Prebiotics • Nitrates • Fibre

USEFUL FOR Heart ①② • Bones ① • Digestion ① • Immunity ① • Skin, hair & nails ①③ • Mind ①② • Fatigue ①⑤ • Women ①

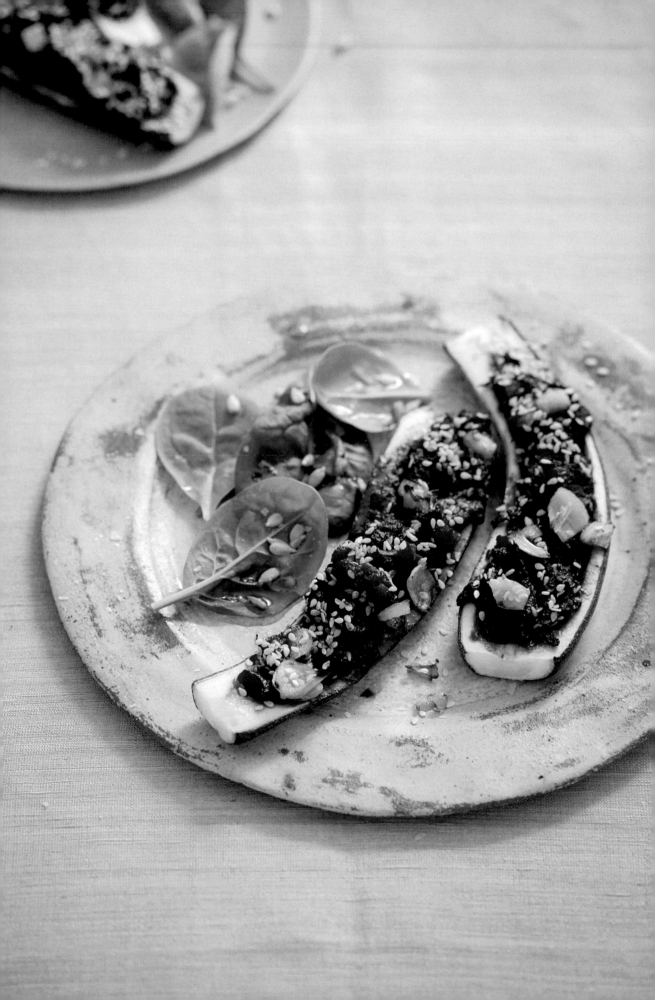

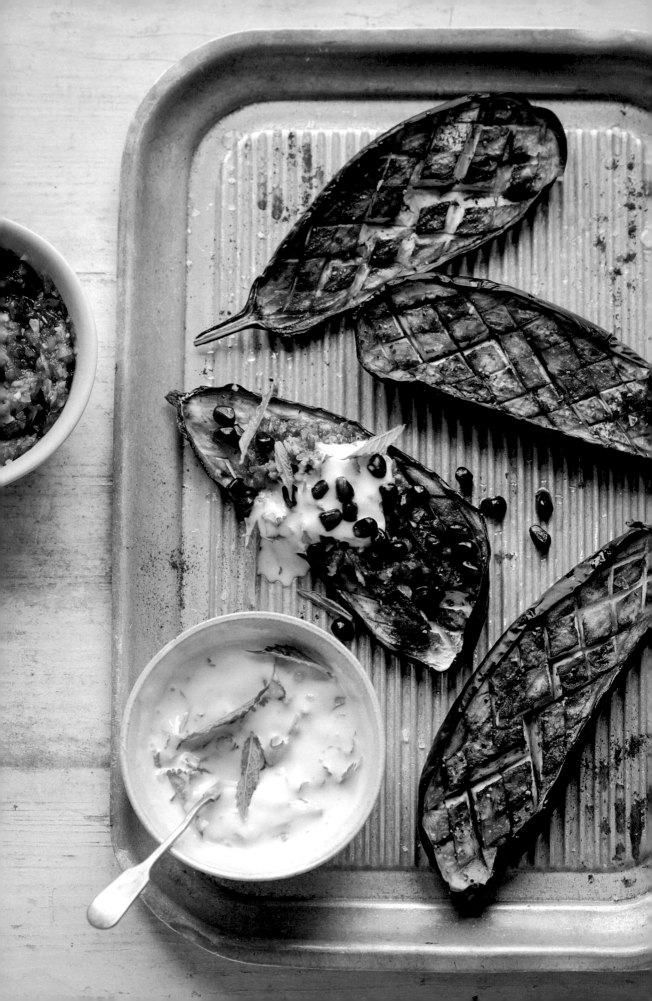

BAKED AUBERGINE WITH POMEGRANATE

SERVES 4 • 145 CALORIES PER SERVING

Middle-Eastern food inspires many of our recipes. The one here is a beautiful dish of contrasts, with the creamy, earthy, slightly bitter aubergine flesh perfectly complemented by the light yogurt, fresh mint and sweet pomegranate seeds. Fresh herbs and spices reduce the need for salt when you're flavouring food, whilst adding an extra nutritional boost to your dishes.

4 aubergines
1 tsp smoked paprika
1 tsp olive oil
1 pomegranate
A pinch of ground sumac, to garnish

FOR THE TOMATO SAUCE
8 ripe vine tomatoes, roughly chopped
4 shallots, roughly chopped
1 fresh red chilli, seeded and roughly chopped
1 celery stick, roughly chopped
5 garlic cloves, roughly chopped
A handful of fresh flat-leaf parsley, roughly chopped
2 sprigs of fresh thyme, leaves picked

FOR THE YOGURT DRESSING
1 tbsp plain soya yogurt
Grated zest and juice of 1 lemon
A handful of fresh coriander, finely chopped
A handful of fresh mint, finely chopped, plus extra leaves to garnish
Salt and pepper

1 Preheat your oven to 200°C/fan 180°C/gas 6.
2 Cut the aubergines lengthways in half. Score the flesh in a diamond pattern, cutting about 1cm deep. Sprinkle with the paprika and some salt and pepper, and drizzle the olive oil over the flesh. Place the aubergine halves, cut side up, on a baking tray and bake in the heated oven for 25 minutes until completely soft.
3 Meanwhile, make the tomato sauce. Combine all the ingredients in a blender and blitz for 30 seconds to create a chunky mixture. Transfer to a medium saucepan. Bring to the boil, then simmer on a medium/low heat for 20 minutes, stirring occasionally.
4 Mix the yogurt with the lemon zest and juice, coriander and mint. Season with salt and pepper to taste.
5 Next remove the seeds from the pomegranate. Cut it in half and place the halves cut side down on some kitchen paper. Gently tap them with a wooden spoon until all the seeds have fallen out. You will have to remove some of the skin that has fallen out too.
6 To serve, place two aubergine halves on each plate. Top with tomato sauce, then yogurt dressing and, finally, pomegranate seeds. Garnish with mint leaves and sumac.

RICH IN Vitamins B6 and C • Folate • Potassium • Lycopene • Fibre

USEFUL FOR Heart ①② • Digestion ① • Immunity ① • Mind ① • Men ① • Women ①

ROASTED BABY AUBERGINE WITH SPINACH SALAD

SERVES 4 • 185 CALORIES PER SERVING

Succulent little aubergines work well with the colourful spinach salad and spicy salsa here. The dish makes a wonderful starter or main course, depending on the portion size, and it could also be served alongside chicken or fish. Baby aubergines can vary in shape: some are small and round, others are long and thin, which is what we use. If you can only find the plump ones, just cut them into quarters. All aubergines are high in fibre, which helps to maintain a healthy digestive system.

20 baby aubergines (preferably the small, thin type)
1 tbsp olive oil
1 tsp flaked sea salt

FOR THE SPINACH SALAD
200g spinach, finely sliced
½ red onion, sliced
Grated zest and juice of ½ lemon
1 tsp rapeseed oil
A handful of fresh coriander
30g home-shelled pistachios
30g cashew nuts

FOR THE TOMATO SALSA
4 ripe tomatoes, finely diced
½ red onion, finely sliced
½ fresh green chilli, seeded and finely chopped
A handful of fresh flat-leaf parsley, finely chopped

1 Preheat your oven to 200°C/fan 180°C/gas 6.
2 Cut the aubergines lengthways in half and place them cut side up on a baking tray. Drizzle the olive oil over them and sprinkle with the sea salt. Roast for 20 minutes until soft.
3 Meanwhile, put the spinach in a bowl with the sliced onion and squeeze over the lemon juice. Place the lemon zest, oil, coriander, pistachios and cashew nuts in a blender and blitz to a coarse texture. Add this mixture to the spinach and onion and mix well.
4 In another bowl, mix together all the ingredients for the salsa.
5 To serve, arrange the aubergine halves, flesh side up, on a large plate and top each one with a spoonful of the spinach salad and a spoonful of the tomato salsa.

RICH IN Vitamins B1 (thiamin), B6 and C • Folate • Potassium • Beta-carotene • Fibre

USEFUL FOR Heart ①② • Bones ① • Digestion ① • Immunity ① • Skin, hair & nails ①③ • Mind ①

AUBERGINE BAKE

SERVES 6 • 380 CALORIES PER SERVING

This simple dish of baked aubergine and tomato is based on the Italian melanzane parmigiana, using a bean mash to create the creaminess that you would get from the cheese in the classic recipe. Wheat-free breadcrumbs and yeast flakes give the same effect as the traditional Parmesan topping. Great for adding a cheesy flavour, yeast flakes are sold in most wholefood shops.

3 aubergines
300g fresh or thawed frozen sweetcorn kernels
50g yeast flakes
300g wheat-free breadcrumbs

FOR THE TOMATO SAUCE
1 tsp olive oil
1 onion, finely chopped
2 garlic cloves, finely chopped
2 celery sticks, finely diced
1 tbsp paprika
1 tsp dried oregano
1 tsp salt
1 tsp pepper
2 x 400g tins chopped tomatoes
100g cherry tomatoes

FOR THE BEAN MASH
2 x 400g tins butter beans, drained and rinsed
200ml rice milk
A pinch of ground cinnamon
1 tsp chilli powder

1 First make the tomato sauce. Heat the oil in a saucepan, add the onion and garlic, and sauté for 5 minutes. Add the celery, paprika, dried oregano, salt and pepper and sauté for a further 2 minutes. Stir in the tinned and fresh tomatoes. Bring to the boil, then turn the heat to low and cook for 20 minutes, stirring occasionally. Add a splash of water if the sauce begins to stick to the pan.
2 Preheat your oven to 200°C/fan 180°C/gas 6.
3 For the bean mash, combine the ingredients in a saucepan and cook on a medium heat for 10 minutes. Transfer to a blender and blitz until smooth. (If you don't have a blender simply mash by hand; you will get a coarser texture but it still works well.)
4 Trim the ends off the aubergines and slice across into 1cm-thick rounds. Lay half of these on the bottom of a 20 x 26cm baking dish.
5 Cover with half of the sweetcorn and half the bean mash, then cover this with half of the tomato sauce. Repeat the layering using up the remaining ingredients. Scatter the yeast flakes and breadcrumbs over the top.
6 Bake for 50 minutes until the top is crispy and the aubergine is tender. Serve hot.

RICH IN Vitamins B1 (thiamin), B6, C and E • Potassium • Magnesium • Iron • Lycopene • Fibre

USEFUL FOR Heart ①② • Digestion ① • Immunity ① • Mind ①② • Fatigue ①③⑤ • Men ① • Women ①③

VEGETABLE LASAGNE

SERVES 4 • 430 CALORIES PER SERVING

We thought it might be impossible to create a meat-, dairy- and wheat-free lasagne, but the substitutes we have found for the key ingredients do the dish complete justice. The creamed butter beans really do give the same effect as the white sauce in a traditional lasagne, bringing the dish together and adding creaminess. Courgette acts as the pasta with a very similar texture. And the chunky vegetables taste and look suitably filling. This dish is high in folate, which helps to break down homocysteine levels in the blood, higher levels of which are linked to heart disease.

8 courgettes
2 tbsp olive oil
1 red onion, finely diced
2 garlic cloves, finely chopped
6 large vine tomatoes, diced
4 sun-dried tomatoes, roughly chopped
1 ear of sweetcorn (corn on the cob), or about 150g thawed frozen sweetcorn kernels
1 red pepper, seeded and finely sliced
1 aubergine, cut into 1cm-thick rounds
1 tbsp dried thyme
2 x 400g tins butter beans, drained and rinsed
250ml rice milk
A handful of fresh flat-leaf parsley, finely chopped
A pinch of crushed dried chilli
Flaked sea salt and cracked black pepper

1 Preheat your oven to 200°C/fan 180°C/gas 6.
2 To make the courgette 'pasta', use a vegetable peeler to shave the courgettes into thin ribbons. Rub 2 teaspoons of the oil and some salt and pepper over the ribbons. You can set them aside now, or griddle them to create charred lines. To do this, heat a ridged griddle/grill pan and griddle the courgette ribbons for 1 minute on each side (you'll probably have to do this in four or five batches, depending on the size of your griddle). Set the ribbons aside.
3 Heat 1 teaspoon of the olive oil in a medium frying pan, add the onion and garlic, and cook for 5 minutes until softened. Remove half of the onion mixture and place in a blender or food processor (this is for the butter bean sauce). Add the diced fresh tomatoes, sun-dried tomatoes and 100ml water to the frying pan and leave to cook on a low heat for 30 minutes, stirring occasionally.

4 Meanwhile, if using fresh sweetcorn, remove the husks and silk, if necessary, then cut the kernels from the cob. To do this, hold the cob at one end, upright at an angle, with the other end in the centre of a kitchen towel on your work surface, and run a knife down the cob to remove the kernels. Do this all the way round. Discard the cob. Spread the sweetcorn kernels on a baking tray with the red pepper and aubergine. Drizzle the remaining tablespoon of olive oil over them and sprinkle with the dried thyme. Roast in the heated oven for 20 minutes.
5 Whilst the vegetables are roasting, make the butter bean sauce. Add the butter beans, rice milk and parsley to the onions and garlic in the blender or food processor and blitz for 5 minutes until very smooth. Transfer to a bowl. Wash the blender or food processor (you'll need it again for the tomato sauce).
6 Season the tomato sauce with salt, pepper and chilli. Transfer to the blender or food processor and blitz to make a coarse-textured sauce. Pour into a large mixing bowl and add the roasted vegetables. (Leave the oven on.)
7 Now you can layer everything up. First, lay a row of courgette ribbons (about a third of them) to cover the bottom of a baking dish. Add a layer of tomato sauce (half of it) followed by a layer of butter bean sauce (half of it). Repeat the layers and finish with a layer of courgette ribbons.
8 Bake for 25 minutes. Serve the lasagne hot with a big green salad.

RICH IN Vitamins B1 (thiamin), B3 (niacin), B6, C and E • Folate • Potassium • Iron • Magnesium • Beta-carotene • Fibre

USEFUL FOR Heart ①②③ • Bones ① • Digestion ① • Immunity ① • Skin, hair & nails ①③ • Mind ①② • Fatigue ①③⑤ • Women ①

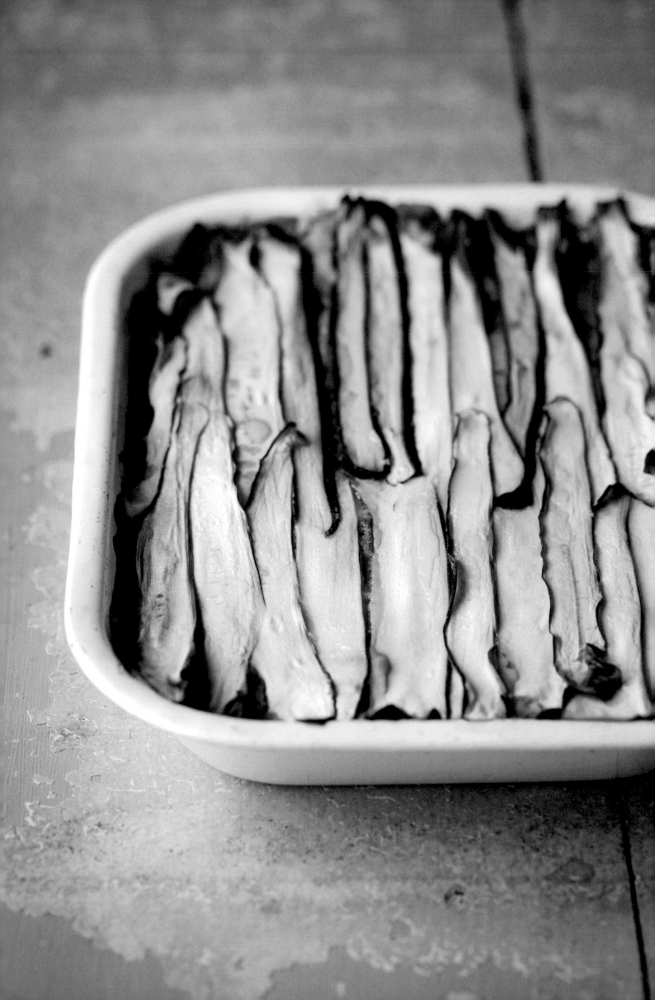

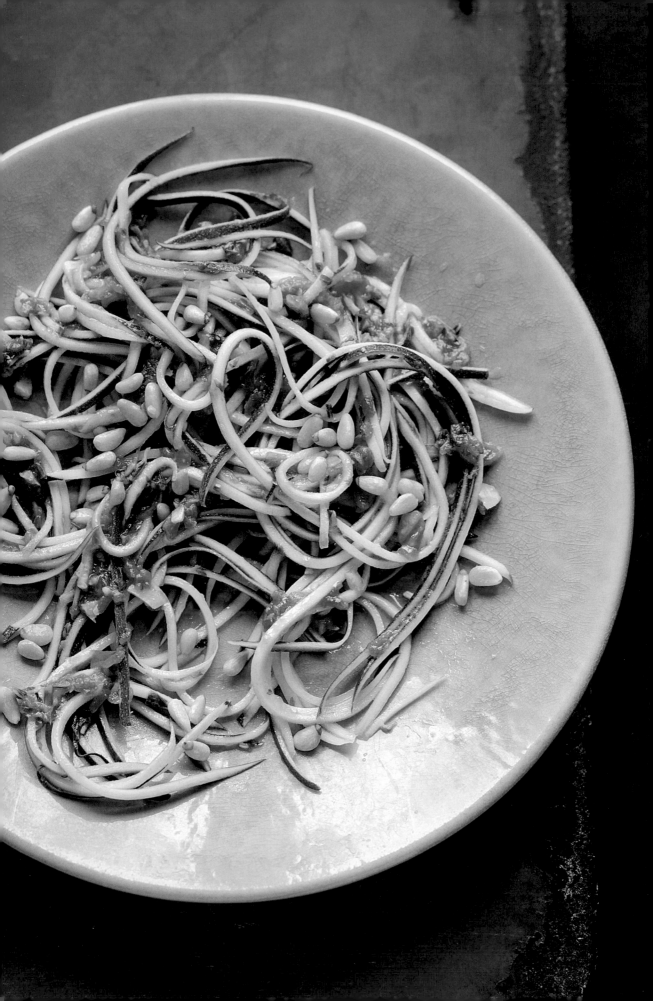

TOMATO PESTO WITH COURGETTE SPAGHETTI

SERVES 2 • 230 CALORIES PER SERVING

Oh, the joy of discovering courgette pasta! You do need to buy a special julienne peeler/cutter to create it, but it is well worth the investment. The best thing about this dish of courgette spaghetti with a fresh tomato sauce is that it is a lower calorie alternative to the traditional pasta dish, so you can eat until you are full. It makes a great lunch if you're trying to lose weight.

4 courgettes
A pinch of flaked sea salt
8 large vine tomatoes
2 handfuls of fresh basil leaves, finely chopped
1 tbsp olive oil
1 garlic clove, crushed
Salt
1 tbsp toasted pine nuts, to garnish

1 Using a julienne peeler/cutter, cut the unpeeled courgettes into long, spaghetti-like strips (stop when you get to the soft seeded centre). Mix with the sea salt and set aside.
2 Bring a pan of water to the boil. Score a cross on the base of each tomato and place in the pan. Boil for 20–30 seconds, then immediately transfer to a bowl of cold water. Peel off the skin.
3 Cut the tomatoes in half and remove the seeds, then finely chop the flesh. Mix with the basil, oil, garlic and salt to taste in a non-stick saucepan.
4 Heat the tomato sauce gently for 2–3 minutes. Add the courgette spaghetti and heat for a further 1–2 minutes. Serve immediately, topped with the toasted pine nuts.

RICH IN Vitamins B6, C and E • Folate • Potassium • Iron • Magnesium • Lycopene • Fibre

USEFUL FOR Heart ①②③ • Bones ① • Digestion ① • Immunity ① • Mind ①② • Fatigue ①③⑤ • Men ① • Women ①③

ROASTED CAULIFLOWER, CARROTS & CARAWAY WITH LEMON YOGURT

SERVES 2 • 210 CALORIES PER SERVING

Cauliflower is wonderfully versatile with myriad guises – as cous cous or rice, in raw shards or in curried florets – each offering a distinct texture and taste. But of all the ways to prepare it, roasting is the best. This method of cooking brings out califlower's savoury, earthy flavour and its creamy, soft texture. The dish is rich in vitamin B1, which is involved in converting carbohydrates into energy.

1 cauliflower

3 large carrots

1 tbsp groundnut oil

Grated zest of 1 lemon

A pinch of flaked sea salt

A pinch of black pepper

1 tsp paprika

1 tsp caraway seeds

1 tsp sesame seeds

FOR THE LEMON AND MINT YOGURT

2 tbsp plain soya yogurt

Grated zest and juice of ½ lemon

A pinch of paprika

3 fresh mint leaves, finely chopped

A pinch of salt

A pinch of black pepper

RICH IN Vitamins B1 (thiamin) and C • Folate • Potassium • Phytoestrogens • Beta-carotene • Fibre

USEFUL FOR Heart ①② • Bones ① • Digestion ① • Immunity ① • Skin, hair & nails ①④ • Men ① • Women ①③④

1 Preheat your oven to 200°C/fan 180°C/gas 6. Line a baking tray with greaseproof paper.

2 Remove the florets from the cauliflower, with as much stalk as possible, and slice them in half. Put them in a large mixing bowl. Peel the carrots and cut them at an angle into slices about 1cm thick. Add these to the bowl.

3 Add the oil, lemon zest, sea salt, pepper, paprika, caraway seeds and sesame seeds. Mix together so that the pieces of vegetable are well coated with the seasonings. Transfer to an ovenproof dish and roast for 20 minutes.

4 Meanwhile, mix the yogurt with the lemon zest and juice, paprika, mint, salt and pepper. Keep in the fridge until needed.

5 Drizzle the lemon and mint yogurt over the cauliflower and carrots before serving.

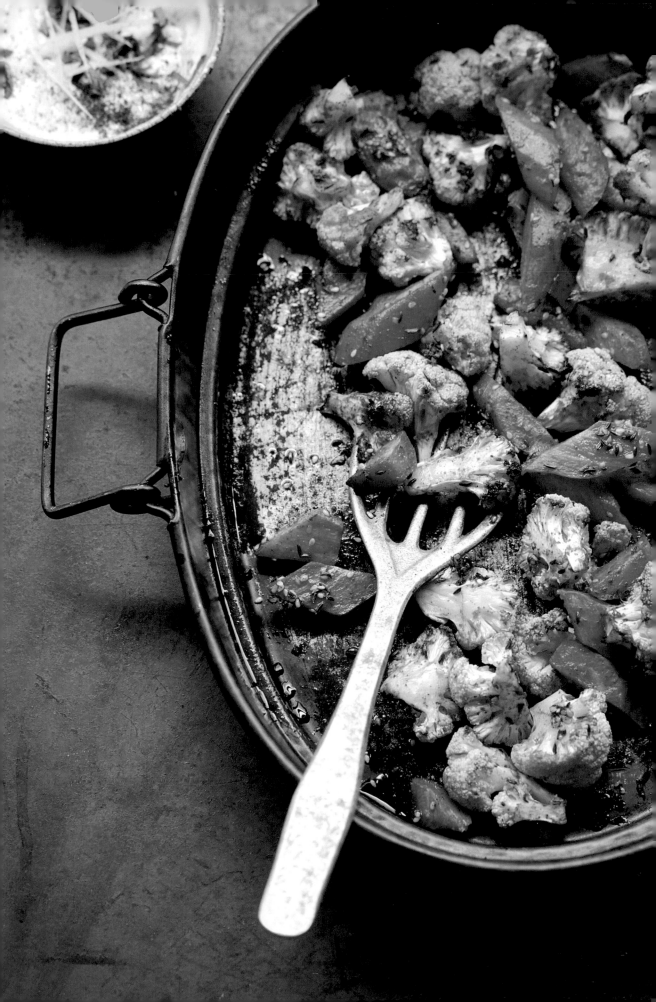

CAULIFLOWER RISOTTO
WITH PISTACHIOS

SERVES 2 • 320 CALORIES PER SERVING

Here we have a risotto … made without rice. Using cauliflower instead really does work. By cooking the core for a long time before adding little rice-shaped pieces of cauliflower floret, you get the creaminess you expect of a risotto along with the slight firmness of the floret. This is a lovely vegetarian dish, finished with chillied pistachios to add extra crunch. Like other nuts, pistachios are a useful source of protein and contain healthy monounsaturated fats.

1 cauliflower

1 tbsp rapeseed oil

3 shallots, finely diced

1 garlic clove, finely chopped

A thumb-sized piece of fresh ginger, peeled and finely grated

2 celery sticks, finely diced

2 carrots, finely diced

600ml vegetable stock (see page 283)

1 tsp crushed dried chilli

1 tsp sesame seeds

30g home-shelled pistachios

1 Remove all the outer leaves from the cauliflower. Cut the florets from their stalks. Put the stalks and core in a blender and blitz to the texture of rice grains. Tip into a bowl. Repeat to blitz the florets to the same texture, then tip into another bowl. Set aside.

2 Heat a little of the oil in a large saucepan and add two of the shallots. Cook on a medium heat for 10 minutes until very lightly browned. Add the garlic and ginger and cook for a further 3 minutes. Now add the blitzed cauliflower core along with the celery, carrots and stock. Bring to the boil, then simmer for 25 minutes.

3 Add the rice-like floret pieces and heat through for 3 minutes.

4 Meanwhile, heat the rest of the oil in a separate pan, add the remaining shallot, the chilli flakes, sesame seeds and pistachios, and gently fry for 2–3 minutes, stirring.

5 Stir the pistachio mix through the cauliflower 'risotto', then serve.

RICH IN Vitamins B1 (thiamin) and C • Folate • Potassium • Iron • Beta-sitosterol • Fibre

USEFUL FOR Heart ①②③ • Digestion ① • Immunity ① • Fatigue ① • Men ①

SPRING VEGETABLE PIE WITH COURGETTE PASTRY

SERVES 4 • 190 CALORIES PER SERVING

This vegetarian dish stands very proudly on its own, but for meat-eaters you can add a chicken breast on the side. It's a great gluten-free pie and you can switch in whichever vegetables are in season. Instead of pastry, the topping is created from long ribbons of courgette. Courgettes have a very high water content, making them one of the lowest calorie vegetables.

5 courgettes
1 tbsp rapeseed oil, plus extra for drizzling
1 red onion, finely chopped
2 garlic cloves, finely chopped
2 sprigs of fresh rosemary
5 sprigs of fresh thyme
2 handfuls of fresh flat-leaf parsley,
finely chopped
Grated zest of 1 lemon
1 tbsp gluten- and wheat-free flour
600ml vegetable stock (see page 283)
½ swede, finely diced
2 carrots, finely diced
1 celery stick, finely diced
1 leek, finely sliced
100g kale, shredded
100g podded fresh or thawed frozen peas

1 Use a vegetable peeler to create long, thin ribbons of courgette. Once you get to the centre of the courgette, stop peeling. (You can dice the courgette centres and add to the stew with the kale, if you like.) Set the ribbons aside.
2 Set a large saucepan on the heat and add the oil. Add the onion and cook for 10 minutes until slightly brown. Add the garlic, rosemary, thyme, parsley and lemon zest and cook for a further 2 minutes. Stir in the flour. Add half the stock and stir well. Bring to the boil, then simmer for 5 minutes, stirring occasionally.
3 Add the swede, carrots, celery, leek and remaining stock and bring back to the boil. Simmer for 20 minutes, then add the kale and peas. Simmer for 5 more minutes.
4 Preheat your grill to medium.
5 Transfer the vegetables to a pie dish (fish out the rosemary stick and discard it). Cover with the courgette ribbons and drizzle a little oil over them. Place under the grill and cook for about 10 minutes until the courgette is crispy. Serve immediately.

RICH IN Vitamins B1 (thiamin), B6 and C • Folate • Potassium • Iron • Beta-carotene • Fibre

USEFUL FOR Heart ①② • Digestion ① • Immunity ① • Skin, hair & nails ①③ • Mind ① • Fatigue ① • Women ①

BEETROOT & CARROT TAGINE WITH CAULIFLOWER COUS COUS

SERVES 4 • 230 CALORIES PER SERVING

It's traditional to make this Moroccan stew in a tagine pot, but as most of us don't have one of those, this recipe uses a standard saucepan. Despite that it does a pretty good job at getting the sweet, savoury, fragrant taste of a classic tagine. Beetroot adds a lovely earthy flavour and, with carrots, a vibrant colour. Carrots are one of the richest sources of beta-carotene, which is converted to vitamin A in the body. This vitamin is essential for healthy skin and eyes.

1 tbsp rapeseed oil

1 onion, finely diced

2 garlic cloves, finely chopped

1 tbsp grated fresh ginger

1 tsp ground turmeric

1 tsp ground coriander

1 tsp ground cinnamon

½ bunch celery, diced

2 raw beetroots, peeled and diced

4 carrots, diced

300ml vegetable stock (see page 283)

400g tin chickpeas, drained and rinsed

Grated zest of 1 lemon

A handful of fresh mint leaves, finely chopped

A handful of fresh coriander, finely chopped

Grated zest of 1 orange

FOR THE CAULIFLOWER COUS COUS

1 large cauliflower

Rapeseed oil, for drizzling

Grated zest and juice of 1 lemon

Salt and cracked black pepper

1 Preheat your oven to 200°C/fan 180°C/gas 6. Line a baking tray with greaseproof paper.

2 To make the cauliflower 'cous cous', remove the outer leaves from the cauliflower. Cut the florets from their stalks. Put the stalks and core in a blender and blitz to the texture of cous cous. Tip on to the baking tray. Repeat to blitz the florets to a cous cous texture, then tip on to the baking tray. Spread out evenly. Set aside.

3 Set a large pan on a medium heat. Add the tablespoon of oil and the onion and cook for 10 minutes. Add the garlic and ginger and cook for 3 minutes. Stir in the turmeric, ground coriander and cinnamon with a splash of water. Turn the heat to low and cook for 3 minutes.

4 Add the celery, beetroot and carrots and cook for 2 minutes, stirring to coat with the spice mixture. Pour in the stock and bring to the boil, then simmer for 20 minutes. All the vegetables should still have a little crunch; you don't want them to be mushy.

5 Meanwhile, drizzle some oil and the lemon zest and juice over the cauliflower cous cous. Cook in the heated oven for 10 minutes. Remove from the oven and season with salt and pepper.

6 While the cous cous is in the oven, add the chickpeas and lemon zest to the tagine and cook for a further 5 minutes. Remove from the heat and leave for 5 minutes before stirring in the chopped mint and coriander, orange zest and seasoning to taste. Serve with the cauliflower cous cous.

RICH IN Vitamins B6 and C • Folate • Potassium • Iron • Beta-carotene • Fibre

USEFUL FOR Heart ①② • Digestion ① • Immunity ① • Skin, hair & nails ①③ • Fatigue ① • Women ①

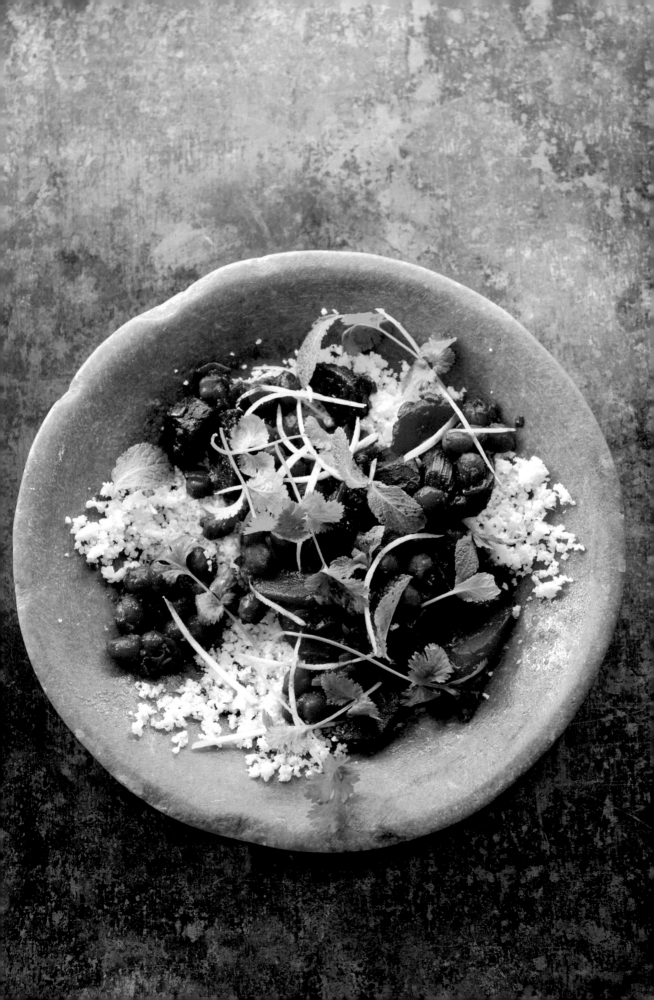

SRI LANKAN BUTTERNUT SQUASH CURRY

SERVES 4 • 535 CALORIES PER SERVING (WITH RICE)

The further south in India you go, the more coconut trees populate the landscape. So it's no surprise that in Sri Lanka, an island just off the coast of the very southernmost point of India, rich creamy coconut is used in abundance. This recipe is an adaptation of a chicken curry, with butternut squash taking the starring role in a fragrant, spicy sauce. If you're looking to reduce your calorie intake, use a reduced-fat coconut milk.

300g brown rice

1 tbsp coconut oil

1 tsp mustard seeds

1 large onion, finely diced

2 garlic cloves, finely chopped

2 tbsp grated fresh ginger

1 fresh red chilli, diced

5 curry leaves

2 tbsp curry powder

1 tsp ground turmeric

2 cardamom pods

4 celery sticks, finely sliced

2 plum tomatoes, seeded and diced

1 butternut squash, peeled, seeded and diced

100g cashew nuts, roughly chopped

600ml vegetable stock (see page 283)

200ml coconut milk

Salt and pepper

Chopped fresh coriander, to garnish

1 Put the rice in a medium-sized saucepan and cover with three times its volume of water. Add a pinch of salt. Set on a high heat and bring to the boil, then cover and simmer for 20 minutes until soft. Drain well and keep hot.

2 While the rice is cooking, prepare the curry. Set a large saucepan on a medium heat and add the coconut oil. Add the mustard seeds and onion and cook for 5 minutes until slightly browned. Add the garlic and ginger, turn the heat to low and cook for a further 2 minutes.

3 Stir in the chilli, curry leaves, curry powder, turmeric and cardamom and cook for 1 more minute; if necessary add a splash of water to prevent the spices from sticking to the bottom of the pan.

4 Add the celery, tomatoes, butternut squash and cashew nuts and mix with the spices and onion. Pour in the vegetable stock and stir, then cover and cook on a medium heat for 15 minutes.

5 Turn the heat to low and add the coconut milk. Simmer gently for a further 5 minutes, stirring occasionally. Season to taste and sprinkle with coriander before serving with the brown rice.

RICH IN Vitamins B3 (niacin), B6 and C • Folate • Potassium • Magnesium • Iron • Zinc • Beta-carotene • Curcuminoids • Fibre

USEFUL FOR Heart ①②③ • Bones ①② • Digestion ① • Immunity ① • Skin, hair & nails ①②③④ • Mind ①② • Fatigue ①③⑤ • Men ①② • Women ①

ROASTED PUMPKIN & TOFU CURRY

SERVES 2 • 515 CALORIES PER SERVING

Roasting a curry is one of the easiest ways to pack flavour into any dinner. Once you have prepped the pumpkin and tomato for this dish, most of the hard work is over. The coconut dressing gives you that classic Asian curry flavour whilst adding a light freshness. It's the perfect dressing for tofu, which is a great dairy-free source of calcium and meat-free protein.

1 small pumpkin
2 tbsp mild curry powder
½ red onion, finely chopped
2 garlic cloves, finely chopped
40ml rapeseed oil
5 under-ripe heirloom tomatoes, cut into quarters
100g firm tofu, cut into small cubes

FOR THE DRESSING
2 tbsp coconut yogurt
1 tbsp rapeseed oil
Grated zest and juice of ½ lemon
A handful of pumpkin seeds, toasted

FOR THE SALAD
100g baby spinach leaves
½ cucumber, peeled and diced
A handful of fresh coriander, finely chopped
Salt and pepper

1 Preheat your oven to 200°C/fan 180°C/gas 6. Line a baking tray with baking parchment.
2 Cut the pumpkin in half and remove the seeds and fibres. Cut into 1cm-thick half-moons.
3 Combine the curry powder, red onion, garlic and oil in a large mixing bowl and mix well. Add the pumpkin, tomatoes and tofu to the bowl and toss to coat with the spice mixture.
4 Tip on to the baking tray and roast in the oven for 25 minutes, shaking the tray frequently to ensure the pumpkin doesn't stick and burn.
5 Meanwhile, make the dressing by mixing together all the ingredients.
6 Finely shred the spinach and mix with the cucumber and coriander. Season to taste. Add half of the dressing and toss.
7 Drizzle the rest of the dressing over the curry and serve with the salad.

RICH IN Vitamins B6, C and E • Folate • Iron • Potassium • Magnesium • Calcium • Tryptophan • Phytoestrogens • Curcuminoids • Beta-carotene • Lycopene • Fibre

USEFUL FOR Heart ①②③ • Bones ①② • Digestion ① • Immunity ① • Skin, hair & nails ①②③ • Mind ①② • Fatigue ①③⑤ • Men ① • Women ①③④

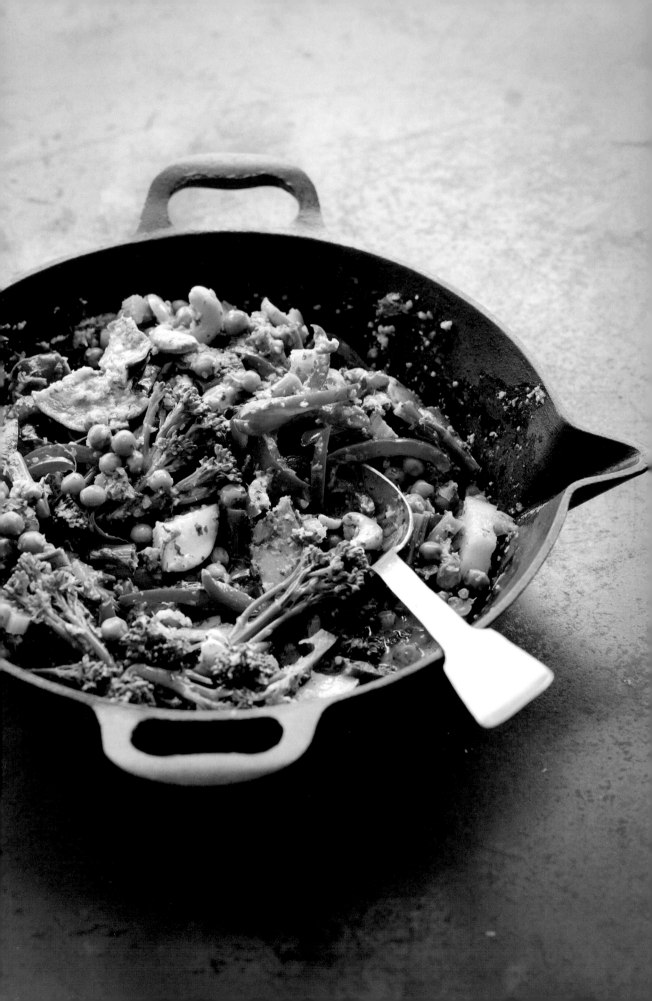

THAI GREEN CURRY

SERVES 4 • 265 CALORIES PER SERVING

When you are in need of spicy comfort food, make this fragrant Thai curry. It's based on a vivid green curry paste made with lots of aromatics, lime and coconut oil. Although coconut oil is high in saturated fat, it contains unique fatty acids that are absorbed and rapidly oxidised for energy.

Grated zest and juice of 1 lime
1 stick of lemongrass, roughly chopped
4 lime leaves
½ fresh red chilli, seeded and roughly chopped
A thumb-sized piece of fresh ginger, roughly chopped with the skin on
2 garlic cloves
A handful of fresh coriander, chopped
1 tbsp tamari
1 tbsp coconut oil
50g cashew nuts
200ml coconut milk
1 aubergine, cut into 2.5cm pieces
2 celery sticks, diced
1 red pepper, seeded and sliced
150g Tenderstem broccoli or broccoli florets
100g podded fresh or thawed frozen peas
1 courgette, finely diced
Salt and pepper

1 To make the curry paste, put the lime zest and juice, lemongrass, lime leaves, chilli, ginger, garlic, coriander, tamari, 1 teaspoon salt and the coconut oil in a blender and blitz to a coarse paste (or very finely chop the ingredients).
2 Set a large saucepan on a high heat and toast the cashew nuts until they are lightly browned. Add the curry paste, reduce the heat to medium and cook for 5 minutes, stirring frequently.
3 Pour in the coconut milk and 200ml water and stir to mix. Add the aubergine, celery and red pepper. Bring to the boil, then simmer for 15 minutes.
4 Add the broccoli, peas and courgette. Simmer for a further 5 minutes. Season well and serve with quinoa or brown rice.

RICH IN Vitamins B1 (thiamin), B6 and C • Folate • Potassium • Chromium • Beta-carotene • Fibre

USEFUL FOR Heart ①② • Digestion ① • Immunity ① • Skin, hair & nails ①③ • Mind ① • Women ①

BEETROOT, TOMATO & COCONUT CURRY

SERVES 2 • 180 CALORIES PER SERVING

This is a light curry with just enough spice to awaken your tastebuds and just enough coconut milk to soothe them afterwards. It combines Indian and Thai flavours to give it its zingy, fragrant taste. The bright yellow colour comes from curcuminoids in turmeric, which are known to have anti-inflammatory properties that may benefit conditions such as psoriasis.

1 tsp coconut oil
1 large onion, finely diced
2 garlic cloves, finely chopped
A thumb-sized piece of fresh ginger, peeled and grated
1 tsp ground cumin
1 tsp ground coriander
1 tsp ground turmeric
A pinch of ground cinnamon
2 cardamom pods
3 cloves
1 fresh green chilli, finely sliced
5 vine tomatoes, finely diced
4 raw beetroots, peeled and diced
100ml coconut milk
A handful of fresh coriander, finely chopped
Juice of ½ lemon

1 Set a large saucepan on a high heat and add the coconut oil, then add the onion and cook for 10 minutes until golden. Turn down the heat, add the garlic and ginger, and cook for a further 3 minutes.
2 Stir in the spices, chilli, 100ml water and the tomatoes. Bring to the boil, then add the diced beetroot. Simmer for 20 minutes until tender.
3 Add the coconut milk, chopped coriander and lemon juice. Stir well, then cook for a further 3 minutes to heat through. Remove from the heat and leave to rest for 10 minutes before serving with quinoa or brown rice.

RICH IN Vitamins B6 and C • Folate • Potassium • Iron • Curcuminoids • Lycopene • Fibre

USEFUL FOR Heart ①② • Bones ② • Digestion ① • Immunity ① • Skin, hair & nails ② • Mind ① • Fatigue ① • Women ①

BUTTERNUT SQUASH & BUTTER BEAN STEW

SERVES 2 · 315 CALORIES PER SERVING

Butternut and rosemary are great companions, the sweet, rich squash being perfectly balanced by the deeply savoury, floral flavour of rosemary. This herb is thought to stimulate the nervous and circulatory system and has been used by herbalists to treat conditions such as Raynaud's phenomenon (cold fingers and toes), so the dish is ideal for the autumn and winter months. Enjoy it as a vegetarian dish or serve as a colourful alternative to mashed potato with meat or fish.

1 red onion, finely sliced

1 tbsp olive oil

1 shallot, finely sliced

2 garlic cloves, chopped

1 sprig of fresh rosemary, leaves picked and finely chopped

½ butternut squash, peeled, seeded and cut into 2.5cm cubes

A pinch of freshly grated nutmeg

150ml vegetable stock (see page 283)

400g tin butter beans, drained and rinsed

Salt and pepper

1 Preheat your oven to 200°C/fan 180°C/gas 6.

2 Spread out the red onion slices on a baking tray and add a drizzle of olive oil and some salt and pepper. Roast in the heated oven for about 15 minutes until browned, then set aside.

3 Meanwhile, sauté the shallot in the rest of the olive oil in a heavy-based pan for 5 minutes until translucent. Add the garlic and rosemary and cook for a further 3 minutes. Stir in the butternut squash and nutmeg and cook for 2–3 minutes, stirring.

4 Pour in the stock and bring to the boil, then simmer for 15 minutes until the butternut squash is completely soft.

5 Mix in the butter beans and heat through for 6 minutes. Season the stew and serve with the red onion on top.

RICH IN Vitamins B6, C and E · Folate · Potassium · Iron · Magnesium · Beta-carotene · Fibre

USEFUL FOR Heart ①② · Bones ① · Digestion ① · Immunity ① · Skin, hair & nails ①③ · Mind ①② · Fatigue ①③⑤ · Women ①③

MEXICAN BEAN STEW

SERVES 4 • 475 CALORIES PER SERVING

This is a re-creation of a vegetarian bean stew I had at La Esquina restaurant in New York. The key is to make sure your beans keep a slight crunch – if they are overcooked, your stew will turn into a bean mash. Add more chillies if you are in the mood, and don't forget to top with lashings of an avocado salad (see a recipe on page 97). Pulses are an essential source of protein for non-meat eaters. To get a full range of amino acids, combine this bean stew with a grain dish.

200g dried black beans
200g dried aduki beans
100g dried chickpeas
1 tbsp rapeseed oil
1 onion, chopped
2 garlic cloves, finely chopped
A handful of sun-dried tomatoes, finely chopped
1 tsp ground cumin
A pinch of smoked paprika
2 carrots, finely diced
4 celery sticks, finely diced
400g tin chopped tomatoes
1 ear sweetcorn (corn on the cob)
A pinch of ground cinnamon
Salt and pepper

1 Place the beans and chickpeas in a large bowl and cover with two to three times their volume of cold water. Leave to soak overnight.
2 Drain the beans and chickpeas and place them in a large pan. Cover with fresh water and bring to the boil, then simmer for about 40 minutes until just tender. Drain and set aside.
3 Set a large pan on a high heat and add the oil. Add the onion and cook for 10 minutes until slightly browned. Add the garlic, sun-dried tomatoes, cumin, smoked paprika, carrots, celery and tinned tomatoes and stir well. Pour in 400ml water and simmer over a low heat for 10 minutes.
4 Add the beans and chickpeas with 200ml more water. Turn the heat up and bring to the boil, then turn the heat down again and leave to simmer for 20 minutes.
5 Meanwhile, shave the sweetcorn kernels off the cob. To do this, hold the cob at one end, upright at an angle, with the other end in the centre of a kitchen towel on your work surface. Run a knife down the cob to remove the kernels. Do this all the way round. Discard the cob.
6 Add the sweetcorn and cinnamon to the chilli and cook for a further 5 minutes. Season well before serving.

RICH IN Vitamins B1 (thiamin) and B6 • Folate • Potassium • Iron • Magnesium • Fibre

USEFUL FOR Heart ①②③ • Bones ① • Digestion ① • Mind ①② • Fatigue ①③⑤ • Women ①

BLACK PEPPER TOFU

SERVES 2 • 310 CALORIES PER SERVING

This dish is inspired by a recipe from Yotam Ottolenghi's cookbook *Plenty*. You might think that tofu is quite tasteless and watery, but this simple yet delicious recipe will change your mind. It makes a great starter, or serve it with some brown rice and stir-fried pak choi for dinner.

400g tofu

1 tbsp brown rice flour

2 tbsp rapeseed oil

1 tbsp groundnut oil

2 red onions, thinly sliced

5 fresh red chillies, thinly sliced

3 garlic cloves, finely chopped

2 tbsp grated fresh ginger

2 tbsp tamari

1 tsp runny honey

2 tbsp crushed black pepper

1 tsp sesame seeds

2 spring onions, finely sliced

1 Cut the tofu into 3cm squares and toss them in the rice flour to coat; shake off the excess flour. Heat the rapeseed oil in a frying pan and fry the tofu until golden on all sides, turning the pieces frequently so that they cook evenly. Transfer the tofu to some kitchen paper and set aside.

2 Wipe out the frying pan with kitchen paper, then set on a medium heat and add the groundnut oil. When it is hot, add the red onions, chillies, garlic and ginger. Cook for 10 minutes until the onions are soft. Add the tamari, honey, black pepper and sesame seeds and stir to mix.

3 Return the tofu to the pan and warm it through, stirring gently to mix with the other ingredients. Serve hot, garnished with the spring onions.

RICH IN Vitamins B6 and C • Folate • Potassium • Calcium • Iron • Phytoestrogens • Tryptophan • Fibre

USEFUL FOR Heart ①②③ • Bones ① • Digestion ① • Immunity ① • Mind ① • Fatigue ①③ • Men ① • Women ①③④

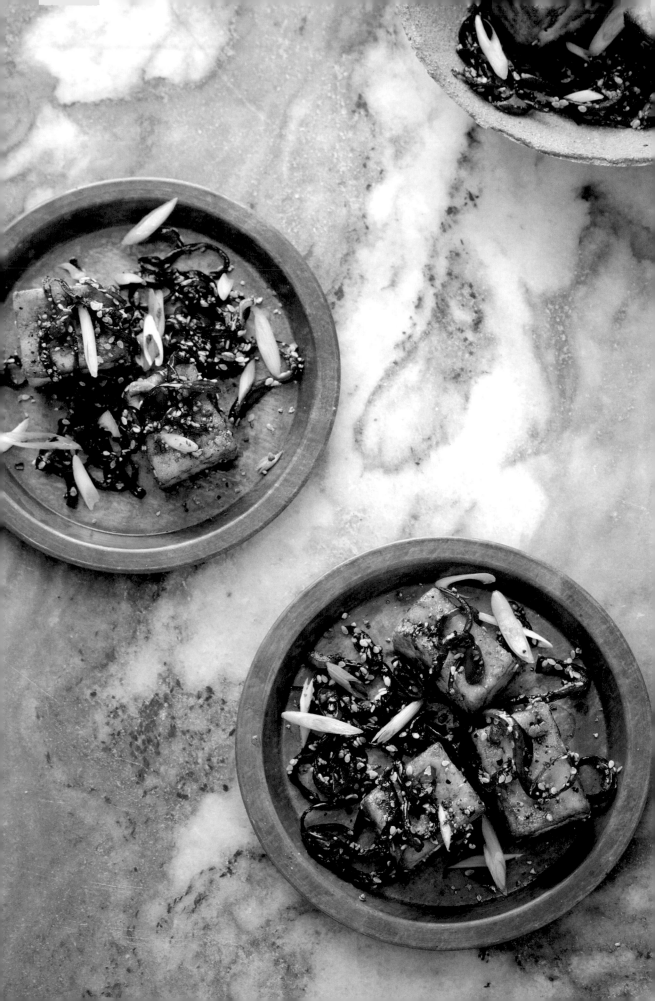

SHIITAKE MUSHROOM & DAIKON STIR-FRY

SERVES 2 • 475 CALORIES PER SERVING

One of the great things about Asian cooking is the ability to pack flavour into vegetarian food. Their key ingredients – garlic, ginger and soy sauce – will make any dish tasty. The type of soy sauce used here is tamari, which is produced during the making of miso paste. Tamari is rich in phytoestrogens and is wheat-free.

6 dried shiitake mushrooms
200g brown rice noodles
2 tbsp rapeseed oil
2 garlic cloves, chopped
1 tsp grated fresh ginger
100g chestnut mushrooms, thinly sliced
3 tbsp tamari
½ fresh green chilli, sliced
2 spring onions, thinly sliced
½ daikon (mooli), peeled and cut into matchsticks
Salt and pepper

1 Soak the shiitake mushrooms in hot water for 45 minutes to rehydrate. Drain, then remove the thick stems (keep for a stock). Slice thinly.
2 Bring a pan of water to the boil, drop in the noodles and cook for 2 minutes until soft. Drain and rinse under cold water. Drizzle a little of the oil over the noodles. Set aside.
3 Heat a teaspoon or so of the oil in a wok. Add the garlic, ginger and mushrooms and stir-fry for 2–3 minutes until the mushrooms start to brown. Add the tamari and chilli and cook for a further 2 minutes. Tip the contents of the wok into a dish and set aside.
4 Wipe the wok clean and add the remaining tablespoon of oil. Add the spring onions and daikon and stir-fry for 2 minutes, then return the mushrooms to the wok along with the noodles. Stir-fry for a further 2 minutes to warm everything through. Season to taste and serve.

RICH IN Vitamins B3 (niacin), B6 and C • Folate • Potassium • Magnesium • Selenium • Zinc • Phytoestrogens • Fibre

USEFUL FOR Heart ①②③ • Bones ① • Digestion ① • Immunity ① • Skin, hair & nails ①④ • Mind ①② • Fatigue ①③⑤ • Men ①②

POINTED CABBAGE & MUSHROOM STIR-FRY

SERVES 2 • 170 CALORIES PER SERVING

Most stir-fry recipes start with onions but this recipe begins with mushrooms, cooking them as Julia Child recommended: without crowding them in the pan. The key is to use a non-stick frying pan with a drop of olive oil and cook the mushrooms in batches so that they can all lie flat – this way they won't steam and become slimy. The dish is rich in vitamin B2 (riboflavin), which may help with migraines.

1 tsp toasted sesame oil
100g chestnut mushrooms, sliced
50g portabellini mushrooms, sliced
50g button mushrooms, halved
1 red onion, finely sliced
2 spring onions, finely sliced
1 garlic clove, finely chopped
1 tbsp tamari
Juice of 1 lime
1 tsp runny honey
A handful of mange tout, finely sliced
1 pointed cabbage, stalk removed and leaves finely shredded
A handful of fresh coriander, finely chopped

1 Set a medium-sized non-stick frying plan on a medium heat. Add the sesame oil with a third of the mushrooms and cook for 5 minutes until lightly crisped. Transfer to a plate. Repeat to cook the rest of the mushrooms in two batches.
2 Return all the mushrooms to the pan and add the red onion, spring onions and garlic. Cook for 2 minutes, then stir in the tamari, lime juice and honey.
3 Add the mange tout and cabbage and cook for a further 3 minutes, stirring – the cabbage should still be slightly crunchy.
4 Remove from the heat and stir in the coriander. Leave to rest for 2 minutes before serving.

RICH IN Vitamins B1 (thiamin), B2 (riboflavin), B6 and C • Folate • Potassium • Fibre

USEFUL FOR Heart ①② • Digestion ① • Immunity ① • Mind ① • Fatigue ⑤

STIR-FRIED CAULIFLOWER RICE WITH SHIITAKE MUSHROOMS & TOFU

SERVES 2 • 620 CALORIES PER SERVING

The cauliflower gives this dish a good crunchy texture and all the flavours are happily married with the egg that is thrown in at the end. But it's the garnish that really makes the dish – salty tamari with cashews and fresh coriander. Shiitake mushrooms contain a type of fibre known as beta-glucan, which may help to strengthen your immune system.

RICH IN B vitamins • Vitamins C and D • Potassium • Magnesium • Zinc • Calcium • Iron • Phytoestrogens • Tryptophan • Fibre

USEFUL FOR Heart ①②③ • Bones ① • Digestion ① • Immunity ① • Skin, hair & nails ①④ • Mind ①② • Fatigue ①③⑤ • Men ①② • Women ①③④

1 cauliflower, outer leaves removed

1 tbsp coconut oil

2 garlic cloves, finely chopped

1 fresh red chilli, finely sliced

5 fresh shiitake mushrooms, sliced

2 tbsp toasted sesame oil

150g firm tofu, cut into 1cm cubes

4 spring onions, sliced

3 eggs

A handful of fresh coriander, roughly chopped

A handful of cashew nuts, toasted and chopped

2 tbsp tamari

1 Cut the cauliflower florets from their stalks. Put the stalks and core in a blender and blitz into little pieces the size of rice grains. Tip into a bowl, then blitz the florets into little pieces in the same way.

2 Line a large bowl with a kitchen towel and pour the cauliflower 'rice' into it. Gather up the corners of the towel to enclose the cauliflower and squeeze to remove any excess liquid.

3 Set a wok on high heat and add the coconut oil, then add the garlic, chilli and shiitake mushrooms and stir-fry for 2 minutes. Tip this mixture into a bowl and set aside.

4 Wipe out the wok with kitchen paper, then set it on a high heat and add the sesame oil. Add the cubes of tofu and lightly fry until golden on each side. Now add the cauliflower rice and the spring onions. Stir-fry for a minute so that the rice is completely coated in oil. Return the shiitake mushroom mixture to the wok and stir to mix.

5 Make a little well in the middle of the mixture in the wok. Crack the eggs into the well and stir them in so that the yolk breaks and the eggs cook through the cauliflower. Serve hot, sprinkled with the coriander, chopped cashew nuts and tamari.

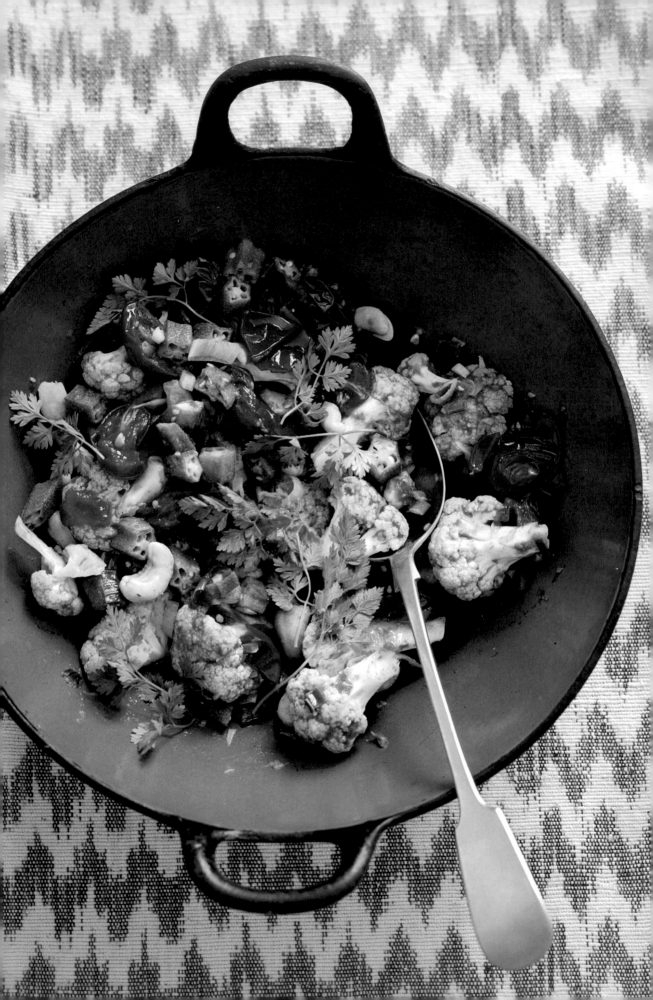

STIR-FRIED OKRA, CAULIFLOWER & TOMATO

SERVES 2 • 215 CALORIES PER SERVING

Okra, often called ladies' fingers, has a unique flavour and texture. Raw, it is slightly furry, but when cooked it has a lovely crunchy texture (or can be very glutinous if cooked longer). The earthy and slightly nutty taste works well in curries and stir-fries.

1 tbsp coconut oil
4 spring onions, finely sliced
2 garlic cloves, finely sliced
200g okra, cut across into pieces
1 fresh green chilli, seeded and finely chopped
A pinch of ground ginger
A pinch of ground cumin
A pinch of ground cinnamon
3 fresh curry leaves
A handful of cashew nuts
½ cauliflower, separated into florets
400g baby plum tomatoes, cut in half
A handful of fresh chervil, roughly chopped
1 lemon, sliced

1 Heat the coconut oil in a medium-sized pan over medium heat for a minute or so, then add the spring onions and garlic and cook for 5 minutes. Add the okra and cook for a further 5 minutes, stirring frequently.

2 Stir in the chilli, all the ground spices, curry leaves and cashews. After a few seconds add the cauliflower and tomatoes and turn the heat to low. Simmer gently for 10 minutes until the tomatoes are soft, stirring occasionally – you want the cauliflower to still be crunchy.

3 Serve garnished with the chervil and lemon.

RICH IN Vitamins B3 (niacin), B6, C and E • Folate • Iron • Potassium • Calcium • Magnesium • Lycopene • Beta-carotene • Fibre

USEFUL FOR Heart ① ② ③ • Bones ① • Digestion ① • Immunity ① • Skin, hair & nails ① ③ • Mind ① ② • Fatigue ① ③ ⑤ • Men ① • Women ① ③

GRAINS & PULSES

The vegetarian dishes based on grains and pulses in this chapter are nourishing enough to satisfy vegetarians and meat-eaters alike. Many take inspiration from other countries' cuisines, reflecting the many exciting ways of preparing these nutritious foods.

Wholegrains and pulses provide a valuable source of fibre, which is essential for maintaining a healthy digestive system. A diet high in fibre offers lots of other health benefits, including a reduction in cholesterol levels and protection against bowel cancer and diabetes, as well as aiding weight control. Wholegrains and pulses also supply a source of protein and other key nutrients, including B vitamins, iron, zinc and potassium.

With most big supermarkets now offering a 'world cuisines' aisle, there are many grains and pulses that you can get your hands on. From quinoa to pearl barley, wild rice to buckwheat, and aduki beans to beluga lentils, these are becoming normal storecupboard ingredients, offering exciting and varied alternatives to wheat- and red meat-based meals.

At the end of most of the recipes, you'll find a list of the main nutrients supplied in a serving as well as a list of health issues that may be benefited by including the recipe in your healthy diet. For more, see page 9.

AVOCADO & QUINOA SALAD

SERVES 4 • 480 CALORIES PER SERVING

Delicious food needs great texture, something that keeps changing as you chew every mouthful, and this dish of crunchy quinoa with creamy avocado does just that. Topped off with spring onions and zingy lemon juice, it will satisfy every tastebud. Quinoa has a low glycaemic load (GL) and is a good source of protein, making it the perfect complex carbohydrate to moderate blood sugar levels.

25g sunflower seeds
200g quinoa
2 avocados
A handful of spinach, roughly chopped
1 tbsp finely chopped fresh coriander
2 spring onions, finely sliced
60g mange tout, sliced
20ml rapeseed oil
Juice of 1 lemon
Salt and pepper

1 Preheat your oven to 200°C/fan 180°C/gas 6. Spread the sunflower seeds on a small baking tray and toast in the oven for 8 minutes until golden. Leave to cool.

2 Put the quinoa in a medium saucepan and cover with three times its volume of water. Place on a high heat and bring to the boil. Once boiling, season the water with salt and continue to boil for a further 6–8 minutes until the quinoa is just tender. Drain in a sieve and rinse under cold water until completely cool. Leave to one side to drain thoroughly.

3 Peel the avocados and remove the stones. Dice the avocado flesh and place in a large mixing bowl. Add the spinach, coriander, spring onions and mange tout and mix gently together.

4 Stir in the toasted sunflower seeds, drained quinoa, rapeseed oil and lemon juice. Season to taste, then serve.

RICH IN Vitamins B2 (riboflavin) and B6 • Potassium • Magnesium • Iron • Zinc • Beta-sitosterol

USEFUL FOR Heart ①②③ • Bones ① • Skin, hair & nails ①④ • Mind ① • Fatigue ⑤ • Men ①② • Women ①

QUINOA PIZZA

SERVES 4 • 664 CALORIES PER SERVING

Using a base made from the same dough as our quinoa bread, this is a healthy and filling version of a gluten- and dairy-free pizza, with yeast flakes creating the cheesy flavour. These are available in most healthfood shops but if you can't find them, the pizza will still be delicious. The sauce will make a little more than you need for the topping, but it is good tossed with some wheat-free pasta or courgette spaghetti (see page 127).

FOR THE PIZZA BASE
1 recipe quantity Quinoa Bread dough
(see page 44)

FOR THE TOPPING
400g tin cherry tomatoes, drained
1 garlic clove
A handful of fresh thyme sprigs, leaves picked
A good pinch of salt
4 large beef tomatoes, sliced
2 handfuls of small broccoli florets
2 tbsp yeast flakes

1 Preheat your oven to 200°C/fan 180°C/gas 6. Line two baking trays with baking parchment (or one large tray if you are going to make one big pizza).
2 Divide the bread dough into four portions. Shape each portion into a disc just under 1cm thick on the lined baking trays. Bake these pizza bases in the heated oven for 40 minutes.
3 Meanwhile, make a tomato sauce by combining the cherry tomatoes, garlic, thyme leaves and salt in a blender or food processor and blitzing until smooth.
4 Remove the pizza bases from the oven and spread the tomato sauce over them in an even layer. Place the tomato slices on the sauce and top with the broccoli florets, then sprinkle with the yeast flakes.
5 Return to the oven and bake for 15 minutes until the broccoli is slightly charred and tender. Serve the pizzas hot.

RICH IN Vitamins B3 (niacin), B6 and C • Folate • Zinc • Potassium • Magnesium • Iron • Chromium • Lycopene • Fibre

USEFUL FOR Heart ①②③ • Bones ① • Digestion ① • Immunity ① • Skin, hair & nails ①④ • Mind ①② • Fatigue ①③⑤ • Men ①② • Women ①④

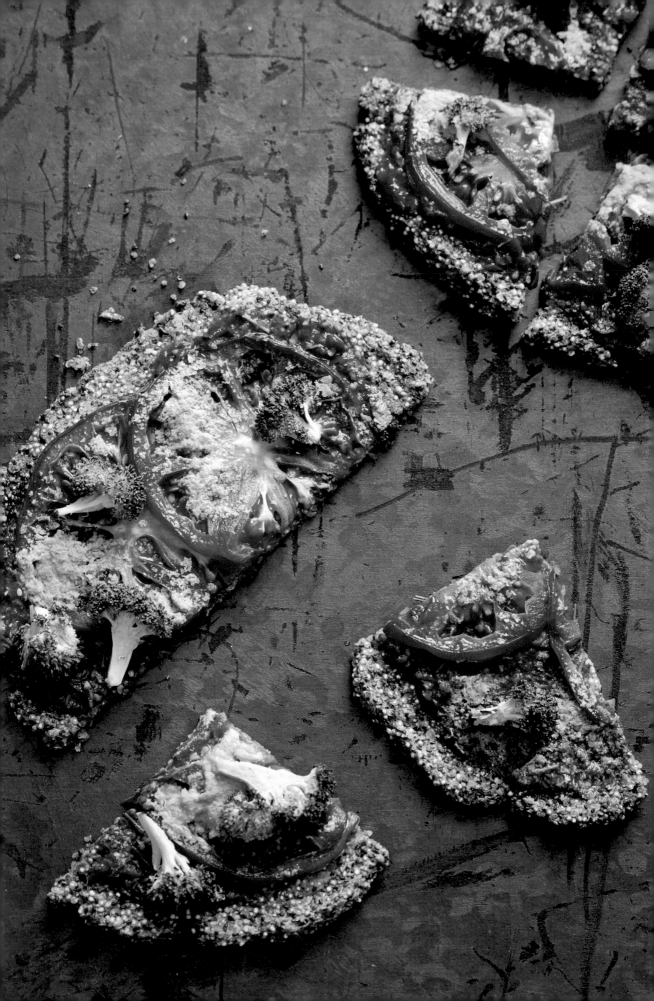

QUINOA & CASHEW SALAD

SERVES 2 • 405 CALORIES PER SERVING

You can throw toasted cashew nuts into any salad and they will transform it, giving it a delicious crunch and depth of flavour. Cashews also improve the nutrient value as they are a good source of magnesium. This salad provides 50 per cent of the RDA for magnesium, a mineral that contributes to good bone health.

40g cashew nuts
100g quinoa
1 red pepper, seeded and finely diced
50g edamame beans, thawed if frozen
2 celery sticks, finely diced
½ red onion, finely sliced
10g sultanas
2 fresh chives, finely chopped
A handful of fresh coriander, finely chopped
1 tsp rapeseed oil
Juice of 1 lemon
1 tsp flaked sea salt
1 tsp cracked black pepper
Salt

1 Preheat your oven to 200°C/fan 180°C/gas 6. Spread the cashew nuts on a small baking tray and toast in the oven for 8 minutes until golden. Leave to cool.
2 Put the quinoa in a medium-sized saucepan and cover with three times its volume of cold water. Bring to the boil. Season the water with salt, then continue to boil for 6–8 minutes until the quinoa is just tender. Drain the quinoa in a sieve and rinse under cold water until completely cool. Leave on one side to drain thoroughly.
3 Tip the quinoa into a large mixing bowl and add the toasted cashews and the rest of the ingredients. Mix together well. (The salad can be made ahead; keep in the fridge.)

RICH IN Vitamins B6 and C • Folate • Magnesium • Potassium • Iron • Zinc • Phytoestrogens • Beta-carotene • Prebiotics

USEFUL FOR Heart ①② • Digestion ② • Immunity ① • Skin, hair & nails ①③④ • Mind ①② • Fatigue ①⑤ • Men ①② • Women ①

QUINOA, ASPARAGUS & ALMOND SALAD

SERVES 4 • 340 CALORIES PER SERVING

Make this zingy little salad when asparagus is in season. This vegetable is a great source of the fibre inulin, which acts as a prebiotic, helping to maintain healthy gut flora.

200g quinoa
8 asparagus spears
1 cauliflower, separated into small florets
40g blanched (skinned) almonds
Grated zest and juice of 2 limes
1 tsp olive oil
5 sprigs of fresh thyme
1 tsp rapeseed oil
A handful of fresh chives, finely chopped
A small handful of sultanas
Salt and pepper

1 Preheat your oven to 200°C/fan 180°C/gas 6. Line a baking tray with greaseproof paper.
2 Put the quinoa in a saucepan, cover with three times its volume of water and bring to the boil. Simmer for 6–8 minutes until the quinoa is just tender. Drain in a sieve and rinse, then allow to cool before tipping into a large mixing bowl.
3 Remove the woody end of the asparagus spears. Cut off the tips in 3.5cm-long pieces and slice the rest of the stalks into 1cm pieces. Spread the asparagus pieces on the baking sheet with the cauliflower florets and almonds.
4 In a small bowl mix together the lime zest, olive oil and thyme. Sprinkle this over the vegetables with a good pinch each of salt and pepper. Roast for 6 minutes – roasting for a short time like this will enhance all the vegetable flavours but keeps everything really crunchy.
5 Add the roasted vegetables and nuts to the quinoa and mix through. Mix in the rapeseed oil, lime juice, chives, sultanas and some salt and pepper, then serve.

RICH IN Vitamins B6, C and E • Folate • Potassium • Magnesium • Iron • Beta-carotene • Asparagine • Prebiotics • Fibre

USEFUL FOR Heart ①②③ • Bones ① • Digestion ①② • Immunity ① • Skin, hair & nails ①③ • Mind ①② • Fatigue ①③⑤ • Women ①③

PEARL BARLEY WITH CANTALOUPE MELON

SERVES 2 • 400 CALORIES PER SERVING

This may sound like an odd combination but it works surprisingly well. The melon adds a sweet flavour and soft texture, which complements the chewy barley. Cantaloupe contains high levels of the antioxidant beta-carotene – this is what gives the flesh its appealing orange colour. It is in season during the summer months, making this the perfect salad for al fresco dining. Serve with grilled fish or meat.

150g pearl barley

1 red onion, finely sliced

3 vine tomatoes, finely sliced

Juice of 2 lemons

A pinch of flaked sea salt

1 tbsp rapeseed oil

½ cantaloupe melon

A pinch of salt

A pinch of cracked black pepper

1 Put the pearl barley in a sieve and give it a good rinse in cold running water. Drain, then tip it into a pan with fresh water – three times the volume of the barley. Set the pan on high heat and bring to the boil, then simmer for 20–25 minutes until soft. Drain and rinse under cold water to cool. Drain thoroughly.

2 Tip the barley into a large mixing bowl. Add the red onion and tomatoes.

3 Combine the lemon juice, sea salt and rapeseed oil in a small bowl and whisk until thickened. Add to the pearl barley and stir through.

4 Cut the melon in half and scoop out the seeds. Cut each half into four wedges. Remove the skin, then cut the flesh into 2.5cm cubes. Put the melon cubes in a separate bowl and season with the salt and cracked black pepper.

5 To serve, spoon the seasoned melon on top of the pearl barley.

RICH IN Vitamins B6, C and E • Potassium • Beta-carotene • Lycopene • Fibre

USEFUL FOR Heart ① ② • Immunity ① • Skin, hair & nails ① ③ • Mind ① • Men ① • Women ③

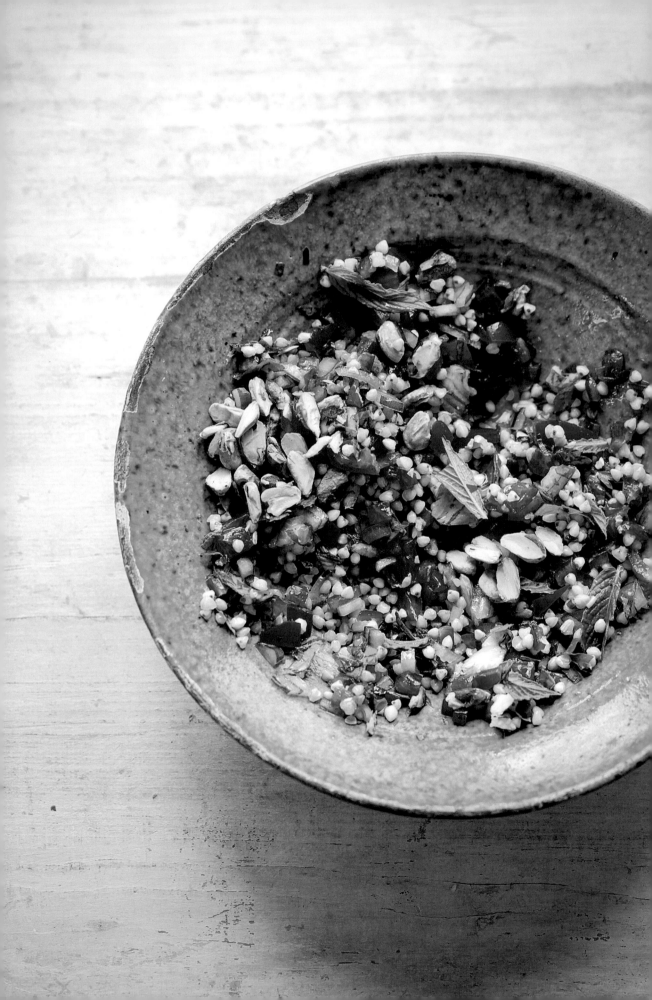

TABOULEH WITH PISTACHIO

SERVES 2 • 350 CALORIES PER SERVING

This Arab dish is traditionally made with bulgur wheat, but we've replaced this with buckwheat, which has a very similar texture and taste, to make a wheat-free version. (Despite its name, buckwheat is no relation to wheat.) The key to a good tabouleh is to use lots of tomatoes and herbs dotted with buckwheat, rather than the other way round. This dish is fresh and delicious, perfect on its own with some good gluten-free bread, or served as a side dish with meat or fish. It's also a great party dish, served with hummus wrapped in lettuce leaves.

100g buckwheat grain
2 handfuls of fresh flat-leaf parsley
A handful of fresh mint
300g ripe vine tomatoes, seeded and very finely chopped
½ red onion, finely chopped
Juice of 1 lemon
1 tbsp olive oil
1 tsp salt
A pinch of black pepper
A handful of home-shelled pistachios, coarsely crushed

1 Put the buckwheat in a saucepan and cover with twice its volume of water. Bring to the boil, then cook for 5 minutes until soft. Drain in a sieve and rinse under cold water to cool, then leave to drain thoroughly.
2 Pull the parsley and mint leaves from their stems and finely chop (keep a few mint leaves for garnish, if you like).
3 Tip the buckwheat into a large mixing bowl and add the tomatoes, onion, parsley, mint, lemon juice, oil, salt and pepper. Mix well.
4 Garnish with the pistachios and mint leaves, and serve.

RICH IN Vitamins B1 (thiamin), B6 and C • Folate • Potassium • Phytoestrogens • Lycopene

USEFUL FOR Heart ① • Immunity ① • Mind ① • Men ① • Women ①③④

WILD RICE SALAD WITH JERUSALEM ARTICHOKE & HEIRLOOM TOMATOES

SERVES 2 • 410 CALORIES PER SERVING

Sweet and crunchy jerusalem artichokes are a great addition to winter salads. Despite their name, they aren't actually artichokes, nor do they come from the Holy Land. They are, in fact, the tubers of a variety of sunflower – 'jerusalem' comes from the Italian word *girasole*, which means sunflower. Jerusalem artichokes contain significant amounts of an insoluble fibre known as inulin, which acts as a prebiotic, keeping the digestive system healthy. In this salad the artichokes are combined with nutty wild rice and heirloom tomatoes, which come in a wide variety of colours, shapes, flavours and sizes. They add real interest and beauty to the dish.

4 jerusalem artichokes, scrubbed

1 tsp olive oil

A pinch of flaked sea salt

A pinch of cracked black pepper

5 heirloom tomatoes, thinly sliced

1 red onion, thinly sliced

Juice of ½ lemon

1 tsp runny honey

100g wild rice

100g rocket, finely chopped

A handful of basil leaves, finely chopped

1 Preheat your oven to 200°C/fan 180°C/gas 6. Slice the artichokes into 1cm-thick discs. Spread them on a baking tray and drizzle the olive oil over them. Season with the sea salt and pepper. Roast for 40 minutes until tender and slightly golden. Leave to cool.

2 Combine the tomatoes and onion in a large mixing bowl and add the lemon juice and honey. Toss gently together.

3 Put the wild rice in a large pan and cover with three times its volume of water. Bring to the boil and simmer for 30–35 minutes until the rice is tender. Drain the rice and rinse thoroughly under cold water to cool.

4 Add the wild rice to the tomato and onion, along with the artichokes, rocket and basil. Fold together gently, then serve.

RICH IN Vitamins B3 (niacin), B6 and C • Potassium • Iron • Magnesium • Beta-carotene • Lycopene • Prebiotics • Fibre

USEFUL FOR Heart ①②③ • Bones ① • Digestion ①② • Skin, hair & nails ①③ • Mind ①② • Fatigue ①③⑤ • Women ①

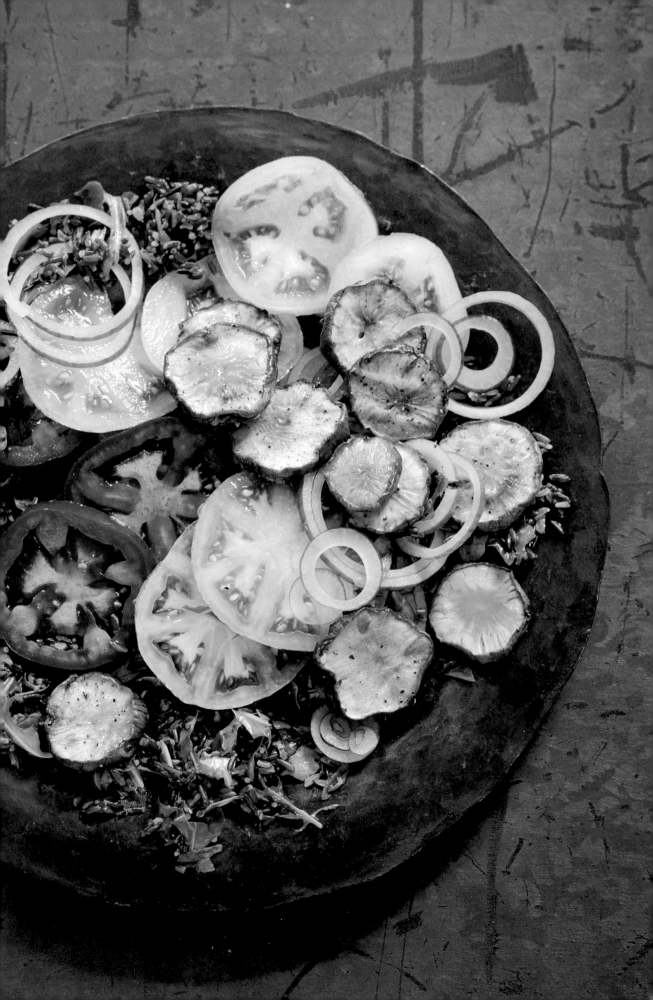

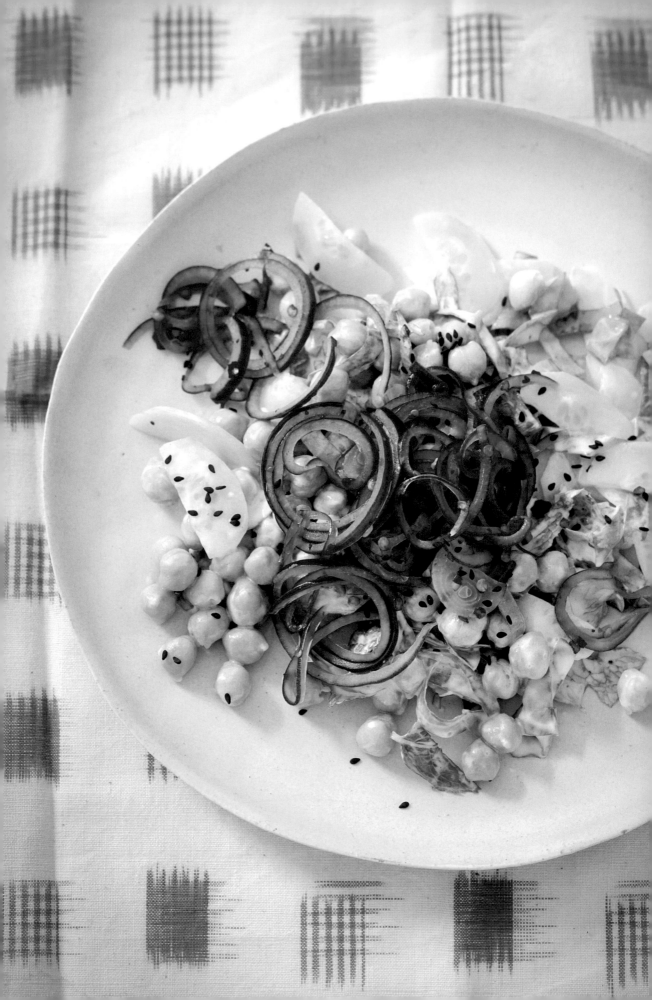

CHICKPEAS & YOGURT

SERVES 2 • 305 CALORIES PER SERVING

You can fling this together very quickly for lunch. The only thing that takes a bit of time is soaking the onion in the lemon juice. You don't have to do this – you can speedily mix and greedily consume – but you will miss out on the beautiful pink colour that the onion turns. It's worth buying good-quality chickpeas as they are most likely to be crunchy. This salad provides phytoestrogens, which may help to relieve symptoms associated with PMS by balancing hormone levels.

1 red onion, finely sliced

1 tsp flaked sea salt

Juice of 1 lemon

A pinch of crushed dried chilli

1 cucumber

400g tin chickpeas, drained, rinsed and patted dry

A handful of fresh mint, finely chopped

A handful of baby spinach leaves

1 tbsp plain soya yogurt

A pinch of black sesame seeds

Salt and pepper

1 Put the red onion slices in a small bowl and add the salt, lemon juice and chilli. Leave to soak for 5 minutes until the onions have turned bright pink.

2 Meanwhile, peel the cucumber. Cut it lengthways in half, then cut across into thin half-moons.

3 Mix together the cucumber, chickpeas, mint, spinach and yogurt in a large bowl. Season to taste. Top with the onion slices and then the black sesame seeds.

RICH IN Vitamin E • Iron • Phytoestrogens • Fibre

USEFUL FOR Heart ① • Digestion ① • Fatigue ① • Women ①③④

FLAGEOLET BEAN SALAD WITH GRIDDLED SWEETCORN

SERVES 2 • 400 CALORIES PER SERVING

Flageolet beans are actually young haricot beans that have been harvested and dried before they are fully ripe. They have a creamy texture and delicate flavour, perfect in any stew. In this salad the flageolets are dressed with a cashew cream and teamed with hot crunchy sweetcorn. Cashew nuts are a good source of magnesium, a deficiency of which may be linked to insomnia. This makes a delicious summer dinner.

A handful of cashew nuts
Juice of ½ lemon
2 tbsp plain soya yogurt
5 fresh mint leaves
A pinch of crushed dried chilli
A pinch of salt
400g tin flageolet beans, drained and rinsed
A handful of spinach, sliced
2 ears of sweetcorn (corn on the cob), with the husks on
A pinch of flaked sea salt
A pinch of ground sumac

1 Soak the cashew nuts in a bowl of hot water for 10 minutes. Drain and transfer to a blender or food processor. Add the lemon juice, soya yogurt, mint, chilli, salt and 50ml cold water, and blitz until smooth.

2 Transfer the cashew cream to a large mixing bowl and add the beans and spinach. Mix well. Chill while you cook the sweetcorn.

3 Heat a ridged griddle/grill pan. Keeping the sweetcorn in their husks, place on the griddle. Cook for about 20 minutes, turning when the husk is browned.

4 Remove the husks and silk, and sprinkle the sweetcorn with the sea salt. Dust the salad with the sumac and serve with the sweetcorn.

RICH IN Vitamins B1 (thiamin) and B6 • Potassium • Magnesium • Selenium • Beta-carotene • Phytoestrogens • Fibre

USEFUL FOR Heart ①②③ • Bones ① • Digestion ① • Skin, hair & nails ①③ • Mind ①② • Fatigue ③⑤ • Men ① • Women ①③④

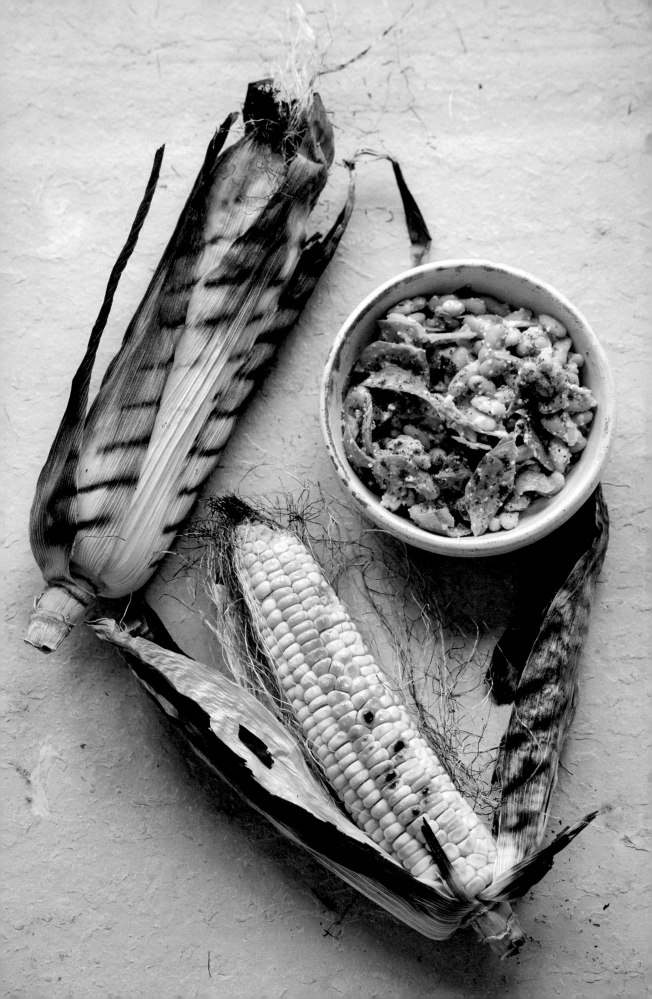

BUTTER BEANS WITH CHERRY TOMATOES & SALSA VERDE

SERVES 2 • 230 CALORIES PER SERVING

Salsa verde, or 'green sauce', should be in everyone's cooking repertoire as it adds so much flavour and colour to all kinds of dishes. The key to a salsa verde is to taste as you go – a little more lemon juice or sprinkle of salt can make all the difference. This is a really simple vegetarian recipe that is packed full of bold flavours. It's high in fibre too, which means it keeps you feeling fuller for longer on fewer calories, so is great if you're trying to lose weight.

400g tin butter beans
A handful of sunflower seeds
200g cherry tomatoes, cut in half
1 tbsp finely chopped fresh chives
A handful of fresh basil leaves
A pinch of flaked sea salt
A pinch of cracked black pepper

FOR THE SALSA VERDE
A handful of fresh flat-leaf parsley
2 sprigs of fresh basil, leaves picked
1 sprig of fresh thyme, leaves picked
½ garlic clove
10 capers
1 tbsp olive oil
A squeeze of lemon juice
Salt and pepper

RICH IN Vitamin C • Potassium • Iron • Lycopene • Fibre

USEFUL FOR Heart ①② • Digestion ① • Immunity ① • Fatigue ① • Men ①

1 Preheat your oven to 200°C/fan 180°C/gas 6.
2 Drain the butter beans, rinse with cold water and pat dry. Spread them on a baking tray with the sunflower seeds. Cook in the heated oven for 10 minutes to slightly dry out the beans and toast the seeds until golden. Leave to cool, then transfer to a large salad bowl. Add the cherry tomatoes, chives, basil, sea salt and cracked black pepper and mix well. Set aside.
3 To make the salsa verde, very finely chop the herb leaves, garlic and capers together with the oil, lemon juice and seasoning on a chopping board, then tip into a large mortar and mash together with the pestle to make a coarse paste. Alternatively, if you are short of time, put all the ingredients in a blender or food processor and pulse to a coarse texture.
4 Serve the butter bean salad with the salsa verde on the side.

PUY LENTILS & ROASTED AUBERGINE WITH BASIL PESTO

SERVES 2 • 465 CALORIES PER SERVING

A delicious, bright green pesto will transform the simplest of salads – here a combination of lentils and aubergine that is hearty and wholesome. Using olive oil in dressings, as in this pesto, is beneficial for your heart health.

1 red onion, sliced
1 aubergine, cut into 1cm cubes
1 tsp olive oil
150g Puy lentils
50g sun-dried tomatoes, finely chopped
10 fresh chives, finely chopped

FOR THE PESTO
A handful of fresh basil leaves
A handful of spinach
A handful of cashew nuts
1 tbsp olive oil
Juice of ½ lemon
Salt and pepper

1 Preheat your oven to 200°C/fan 180°C/gas 6. Line a baking tray with greaseproof paper.
2 Spread the onion and aubergine on the baking tray. Drizzle the oil over them and season with salt and pepper. Roast for 15 minutes.
3 Meanwhile, put the lentils in a large pan of cold water, set on a high heat and bring to the boil. Once boiling, cook for 10 minutes until the lentils are tender but still slightly firm. Drain well, leaving them in the colander for at least 5 minutes, then tip into a large mixing bowl.
4 Add the roasted aubergine and onion, sun-dried tomatoes and chives to the lentils. Season to taste, then mix gently together. Leave to cool.
5 Now make the pesto. Reserve a few basil leaves to garnish. Finely chop the rest of the basil with the remaining ingredients and some seasoning, then transfer to a large mortar and pound to a coarse texture. (Alternatively, blitz everything together in a food processor.)
6 Serve the pesto on top of the lentils, garnished with basil leaves.

RICH IN Potassium • Zinc • Lycopene • Fibre

USEFUL FOR Heart ①② • Digestion ① •
Immunity ① • Skin, hair & nails ①④ • Men ①②

LENTIL SPROUT & CELERY SALAD

SERVES 2 • 295 CALORIES PER SERVING

The key to getting big bold flavours into salads is, first, to start by frying some onion and garlic; and, second, to always include seeds or nuts. The salad here does both, plus it contains lentil sprouts, which are a great addition, either raw or lightly sautéed, adding crunchiness and earthy flavour. It is really easy to sprout lentils. You can use any type. Simply soak them in water overnight, then drain and transfer to a large flat dish. Cover them and leave in a cool, dark place until they begin to sprout. This usually takes 1–2 days. Rinse them thoroughly before using. Alternatively, you can buy lentil sprouts from good greengrocers.

1 tsp olive oil
1 tsp sunflower seeds
1 red onion, finely sliced
2 garlic cloves, finely sliced
200g lentil sprouts
Juice of ½ lemon
A pinch of flaked sea salt
A pinch of cracked black pepper
4 celery sticks, very finely sliced
1 yellow pepper, seeded and finely sliced
A handful of radishes, cut into quarters
50g edamame beans, thawed if frozen
100g mange tout, finely sliced

1 Set a non-stick frying pan on a high heat, add the olive oil and then add the sunflower seeds, onion and garlic. Cook for 3 minutes, stirring occasionally.
2 Add the lentil sprouts and cook for a further 1 minute. Tip the sprouts mixture into a large mixing bowl. Add the lemon juice, sea salt and pepper and toss to mix. Leave to cool.
3 Now add the rest of the ingredients. Mix thoroughly and serve.

RICH IN Vitamins B6, C and E • Folate • Potassium • Beta-carotene • Phytoestrogens • Fibre

USEFUL FOR Heart ①② • Bones ① • Immunity ① • Skin, hair & nails ①③ • Mind ① • Men ① • Women ①③④

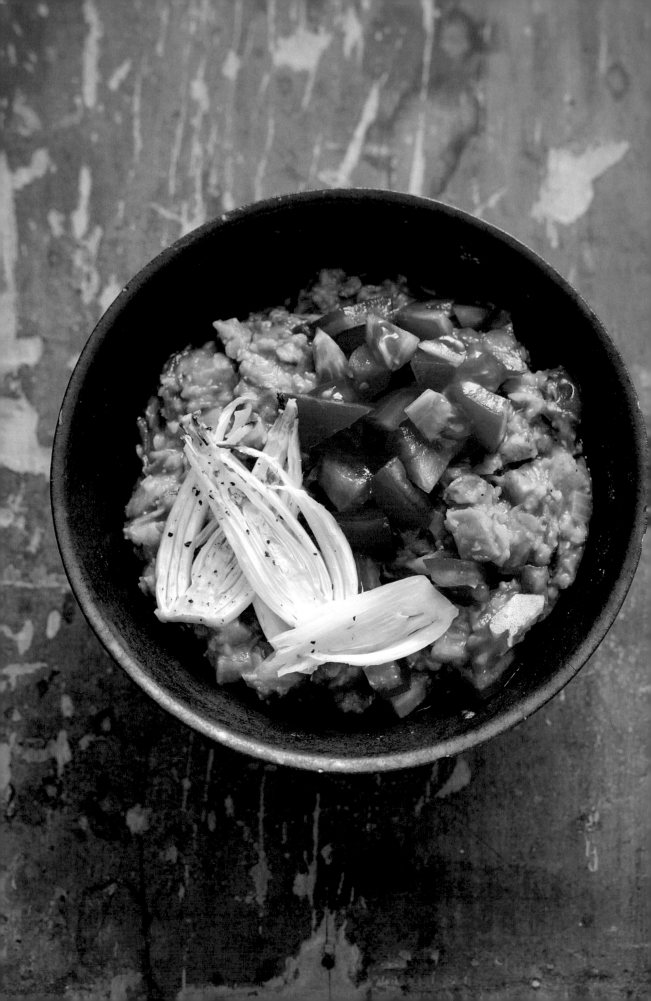

DAL WITH ROASTED FENNEL

SERVES 2 • 430 CALORIES PER SERVING

Every restaurant and home in India has its own version of dal. Some use red lentils with the classic ginger and onion base, giving a yellow colour and earthy taste. Some add tomatoes, for richer flavour and a bright red colour. This dal is a boldly spiced, thick soup that is more-ish and totally comforting. A garnish of crunchy roasted fennel and chopped tomatoes provide a sharp contrast to the smooth lentils.

1 tsp rapeseed oil

1 tsp mustard seeds

1 red onion, finely chopped

1 garlic clove, finely chopped

A large thumb-sized piece of fresh ginger, grated with the skin on

150g red lentils

1 carrot, finely diced

2 celery sticks, finely diced

1 bay leaf

1 tsp ground cumin

600ml vegetable stock (see page 283)

1 fennel bulb

1 tsp crushed dried chilli

Grated zest and juice of 1 lemon

A handful of fresh coriander, finely chopped

3 ripe vine tomatoes, roughly chopped

Flaked sea salt and cracked black pepper

1 Preheat your oven to 200°C/fan 180°C/gas 6. Line a baking tray with greaseproof paper.

2 Set a large saucepan on a high heat. Add the oil and then the mustard seeds and cook for 2 minutes. Add the onion and cook on a high heat until slightly browned. Stir in the garlic and ginger and continue to cook on a high heat, stirring, for 2 minutes.

3 Add the lentils, carrot, celery, bay leaf, cumin and stock. Season with sea salt and pepper. Bring to the boil, then turn the heat to low and simmer for 20 minutes until the lentils have completely broken up, stirring occasionally.

4 Meanwhile, cut the root or core out of the fennel bulb, then thinly slice lengthways. Spread the fennel slices on the baking tray and sprinkle with the chilli flakes, lemon zest, sea salt and pepper. Roast in the heated oven for 15 minutes. Remove from the oven and set aside.

5 Once the lentils are cooked, remove the bay leaf and add a squeeze of lemon juice and the coriander. Blitz with a hand blender (or tip into a blender or food processor, then blitz). You don't want to create a really smooth, soupy texture – there should still be visible lentils.

6 Serve the dal in pasta or soup bowls with the tomatoes and roasted fennel on top.

RICH IN Vitamins B3 (niacin) and C • Folate • Potassium • Iron • Magnesium • Calcium • Zinc • Beta-carotene • Fibre

USEFUL FOR Heart ①②③ • Bones ① • Digestion ① • Immunity ① • Skin, hair & nails ①②④ • Mind ② • Fatigue ①③⑤ • Men ①② • Women ①

CHICKPEA, POMEGRANATE & PUMPKIN CURRY

SERVES 4 • 285 CALORIES PER SERVING

Chickpeas seem to have been made for vegetable curries as they have a wonderfully satisfying texture and they soak up all the spicy flavours. This recipe combines Indian spices with some Middle-Eastern influences in the pomegranate seeds and mint. The curry makes the perfect nourishing meal when you've been hit with the flu – iron and vitamin C are essential for a strong immune system, and coconut contains lauric acid, which has anti-viral properties.

½ large pumpkin
1 tsp coconut oil
1 large onion, finely diced
2 garlic cloves, finely sliced
A thumb-sized piece of ginger, grated with the skin on
5 curry leaves (preferably fresh)
1 tbsp curry powder
3 cardamom pods
1 fresh red chilli, seeded and finely sliced
1 tsp salt
1 tsp ground black pepper
1 pomegranate
400g tin chickpeas, drained and rinsed
200ml coconut milk
Juice of 1 lime
A handful of fresh mint leaves, finely chopped, plus extra leaves to garnish

1 To prepare the pumpkin, cut the piece in half and scoop out the seeds and fibres. Cut each half into four pieces, then peel off the skin and discard. Cut the flesh into 1cm-thick wedges or half-moons.

2 Set a large pan on a high heat and add the oil. Add the onion and cook for 5 minutes. Turn the heat to low and cook for another 5 minutes. Now stir in the garlic, ginger and curry leaves and cook for 3 more minutes. Mix in the curry powder, cardamom, chilli, 100ml water, the salt and the pepper. Cook for another 3 minutes.

3 Add the pumpkin to the pan with 150ml water. Stir well. Simmer for 20–25 minutes until tender.

4 Meanwhile, cut the pomegranate in half and place the halves cut side down on some kitchen paper. Gently tap them with a wooden spoon until all the seeds have fallen out. You will have to remove some of the skin that has fallen out too. Set the seeds aside.

5 Add the chickpeas and coconut milk to the curry and simmer for a further 5 minutes. Finally, add the lime juice and chopped mint and stir through. Serve hot, garnished with the pomegranate seeds and mint leaves.

RICH IN Vitamins B1 (thiamin), C and E • Iron • Potassium • Phytoestrogens • Fibre

USEFUL FOR Heart ①② • Digestion ① • Immunity ① • Fatigue ① • Women ①③④

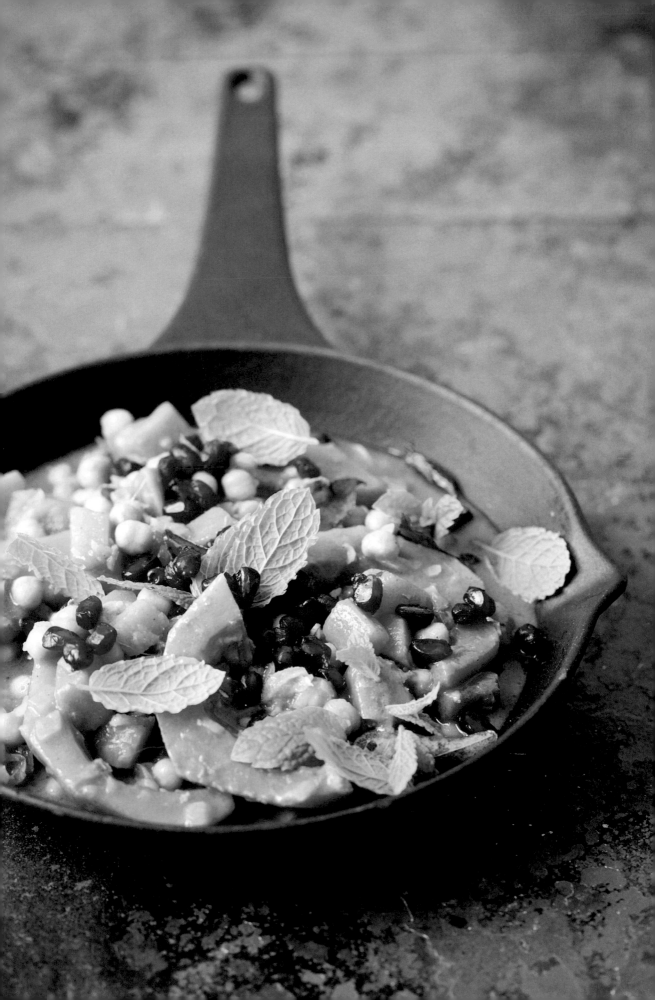

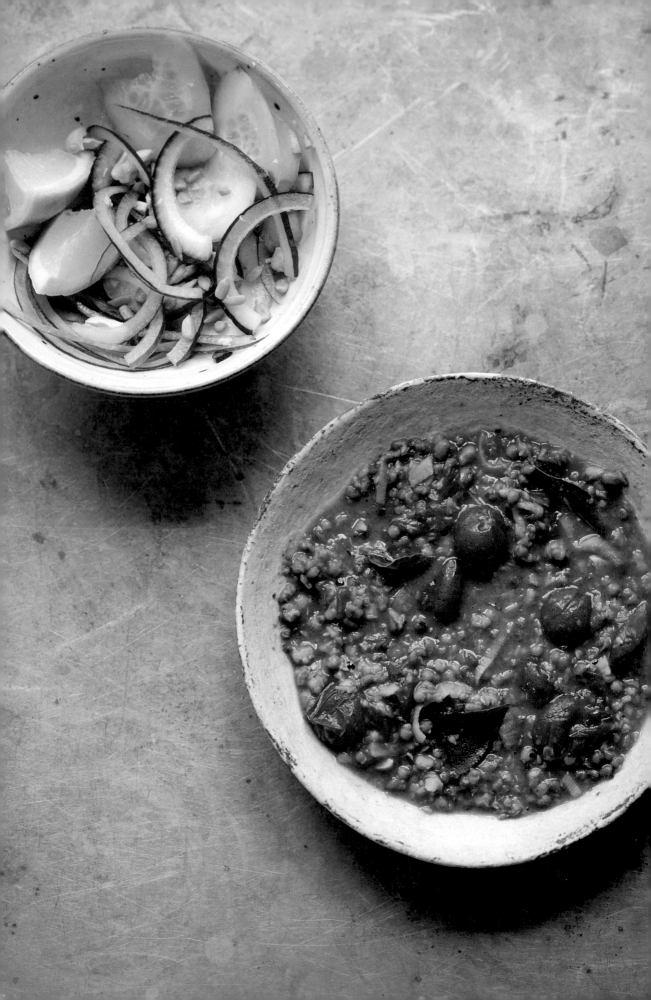

MUNG BEAN CURRY WITH ONION, CUCUMBER & CASHEW NUT SALAD

SERVES 2 • 480 CALORIES PER SERVING

Mung beans are becoming ever more popular, which means that they can be found in most supermarkets. They are unique little beans, earthy and slightly nutty in flavour with a crunchy texture. They work really well in a curry, acting as the perfect backdrop for the spicing. Spices offer a concentrated source of iron, with this dish providing nearly half the RDA of this fatigue-fighting mineral.

100g dried mung beans

1 tsp olive oil

1 red onion, finely diced

A thumb-sized piece of fresh ginger, peeled and finely chopped

1 garlic clove, finely chopped

5 curry leaves (preferably fresh)

1 tsp curry powder

1 tsp ground turmeric

½ tsp ground coriander

1 tsp ground cumin

1 tsp garam masala

150g cherry tomatoes or 6 vine tomatoes, finely diced

A pinch of salt

100ml coconut milk

Juice of 1 lime

FOR THE SALAD

½ red onion, finely sliced

1 cucumber, peeled and sliced

A handful of cashew nuts, toasted

A handful of sunflower seeds, toasted

Juice of ½ lemon

1 tsp rapeseed oil

1 Put the mung beans in a large pan and cover with three times their volume of water. Set on a high heat and bring to the boil. Continue to boil for 20 minutes until the beans are almost cooked. Drain and set aside.

2 Set a medium-sized saucepan on a high heat and add the olive oil, then add the onion, ginger and garlic. Cook, stirring, for 4 minutes. Add all the spices with a splash of water and stir in, then add the tomatoes and continue to cook on a high heat, stirring frequently, until the tomatoes have softened. Reduce the heat, add 50ml of water and simmer for 10 minutes, stirring occasionally.

3 Meanwhile, mix together all the ingredients for the salad.

4 Stir the salt, coconut milk and a good squeeze of lime into the curry along with the cooked mung beans. Simmer for a further 5 minutes. Serve the curry hot, with the salad and some brown rice or quinoa.

RICH IN Vitamins B1 (thiamin), B6, C and E • Folate • Potassium • Iron • Curcuminoids • Fibre

USEFUL FOR Heart ①② • Bones ② • Digestion ① • Immunity ① • Skin, hair & nails ② • Mind ① • Fatigue ① • Women ③

PINTO BEAN CHILLI

SERVES 4 • 380 CALORIES PER SERVING

Most cooks' idea of heaven is putting lots of
ingredients in a pot and leaving them to work their
magic, then coming back to a delicious hot meal.
This recipe is just like that. It's also economical,
satisfying and nourishing, offering a valuable
source of protein. Dried beans, soaked overnight,
give a much better texture to the chilli than tinned
beans, and cooking them gently for 2 hours means
they have time to soak up all the delicious flavours
in the sauce.

200g dried pinto beans
100g dried black beans
100g dried red kidney beans
1 tsp rapeseed oil
1 large onion, finely chopped
1 carrot, finely diced
2 celery sticks, finely diced
1 red pepper, seeded and finely diced
2 garlic cloves, finely chopped
1 tbsp grated fresh ginger
½ fresh red chilli, seeded and finely chopped
400g tin cherry tomatoes
1 tsp chilli powder
1 tsp paprika
Chervil, to garnish
Lime wedges, to serve

FOR THE GUACAMOLE
2 avocados
½ red onion, finely chopped
½ fresh green chilli, seeded and roughly
chopped
Juice of 1 lime
Salt and pepper

1 Put all the beans in a large bowl, cover with
plenty of cold water and leave to soak overnight.
Drain in a colander and rinse. Tip the beans into
a saucepan, cover with fresh cold water and
bring to the boil. Boil for 10 minutes, then drain
and set aside.
2 Heat the oil in a large saucepan and cook the
onion for 10 minutes on a medium heat until
lightly browned. Add the carrot, celery and red
pepper and cook for a further 5 minutes. Stir in
the garlic, ginger and chilli and cook for another
5 minutes.
3 Add the beans, tin of tomatoes, chilli powder,
paprika and 250ml water. Simmer gently for
2 hours, stirring from time to time.

4 Meanwhile, make the guacamole. Halve the
avocados and remove the stone, then scoop
the flesh into a bowl. Mash roughly with a fork.
Mix in the red onion, chilli, lime juice and a
pinch of salt.
5 Season the chilli. Serve in bowls, each topped
with chervil and a big dollop of guacamole, with
lime wedges for squeezing over.

RICH IN Vitamins B1 (thiamin), B6, C and E • Folate •
Potassium • Magnesium • Iron • Beta-carotene •
Lycopene • Beta-sitosterol • Fibre

USEFUL FOR Heart ①②③ • Bones ① •
Digestion ① • Immunity ① •
Skin, hair & nails ①③④ • Mind ①② •
Fatigue ①③⑤ • Men ① • Women ①③

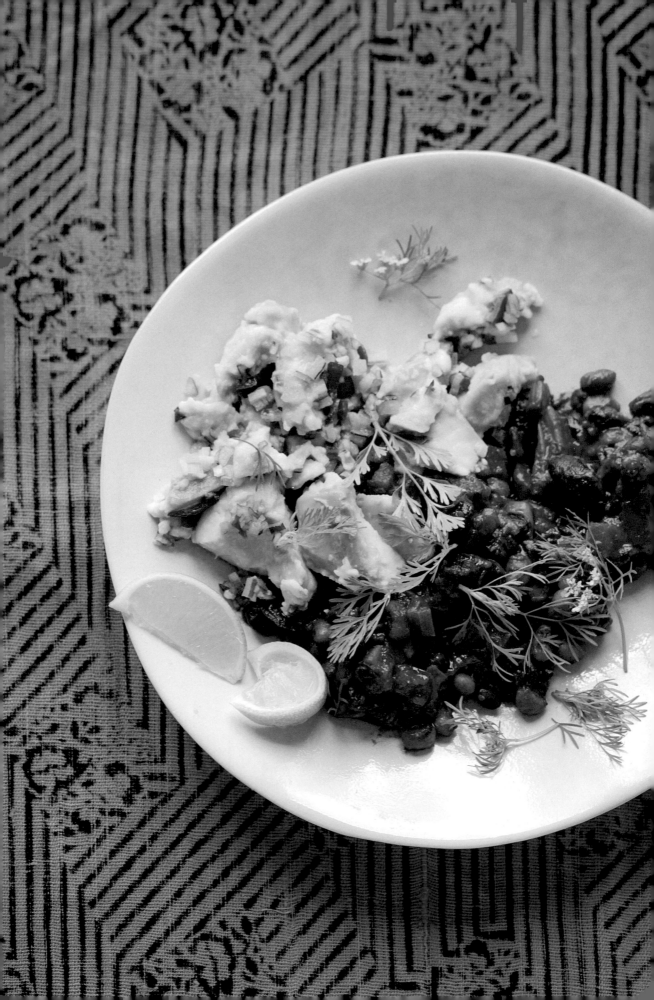

ADUKI BEAN STEW

SERVES 2 • 350 CALORIES PER SERVING

Small and dark red, with a sweet nutty taste, aduki beans are widely used in Japanese cooking because of their health benefits. Compared to other beans they are easy to digest, which means they are less gassy. All beans and pulses are a good source of protein, and if you swap meat for pulses across the week, you'll get an additional boost of fibre too. This is a hearty recipe that's quick and easy to put together.

1 tbsp rapeseed oil
1 red onion, diced
A 2.5cm piece of fresh ginger, peeled and grated
1 garlic clove, finely chopped
400ml vegetable stock (see page 283)
3 celery sticks, diced
1 carrot, diced
1 fennel bulb, sliced
400g tin aduki beans, drained and rinsed
1 courgette, diced
Grated zest of 1 lemon
A handful of fresh coriander, finely chopped
Salt and cracked black pepper

1 Set a large saucepan on a high heat, add the oil and then add the onion, ginger and garlic. Cook for 5 minutes. Pour in the stock and add the celery, carrot and fennel. Cook for 12 minutes until the vegetables are tender.
2 Add the aduki beans and the courgette and cook for 5 more minutes. Mix through the lemon zest and coriander, season well and serve.

RICH IN Vitamins B6 and C • Folate • Potassium • Iron • Magnesium • Calcium • Zinc • Beta-carotene • Fibre

USEFUL FOR Heart ①②③ • Bones ① • Digestion ① • Immunity ① • Skin, hair & nails ①③④ • Mind ①② • Fatigue ①③⑤ • Men ①② • Women ①

LENTIL BAKE

SERVES 4 • 305 CALORIES PER SERVING

A rustic, wholesome dish, this is just what you want on a winter's day. All the work is in the chopping, so once the dish is in the oven, you can sit back and enjoy the spicy aromas filling your kitchen. The bake is rich in selenium (lentils are a valuable source of this mineral), which has a key role to play in regulating the immune system.

250g Puy lentils
1 tbsp olive oil
1 red onion, finely chopped
1 aubergine, diced
3 garlic cloves, roasted for 30 minutes
(see Creamy Cauliflower & Roasted Garlic Soup, page 90)
1 tsp flaked sea salt
1 tsp cracked black pepper
1 courgette, diced
1 red pepper, seeded and diced
400g tin cherry tomatoes
1 tsp ground cumin
A pinch of ground cinnamon
A handful of fresh thyme sprigs
2 bay leaves
200ml vegetable stock (see page 283)
A handful of fresh coriander, finely chopped
Grated zest and juice of ½ lemon

1 Preheat your oven to 200°C/fan 180°C/gas 6.
2 Put the lentils in a large saucepan, cover with cold water and bring to the boil, then simmer for 5 minutes to part-cook. Drain and tip into a large mixing bowl.
3 Heat the oil in a frying pan and gently fry the onion for 8 minutes until softened. Add the aubergine and cook for 5 minutes until lightly golden, stirring occasionally. Add to the mixing bowl along with the rest of the ingredients. Mix well with the lentils.
4 Transfer the mixture to an ovenproof dish and cover with foil. Bake in the heated oven for 50–60 minutes, giving the mix a little stir after 20 minutes. When the lentils and vegetables are tender, serve hot with a spinach salad.

RICH IN Vitamin C • Folate • Selenium • Potassium • Iron • Zinc • Beta-carotene • Lycopene • Fibre

USEFUL FOR Heart ①②③ • Digestion ① • Immunity ① • Skin, hair & nails ①③④ • Fatigue ① • Men ①②

LENTIL BURGERS WITH WHITE CABBAGE & MANGE TOUT SALAD

SERVES 2 • 600 CALORIES PER SERVING

This dish is really simple to make and cheap with it. One of the very best things about white cabbage is that if you buy a big one, it can last you a whole week – use it in salads like this one or throw it into stews and soups to add an extra crunch. This cabbage salad works perfectly with these smooth-textured lentil burgers. Two kinds of lentils are used – both beluga and red. Lentils are a good source of iron and a key provider of this mineral in meat-free diets.

FOR THE BURGERS

100g beluga lentils

100g red lentils

1 tsp ground cumin

1 spring onion, finely chopped

A handful of fresh coriander, finely chopped

A handful of fresh mint leaves, finely chopped

Grated zest of 1 lemon

20g cashew nuts, roughly chopped

1 tsp groundnut oil

1 egg, beaten to mix

1 tbsp gluten- and wheat-free flour

A handful of pumpkin seeds

FOR THE SALAD

20g sunflower seeds

½ small white cabbage

100g mange tout

2 spring onions, finely chopped

1 tbsp finely chopped fresh coriander

4 fresh mint leaves, finely chopped

1 tbsp lemon juice

1 tsp rapeseed oil

1 Put the beluga and red lentils in a saucepan of cold water with a pinch of salt and bring to the boil. Simmer for 15 minutes until tender but still firm. Drain and leave to cool completely.

2 While the lentils are cooling, make the salad. First, toast the sunflower seeds in a dry frying pan for 4 minutes, shaking the pan constantly; leave to cool. Thinly slice the cabbage into long strips (or shred it, if you prefer) and place in a large mixing bowl. Thinly slice the mange tout into strips and add to the bowl. Add the spring onions, coriander, mint and toasted seeds. Toss with the lemon juice and rapeseed oil. Set aside (chill if you like).

3 Preheat your oven to 200°C/fan 180°C/gas 6. Line a small baking tray with baking parchment.

4 Once the lentils are cool, tip them into a large mixing bowl. Add the cumin, spring onion, coriander, mint, lemon zest, cashew nuts, oil, beaten egg and flour. Mix together well, then shape into four medium-sized burgers. Sprinkle the pumpkin seeds on top and press them into the burgers.

5 Place the burgers on the lined baking tray and bake in the heated oven for 20 minutes until golden. Serve warm with the cabbage salad.

RICH IN Vitamins B6, B12 and C • Iron • Potassium • Zinc • Magnesium • Selenium • Tryptophan • Fibre

USEFUL FOR Heart ①② • Bones ① • Digestion ① • Immunity ① • Skin, hair & nails ①④ • Mind ①② • Fatigue ①③⑤ • Men ①② • Women ①

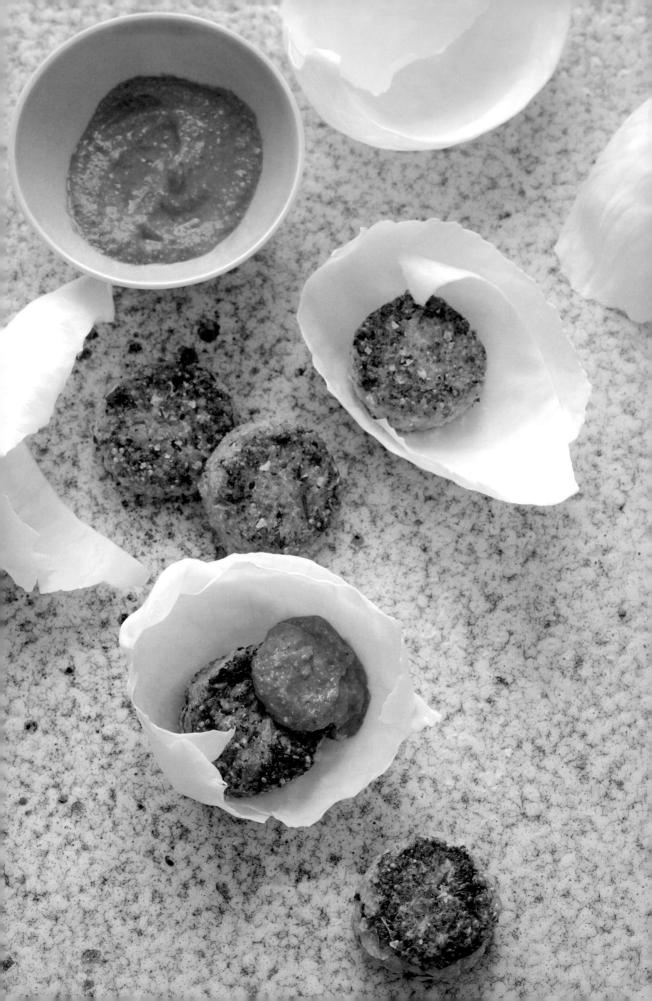

QUINOA, KALE & PISTACHIO BURGERS

MAKES 8 BURGERS TO SERVE 4 • 315 CALORIES PER SERVING

If you have cooked from this book, you may by now have realised that we are mad about cauliflower. Recently our greengrocer has started to stock Romanesco, a lime green cauliflower with pointed cone-shaped knobbles, and Purple Cape, whose vibrant colour you can guess from its name. Either of these or regular cauliflower will work for this recipe. If you are making lots and you have time, make batches in three different colours for that extra wow! Served with salads, these burgers are great for supper on a summer's day.

150g quinoa
30g home-shelled pistachios
1 cauliflower, separated into florets
1 garlic clove, finely chopped
1 spring onion, finely sliced
1 egg, beaten to mix
A handful of kale, finely chopped
A handful of fresh coriander, finely chopped
A handful of fresh flat-leaf parsley, finely chopped
1 tsp onion seeds
1 tbsp rapeseed oil, plus extra for optional frying
2 tbsp porridge oats
2 tbsp gluten- and wheat-free flour
A pinch of salt
A pinch of pepper

TO SERVE
8 large cabbage leaves
100g Tomato & Cashew Cream (see page 62)

1 Put the quinoa in a saucepan with three times its volume of water and bring to the boil. You want the quinoa to be slightly overcooked for this recipe, so cook for 12 minutes. Drain in a sieve, then rinse under cold water to cool. Leave to drain well.
2 Place the pistachios and cauliflower florets in a food processor and blitz to a crumbly texture. Transfer to a large bowl and add the quinoa as well as the rest of the ingredients. Mix together.
3 Spread out the mixture on a baking tray and chill for 1 hour to allow it to firm up. Then form the mixture into eight small burgers.
4 Preheat the grill to medium. Line a baking tray with baking parchment.
5 Place the burgers on the lined baking tray and grill, turning often, for about 12 minutes until golden brown and crisp on both sides. (You can also fry the burgers in a little rapeseed oil for 5 minutes on each side, but grilling is a healthier cooking method.)
6 Serve each burger in a cabbage leaf topped with a dollop of tomato and cashew cream.

RICH IN Vitamins B1 (thiamin), B6 and C • Folate • Potassium • Magnesium

USEFUL FOR Heart ②③ • Bones ① • Immunity ① • Mind ①② • Fatigue ⑤ • Women ①

WHOLE ROASTED CAULIFLOWER

SERVES 2 • 350 CALORIES PER SERVING

My enthusiasm for this humble vegetable knows no bounds: I often used to think that when I walked down the aisle I should have a cauliflower as my bridal bouquet – perhaps a step too far. But there's no doubt that cauliflower is incredibly versatile (bouquets aside) and roasting it whole is only one of the great ways to cook it. The key is to ensure that the cauliflower is held up straight in the roasting tin while it's in the oven. Cauliflower is one of the richest vegetable sources of vitamin C, which is needed to make collagen, a key component of healthy skin.

1 large cauliflower
1 tbsp rapeseed oil
1 tbsp runny honey
A pinch of ground cinnamon
A pinch of paprika
5 cloves

FOR THE PEARL BARLEY
100g pearl barley
A handful of fresh mint leaves, finely chopped
A handful of fresh flat-leaf parsley, finely chopped
½ red onion, chopped
Juice of 1 lemon
Salt and pepper

1 Preheat your oven to 200°C/fan 180°C/gas 6.
2 Make a large sausage shape out of foil. It needs to be solid, so scrunch the foil up tightly, and it should be about 30cm long and 7cm high. Curl the foil sausage into a ring shape and place it in the middle of a baking tray.
3 Remove the outer leaves of the cauliflower, then set it on the foil ring – the foil will ensure that the cauliflower doesn't touch the tray.
4 Mix together the oil, honey, cinnamon, paprika and a pinch each of salt and pepper in a bowl. Cover the cauliflower with this mixture. Stick the cloves into the cauliflower so that they are secure. Roast for 30 minutes. Remove from the oven and leave to cool.
5 While the cauliflower is cooling, put the pearl barley in a large pan and cover with three times its volume of water. Bring to the boil, then leave to simmer for 25–30 minutes until the pearl barley is soft. Drain in a sieve and rinse under cold running water.

6 Tip the pearl barley into a large mixing bowl and add the mint, parsley, red onion, lemon juice and a pinch each of salt and pepper. Keep warm.
7 Once the cauliflower is cool, slice it and serve with the pearl barley.

RICH IN Vitamins B1 (thiamin), B6 and C • Folate • Potassium • Iron • Fibre

USEFUL FOR Heart ② • Digestion ① • Immunity ① • Mind ① • Fatigue ① • Women ①

QUINOA, BRUSSELS SPROUTS & CASHEWS

SERVES 2 • 594 CALORIES PER SERVING

We served this during a Christmas food festival called Feast. We wanted to create something warming, spicy and Christmassy, hence the trusty Brussels sprouts with a hint of chilli. The dish was served with a thick red lentil soup (see recipe on page 89) as a gravy, which worked really well. Quinoa is a favourite at the Detox Kitchen, being a great protein source for non-meat eaters as it contains all of the essential amino acids.

200g quinoa

1 tsp rapeseed oil

3 shallots, finely sliced

1 garlic clove, finely chopped

50g cashew nuts

A pinch of crushed dried chilli

250g Brussels sprouts, cut in half

A handful of fresh coriander, finely chopped

Salt and pepper

1 Put the quinoa in a medium-sized saucepan and cover with three times its volume of water. Set the pan on a high heat and bring to the boil. Once boiling, cook for 6–8 minutes until just tender, then drain in a sieve and rinse.

2 Set a medium-sized, non-stick frying pan on a high heat. Add the oil and then the shallots and cook for 3 minutes. Add the garlic and cashew nuts and cook for another 3 minutes until the nuts start to turn golden.

3 Stir in the chilli flakes and 2 tablespoons water and add the Brussels sprouts. Cook for about 3 minutes until the sprouts are tender but still crunchy. Now add the quinoa back in to warm through for 3 minutes. Remove from the heat and mix in the coriander. Season and serve.

RICH IN Vitamins B1 (thiamin), B6 and C • Folate • Potassium • Magnesium • Fibre

USEFUL FOR Heart ①②③ • Bones ① • Digestion ① • Immunity ① • Mind ①② • Fatigue ③⑤ • Women ①

PEARL BARLEY, PEAS, SPINACH, BROAD BEANS & HAZELNUTS

SERVES 4 • 305 CALORIES PER SERVING

We served this dish at our first-ever pop-up restaurant in London. Pearl barley is always a crowd-pleaser, and combined with bright green vegetables and lightly toasted hazelnuts, it is wonderfully wholesome as well as looking impressive and tasting superb. The pop-up also happened to fall on the first day of spring, so we wanted to use the new season's fresh, beautiful green ingredients.

30g blanched (skinned) hazelnuts
200g pearl barley
200g frozen peas
100g podded fresh or thawed frozen broad beans
A handful of spinach, roughly chopped
1 tbsp rapeseed oil
1 spring onion, sliced
10 fresh mint leaves, plus extra leaves to garnish
Pinch of flaked sea salt
Pinch of cracked black pepper
Lemon wedges, to serve

1 Preheat your oven to 200°C/fan 180°C/gas 6. Spread the hazelnuts on a small baking tray and toast in the oven for 8 minutes until golden.

2 Tip the hazelnuts into a blender and pulse for a few seconds just to break them up a little.

3 Rinse the pearl barley in cold running water, then put it in a large pan and cover with four times its volume of water. Set the pan on a high heat and bring to the boil, then reduce the heat to medium and cook for 20 minutes. Add the peas, turn up the heat to high again and bring back to the boil. Once boiling, cook for a further 2 minutes, then drain.

4 Meanwhile, tip the broad beans into a blender or food processor and add the spinach, rapeseed oil, spring onion and mint. Blitz to a rough paste (you want to keep it quite chunky so the dish has some crunch).

5 Now mix all the ingredients together. Serve garnished with mint leaves and with wedges of lemon for squeezing over. This dish is great either hot or cold.

RICH IN Vitamins C and E • Folate • Fibre

USEFUL FOR Heart ① • Bones ① • Immunity ① • Women ③

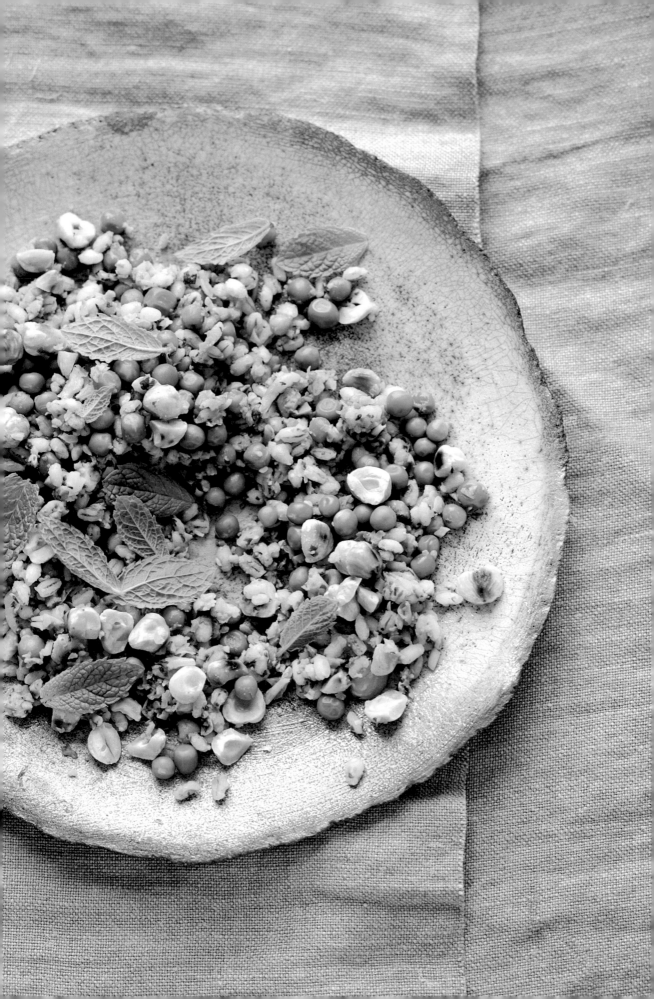

PASTA WITH BROAD BEANS & MINT PESTO

SERVES 2 • 465 CALORIES PER SERVING

This dish is a celebration of green, from the almost luminous grass-green colour of peeled broad beans and a fresh mint and spinach pesto. Combining these with comforting pasta makes a very appealing summery dish. Broad beans are high in potassium, which is beneficial for healthy blood pressure.

30g pine nuts
100g podded broad beans
150g gluten-free fusilli pasta
100g frozen peas

FOR THE PESTO

100g spinach
A handful of fresh mint leaves
A handful of fresh chives
A handful of fresh flat-leaf parsley
Juice of ½ lemon
1 tbsp rapeseed oil
1 tsp flaked sea salt

RICH IN Vitamins B3 (niacin), C and E • Folate • Magnesium • Potassium • Zinc • Iron • Beta-carotene • Fibre

USEFUL FOR Heart ①②③ • Bones ① • Digestion ① • Immunity ① • Skin, hair & nails ①③④ • Mind ② • Fatigue ①③⑤ • Men ①② • Women ①③

1 Preheat your oven to 200°C/fan 180°C/gas 6. Line a small baking tray with greaseproof paper.

2 Spread the pine nuts on the baking tray and toast in the oven for 6 minutes until golden. Set aside.

3 Bring a saucepan of water to the boil, add the broad beans and cook for 4 minutes. Drain and rinse under cold running water, then slip the beans out of their skins. Set aside.

3 Bring a medium-sized pan of water to the boil. Add the pasta and cook for 8 minutes, then add the peas and cook for a further 3 minutes (or according to the timing on the packet) until the pasta is tender.

4 While the pasta is cooking, very finely chop the spinach and herbs for the pesto, then pound together with the lemon juice, oil and sea salt using a pestle and mortar to make a coarse paste. (Alternatively, blitz all the ingredients together in a food processor.)

5 Once the pasta is cooked, scoop out a cupful of the cooking water, then drain the pasta – try to keep it quite wet as this will help the pesto to coat it. Tip the pasta back into the empty pan and return to the heat. Add the pesto and broad beans and heat through for 3 minutes, stirring in the reserved pasta cooking water as needed. Sprinkle with the toasted pine nuts to finish.

GRIDDLED BROCCOLI & PASTA

SERVES 2 • 445 CALORIES PER SERVING

Here is a simple dish that is filling and wholesome. Broccoli is the richest food source of chromium, a mineral that is involved in maintaining normal blood sugar levels. Griddling this vegetable gives it a greater depth of flavour and retains its essential crunchiness. Here it's combined with gluten-free pasta but it works just as well with brown rice, quinoa or buckwheat.

A handful of cashew nuts
2 handfuls of broccoli florets
200g gluten-free pasta
1 tsp crushed dried chilli
1 tsp toasted sesame seeds
2 spring onions, finely sliced
A pinch of flaked sea salt
A pinch of cracked black pepper
1 tsp olive oil

1 Preheat your oven to 200°C/fan 180°C/gas 6. Spread the cashew nuts on a small baking tray and toast in the oven for 8 minutes until golden. Set aside.
2 Cut off the broccoli florets, then cut the stalk into long thin strips. Bring a pan of water to the boil and blanch the broccoli florets and strips of stalk for 1 minute. Drain and rinse with cold water.
3 Bring another pan of water to the boil, add the pasta and cook for 8–12 mintues until tender, then drain.
4 While the pasta is cooking, set a ridged griddle/grill pan on a medium heat. When the griddle is hot, place the broccoli florets on it and cook for 2 minutes. Turn over and cook for another 2 minutes. The florets should be slightly charred. Transfer to a bowl, then cook the broccoli stalks in the same way.
5 Add the chilli, cashew nuts, toasted sesame seeds, spring onions, salt and pepper to the broccoli. Mix in the pasta and serve with a drizzle of olive oil.

RICH IN Vitamins B1 (thiamin) and C • Folate • Potassium • Magnesium • Chromium • Fibre

USEFUL FOR Heart ①②③ • Bones ① • Digestion ① • Mind ② • Fatigue ⑤ • Women ①

WARM QUINOA, SQUASH & SPINACH RISOTTO

SERVES 2 • 255 CALORIES PER SERVING

Try this for a really warming yet light lunch. The basil pesto gives it a delicious intense flavour that brings out the sweetness of the butternut squash. Risotto is typically served with Parmesan, to add an essential saltiness that brings all the flavours together, so add a sprinkling of flaked sea salt at the end of cooking. The dish is suitable for vegans and provides a good source of iron and some omega 3 fatty acids, which can be difficult to obtain from a vegan diet.

½ butternut squash, peeled and cut into 1cm cubes
200g quinoa
A large handful of fresh basil leaves
A handful of sunflower seeds
1 tbsp rapeseed oil
1 tsp salt
A handful of spinach, roughly chopped
1 large plump tomato, finely diced
Flaked sea salt, to finish

1 Preheat your oven to 200°C/fan 180°C/gas 6. Spread the squash cubes on a baking tray and roast for 20 minutes until tender.
2 Meanwhile, put the quinoa in a saucepan and cover with three times its volume of cold water. Place on a high heat and bring to the boil. Cook for 6–8 minutes until just tender, then drain in a sieve and rinse under cold water. Set aside.
3 Place most of the basil leaves, the sunflower seeds, rapeseed oil and salt in a blender and blitz to a smooth paste. Transfer the paste to a saucepan and heat gently. Add the roasted squash, spinach and quinoa and heat for about 3 minutes until piping hot, stirring gently to mix. Season with sea salt.
4 Serve topped with the diced tomato and remaining fresh basil leaves.

RICH IN Magnesium • Iron • Potassium • Omega 3 • Beta-carotene

USEFUL FOR Heart ②③ • Bones ① • Skin, hair & nails ①④ • Fatigue ①③

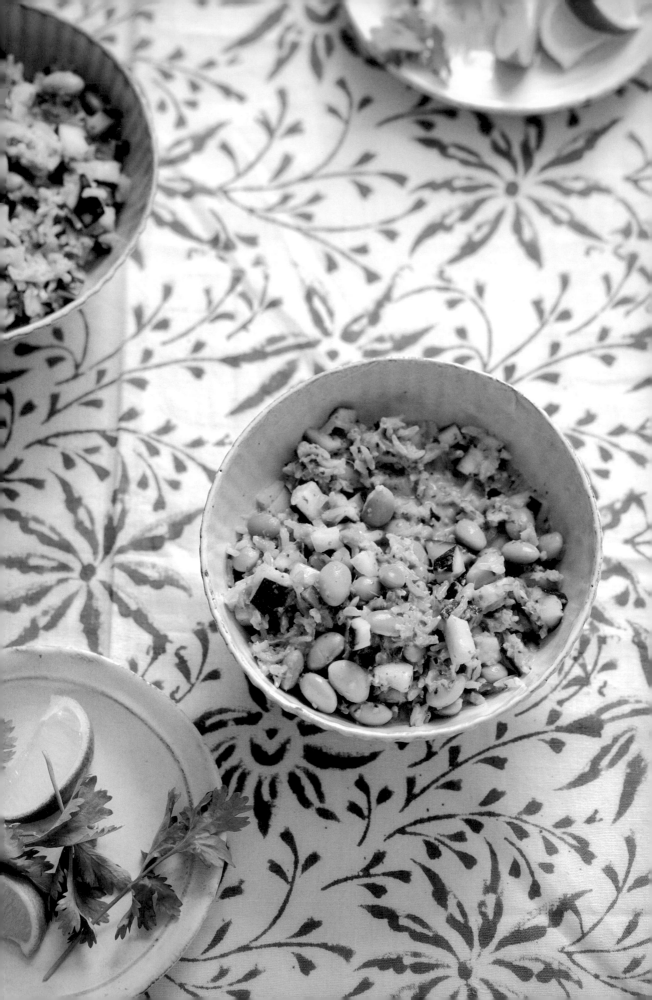

LEMONGRASS & COCONUT RICE WITH EDAMAME

SERVES 2 • 520 CALORIES PER SERVING

This could be described as an Asian-flavoured risotto. Lemongrass gives it a strong citrus fragrance and taste, with coconut mellowing the flavours and creating a lovely creamy texture. Topped with crunchy edamame beans, the dish is packed full of interesting textures and tastes. Edamame, with their soy isoflavones (a type of phytoestrogen), are worth including in your diet if you want to reduce your cholesterol levels.

150g brown rice

1 stick of lemongrass, roughly sliced

2 lime leaves

½ fresh green chilli, seeded

A thumb-sized piece of fresh ginger, roughly chopped with the skin on

1 shallot, roughly chopped

A handful of fresh coriander, finely chopped, plus extra to garnish

1 tbsp coconut oil

150ml coconut milk

200g edamame beans, thawed if frozen

1 courgette, finely diced

Salt

Lime wedges, to serve

1 Put the brown rice in a pan of cold water and bring to the boil, then part-cook for 15 minutes. Drain and set aside.

2 Place the lemongrass, lime leaves, chilli, ginger, shallot, coriander and coconut oil in a blender and blitz to a coarse paste. If you don't have a blender, you can finely chop the ingredients, then bash them together using a pestle and mortar.

3 Set a wide, deep frying pan on the hob, add the spice paste and cook for 2 minutes, stirring. Add the part-cooked rice and mix well with the paste. Pour in the coconut milk and 100ml water and add a pinch of salt. Bring to the boil, then simmer for 10 minutes.

4 Add the edamame and courgette and cook for a further 3 minutes. Garnish with extra coriander and serve with wedges of lime.

RICH IN Vitamins B3 (niacin), B6 and C • Folate • Potassium • Magnesium • Iron • Zinc • Phytoestrogens • Fibre

USEFUL FOR Heart ①②③ • Bones ① • Digestion ① • Immunity ① • Skin, hair & nails ①④ • Mind ①② • Fatigue ①③⑤ • Men ①② • Women ①③④

BROWN RICE & MUSHROOM RISOTTO

SERVES 2 • 425 CALORIES PER SERVING

Mushroom risotto is a vegetarian classic that can be quite stodgy. Using brown rice instead of the starchier risotto rice gives a lighter, coarser texture. Brown rice also makes this risotto a rich source of B vitamins, which are involved in converting food into energy. We've packed this recipe full of mushrooms, using a mixture of closed cup and wild to give a deep, nutty mushroom flavour.

1.2 litres vegetable stock (see page 283)
1 tsp groundnut oil
300g button or chestnut mushrooms, finely sliced
100g fresh wild mushrooms, finely sliced
3 shallots, finely diced
2 garlic cloves, finely chopped
1 sprig of fresh rosemary
150g brown rice
A pinch of salt
A handful of fresh flat-leaf parsley, finely chopped
1 tsp truffle oil

1 Pour the stock into a large pan and bring to the boil on a high heat. Reduce the heat to low so the stock is just simmering.
2 Set a large non-stick frying pan on a high heat, add the oil and then add the mushroom. Cook for 5 minutes until browned. Add the shallots and cook for 5 minutes until soft, then add the garlic and rosemary sprig. Turn the heat to medium and cook for a further 3 minutes.
3 Add the brown rice and salt and mix well. Now start adding the hot stock, one ladleful at a time. Once each addition has been absorbed, add another ladleful. Keep stirring as the risotto bubbles. It should take about 20 minutes to add the stock and cook the rice until tender.
4 Mix through the parsley and serve immediately, with a few drops of truffle oil on top.

RICH IN Vitamins B1 (thiamin), B2 (riboflavin), B3 (niacin), B6 and C • Folate • Potassium • Selenium • Iron • Beta-carotene • Fibre

USEFUL FOR Heart ①② • Digestion ① • Immunity ① • Skin, hair & nails ①③ • Mind ① • Fatigue ①⑤ • Men ① • Women ①

BUTTERNUT SQUASH & SAGE RISOTTO

SERVES 4 • 315 CALORIES PER SERVING

In this recipe it is the starch in pearl barley that creates the creaminess of a classic risotto made with rice. The key is to cook the barley slowly, adding the hot liquid gradually.

30g sunflower seeds
1 litre vegetable stock (see page 283)
3 sprigs of fresh sage, leaves picked
1 tsp rapeseed oil
3 banana shallots, finely sliced
3 garlic cloves, finely diced
200g pearl barley
1 butternut squash, peeled and cut into 1cm cubes
A handful of green beans, finely chopped
A small bunch of fresh chives, finely chopped
Grated zest of 1 lemon
Salt and pepper

1 Preheat your oven to 200°C/fan 180°C/gas 6.
2 Spread the sunflower seeds on a baking tray. Toast in the oven for 10 minutes until golden.
3 Pour the stock into a medium-sized pan, add the sage leaves and bring to a simmer.
4 Meanwhile, heat the oil in a large frying pan. Add the shallots and cook for 6 minutes. Add the garlic and cook for 3 minutes.
5 Now add the pearl barley and stir until all the grains are coated with oil. Add two ladles of the hot stock and simmer, stirring, until all the liquid has been absorbed – this will take 4–5 minutes.
6 Add the butternut squash with another ladle of stock. Once this stock is absorbed, add another ladleful, continuing to stir regularly. Keep adding the stock in this way, adding the green beans with the final ladleful. Once this final addition of stock has been absorbed, remove from the heat.
7 Season and stir in the chives and lemon zest. Leave for 5 minutes before serving, sprinkled with the toasted sunflower seeds.

RICH IN Vitamins B1 (thiamin), C and E • Folate • Potassium • Magnesium • Iron • Beta-carotene • Fibre

USEFUL FOR Heart ①②③ • Bones ① • Digestion ① • Immunity ① • Skin, hair & nails ①③ • Mind ② • Fatigue ⑤ • Women ①③

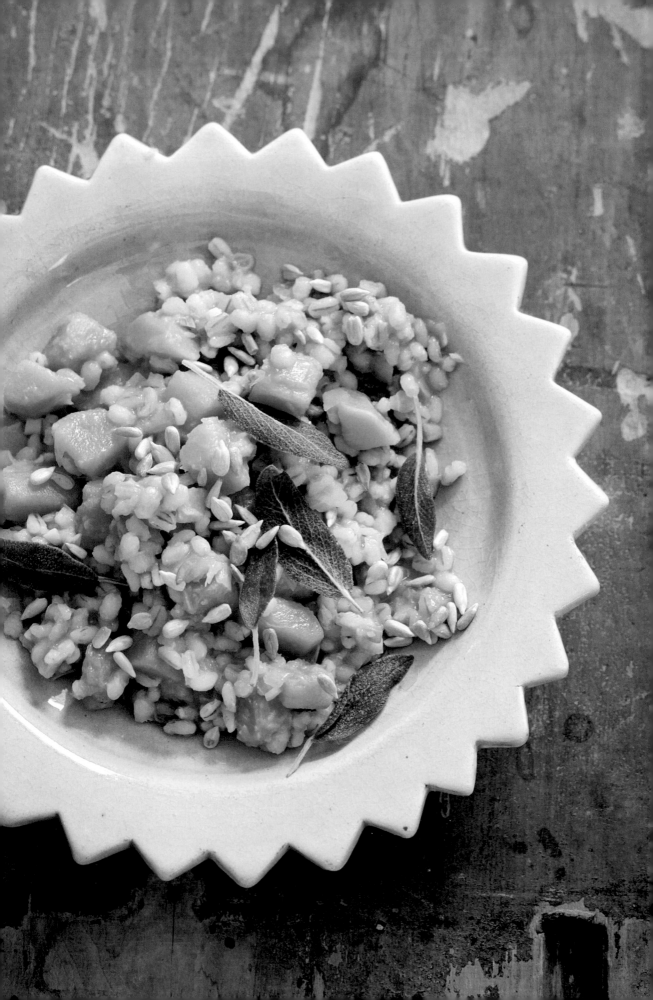

EGGS

Eggs have been given a bad rap over the years, mainly because of their high cholesterol content and suspected links to heart disease. This is undeserved: it is now clear that the cholesterol found naturally in eggs (and other foods) makes very little impact on cholesterol levels in the blood and does not contribute to the risk of heart disease, so there is no limit to the number of eggs you can safely have each week.

This is good news for your health because eggs are one of the most nutritious foods you can eat. A great source of protein, they are also rich in vitamins B2 and B12, selenium and iodine, and are one of the few food sources of vitamin D. In addition, eggs are a rich source of the antioxidants lutein and zeaxanthin, which have been linked to a reduced risk of eye diseases.

Wonderfully versatile, eggs are perfect for making quick, satisfying meals, and dishes such as omelettes and frittatas are ideal vehicles for an array of tasty vegetables. In the pages that follow, we've given the recipes we turn to again and again for weekday lunches and suppers.

At the end of most of the recipes, you'll find a list of the main nutrients supplied in a serving as well as a list of health issues that may be benefited by including the recipe in your healthy diet. For more, see page 9.

ASPARAGUS & EGG SMASH

SERVES 2 • 248 CALORIES PER SERVING

At the height of the English asparagus season it is very common for us to over-order. This delicious vegetable is here for such a short time that it seems criminal not to take full advantage. As a result, there is always some asparagus left over for us chefs in the kitchen. So we turn the griddle up high, put on some water for the eggs and in less than 10 minutes we have this rich, tasty dish for our lunch. It is rich in vitamin B12, which is essential for making healthy red blood cells and for fighting tiredness and fatigue.

4 eggs
8 asparagus spears
1 tbsp rapeseed oil, plus extra for drizzling
A squeeze of lemon juice
A handful of cress
Salt and pepper

1 Bring a medium-sized pan of water to the boil, then gently place the eggs in the pan. Simmer for 8–10 minutes (the eggs will be hard-boiled; cook for a shorter time if you prefer your eggs to be less well cooked). Cool the eggs under cold running water before peeling.
2 Meanwhile, set a ridged griddle/grill pan on a high heat to warm up.
3 Break the woody ends off the asparagus spears (this is usually the bottom 2.5–5cm and has a lighter colour than the tip – it should break off naturally if you apply gentle pressure). Put the asparagus in a bowl and drizzle some rapeseed oil over the spears. Once the griddle is hot, place the asparagus on it and cook for 5 minutes, turning occasionally. Remove the asparagus from the pan and set aside.
4 Combine the tablespoon of rapeseed oil, lemon juice and some salt and pepper in a bowl and whisk together thoroughly. Add the eggs and crush them into the dressing with a fork. You want to create a smooth texture with chunks running through.
5 Serve the egg smash with the cress on top and with the asparagus on the side.

RICH IN Vitamins B2 (riboflavin), B12 and D • Folate • Asparagine

USEFUL FOR Bones ① • Mind ① • Fatigue ⑤ • Women ①

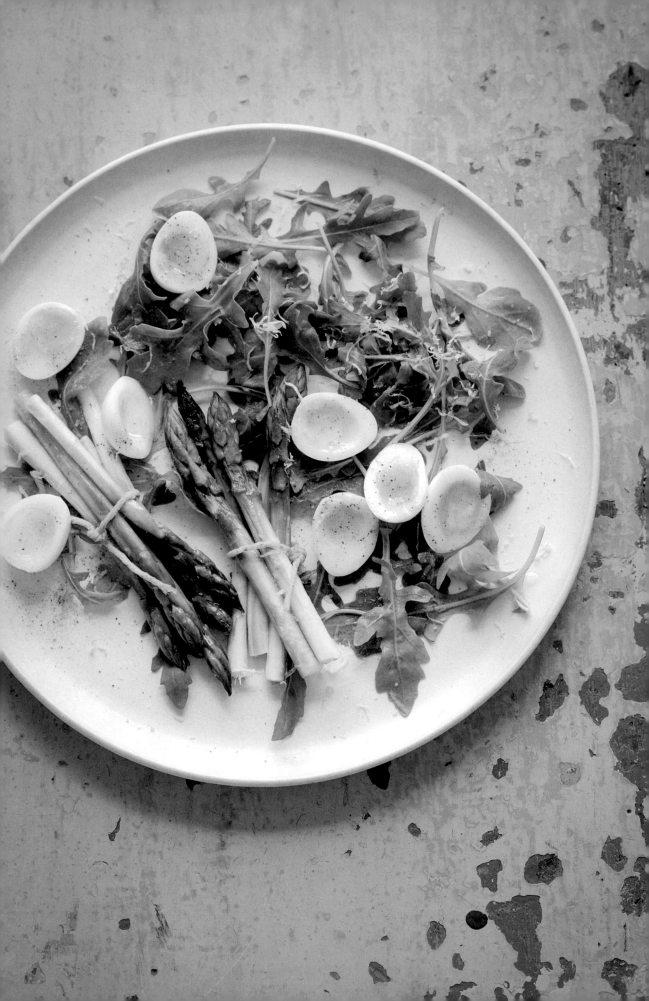

OVEN-BAKED ASPARAGUS & QUAIL'S EGGS

SERVES 2 • 310 CALORIES PER SERVING

The day that our grocer delivers the first asparagus of the season, this is the recipe we make. It is seasonal cooking at its most perfect. Asparagus is a good source of glutathione, a detoxifying compound that helps break down carcinogens and helps protect cells from free radicals. If you cannot get quail's eggs, regular eggs are fine – you just need fewer.

10 large asparagus spears
Grated zest of 1 lemon
1 tsp rapeseed oil
2 garlic cloves, gently crushed with the skin on
2 sprigs of fresh thyme
2 pinches of flaked sea salt
8 quail's eggs
A pinch of celery salt

TO SERVE
100g rocket
Rapeseed oil
Lemon juice

RICH IN Vitamins B2 (riboflavin), B3 (niacin), B6, C and D • Folate • Iron • Potassium • Calcium • Tryptophan • Asparagine • Beta-carotene • Fibre

USEFUL FOR Heart ②③ • Bones ① • Digestion ① • Immunity ① • Fatigue ①③ • Women ①④

1 Preheat your oven to 200°C/fan 180°C/gas 6. Lay out two 20cm-square pieces of baking parchment.

2 Snap off the woody end from each asparagus spear, then thinly peel the remaining stalk. Divide the spears in half and tie each bundle of five together with kitchen string. Place a bundle in the middle of each piece of baking parchment. Sprinkle the asparagus with the lemon zest, oil, garlic, thyme and sea salt, dividing the seasonings equally.

3 Fold the parchment around the asparagus to seal. Place the parcels on a baking sheet and cook in the heated oven for 10 minutes.

4 Meanwhile, bring a large pan of water to the boil. Turn down to a simmer and gently lower the quail's eggs into the water using a large spoon. Simmer for 4 minutes. Remove the eggs and run under cold water to stop them cooking further (the yolks will be soft, but not too runny). Peel the eggs and sprinkle with celery salt.

5 Toss the rocket with a little rapeseed oil and lemon juice, then spread out on two plates. Set the asparagus bundles on top and scatter the eggs (whole or halved) around.

BOILED EGGS & CAPER SALAD

SERVES 2 • 220 CALORIES PER SERVING

Salty, sharp capers with hard-boiled eggs is
a delightful combination that packs a punch.
The salad may seem frugal but it's delicious and
filling. You can gently toss everything together
or very finely chop the ingredients and mix them
thoroughly. Sweet red and yellow peppers are the
richest vegetable source of vitamin C.

4 eggs, at room temperature

1 yellow pepper, seeded and sliced

100g baby spinach leaves

A handful of capers, rinsed

A pinch of flaked sea salt

A pinch of cracked black pepper

Fresh chives, to garnish

Olive oil, for drizzling

1 Bring a medium-sized pan of water to the boil.
  Gently place the eggs in the water and simmer
  for 8–10 minutes. They will be hard-boiled (cook
  for a shorter time if you prefer your eggs to be
  less well cooked). Drain the eggs and run under
  cold water to stop them cooking further.

2 Peel the eggs and cut them lengthways
  into quarters.

3 Combine the yellow pepper, spinach, capers,
  salt and pepper in a bowl and mix together
  gently but thoroughly.

4 Divide among individual serving bowls and place
  the eggs on top. Finish each serving with chives
  and a drizzle of olive oil.

RICH IN Vitamins B6, B12, C and D • Folate •
Potassium • Beta-carotene • Tryptophan

USEFUL FOR Heart ② • Bones ① •
Skin, hair & nails ① • Mind ① •
Fatigue ③ • Men ① • Women ①

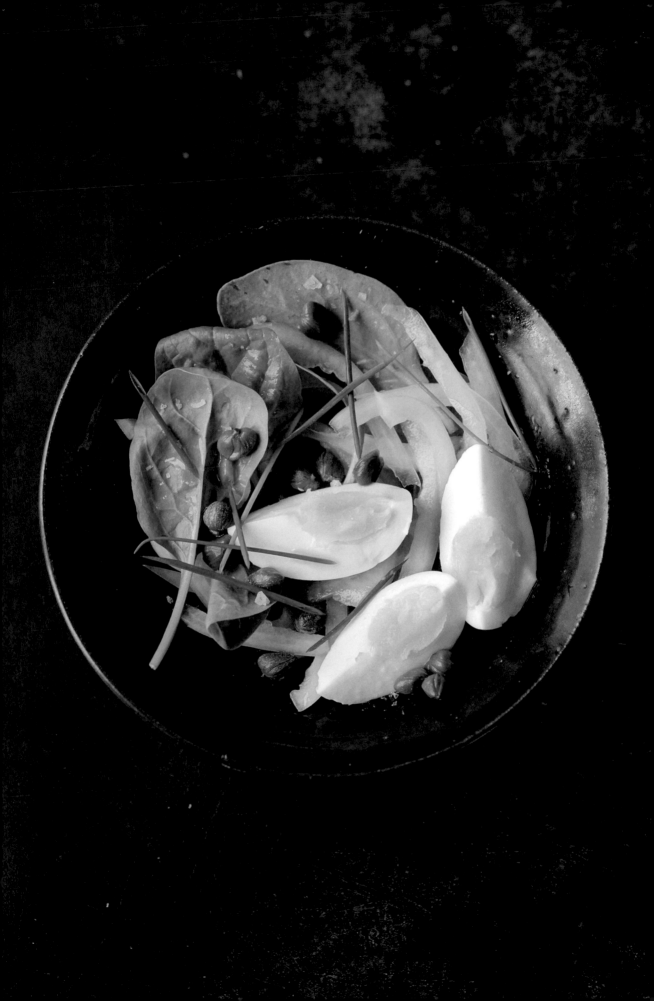

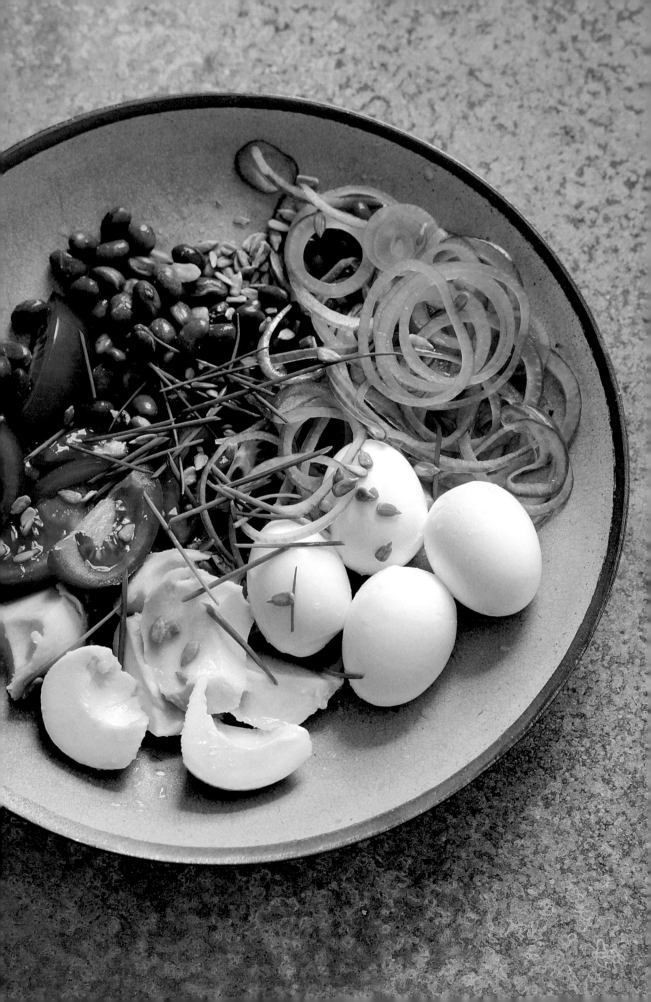

BORLOTTI BEAN, AVOCADO, TOMATO & ONION SALAD WITH HARD-BOILED EGGS

SERVES 2 • 460 CALORIES PER SERVING

The flavours of this colourful salad are bold and robust. The eggs bring a richness, and with the beans make this salad ideal for a quick, satisfying dinner. It's perfect for vegetarians as it contains a full range of amino acids and offers a good source of iron.

4 eggs
1 avocado
½ red onion, sliced
Juice of 1 lemon
400g tin borlotti beans, drained and rinsed
4 ripe plum tomatoes, cut into quarters
1 tsp runny honey
A handful of fresh chives, snipped
1 tbsp sunflower seeds, toasted
Salt and cracked black pepper

1 Bring a medium-sized pan of water to the boil, then gently place the eggs in the pan. Simmer for 8–10 minutes (the eggs will be hard-boiled; cook for a shorter time if you prefer your eggs to be less well cooked). Cool the eggs under cold running water before peeling.
2 Meanwhile, peel the avocado and remove the stone, then cut up the flesh. Put it in a bowl with the onion and cover with the lemon juice. Leave for 5 minutes. (The lemon will prevent the avocado from browning, and will also change the colour of the onion to bright pink.)
3 Add the borlotti beans to the bowl along with the tomatoes, honey, chives and sunflower seeds. Mix well.
4 Cut the eggs into quarters and serve on top of the salad with a sprinkle of salt and cracked black pepper.

RICH IN Vitamins B1 (thiamin), B6, C and E • Folate • Potassium • Iron • Phytoestrogens • Fibre

USEFUL FOR Heart ① ② • Bones ① • Digestion ① • Immunity ① • Mind ① • Fatigue ① • Women ① ③ ④

EGG-FRIED BROWN RICE & PEAS

SERVES 4 • 430 CALORIES PER SERVING

Traditionally made from leftovers, egg-fried rice is a simple dish, but don't be fooled. There is a big difference between a deliciously crunchy, rich golden rice and a pale, mushy mess. The key is to use very cold rice – if it is warm it will lead to a soft texture. A salad of sweet juicy tomatoes complements the rice perfectly.

400g brown rice
150g frozen peas
1 tbsp rapeseed oil
2 large eggs
1 tbsp tamari
2 spring onions, sliced

TO SERVE
2 ripe vine tomatoes, roughly chopped
salt and pepper

1 Put the rice in a pan of cold water and bring to the boil, then cook for 20 minutes until tender. Drain the rice and run under cold water until completely cooled. Tip the rice into a bowl, cover with clingfilm and chill for 20 minutes.
2 Meanwhile, cook the peas in a pan of boiling water according to the instructions on the packet. Drain and set aside.
3 Once the rice is very cold, add the rapeseed oil to a wok set on a high heat. Add the rice and move it around in the wok so that all the grains become coated with oil, then continue to fry for 3 minutes, stirring constantly. You want the rice to become slightly golden.
4 Add the eggs and mix very quickly into the rice. Continue to cook for 2 minutes, then throw in the tamari, spring onions and peas and stir through the rice. Serve immediately, with the seasoned tomatoes.

RICH IN Vitamins B1 (thiamin), B3 (niacin) and B12 • Folate • Magnesium

USEFUL FOR Heart ③ • Mind ① • Fatigue ③ ⑤

EGG WHITE & BROCCOLI OMELETTE

MAKES 2 OMELETTES • 120 CALORIES EACH

Egg white omelettes may sound a bit boring – both to taste and to look at – but try one and you'll change your mind. This wonderfully light, fluffy dish is a lower calorie alternative to the traditional omelette made with whole eggs. Broccoli is used here, but the omelette is also delicious made with roasted or fresh peppers, spinach or tomatoes.

A large handful of very small broccoli florets
½ onion, finely sliced
1 tbsp sunflower seeds
2 tsp rapeseed oil
3 large egg whites
Salt and white pepper
Fresh coriander, to garnish

1 Preheat your oven to 180°C/fan 160°C/gas 4.
2 Spread out the broccoli florets on a baking tray with the onion and sunflower seeds. Drizzle 1 teaspoon of the rapeseed oil over them. Roast for 10 minutes.
3 Meanwhile, put the egg whites in a bowl with a pinch each of salt and pepper and whisk together until frothy.
4 Heat a medium-sized frying pan and add the remaining rapeseed oil. Pour in the egg whites and top with the roasted broccoli, onion and sunflower seeds. Cook on a medium heat for about 3 minutes until the bottom of the omelette is golden and the top is almost set.
5 Fold the omelette over in half and serve, garnished with fresh coriander.

RICH IN Vitamins C and E

USEFUL FOR Immunity ① • Women ③

SHALLOT OMELETTE

MAKES 1 OMELETTE • 330 CALORIES

The inspiration for this recipe has come all the way from the Taj Mahal Palace hotel in Mumbai. Such a simple dish – a plain omelette with sweet shallots and a kick from chilli flakes. It's often the simplest dishes that stay in your memory.

3 eggs
50ml rice milk
A pinch of crushed dried chilli
A pinch of flaked sea salt
A pinch of white pepper
1 tbsp rapeseed oil
2 shallots, finely sliced

1 Mix together the eggs and rice milk in a large bowl using a whisk. Add the chilli flakes, sea salt and pepper and whisk again. Put to one side.
2 Set a non-stick frying pan, about 20cm in diameter, on a high heat. Add a drop of oil and then add the shallots. Cook on a high heat for a few minutes, then turn the heat to low and cook for a further 6 minutes until the shallots are lightly browned. Transfer them to a bowl and set to one side.
3 Add a drop more oil to the pan and turn the heat back up to high, then pour in the egg mixture. Cook on a high heat for a minute, then turn the heat to medium. Add the shallots to the omelette, scattering them over evenly, and cook for a further 2 minutes until the egg mixture begins to set on top.
4 Fold the omelette over in half and press down to firm it up before tipping on to a plate. Serve immediately, sprinkled with a few more chilli flakes if you can take the heat.

RICH IN Vitamins B2 (riboflavin), B12 and D • Folate • Selenium • Iron • Tryptophan

USEFUL FOR Bones ① • Mind ① • Fatigue ①③⑤ • Men ①

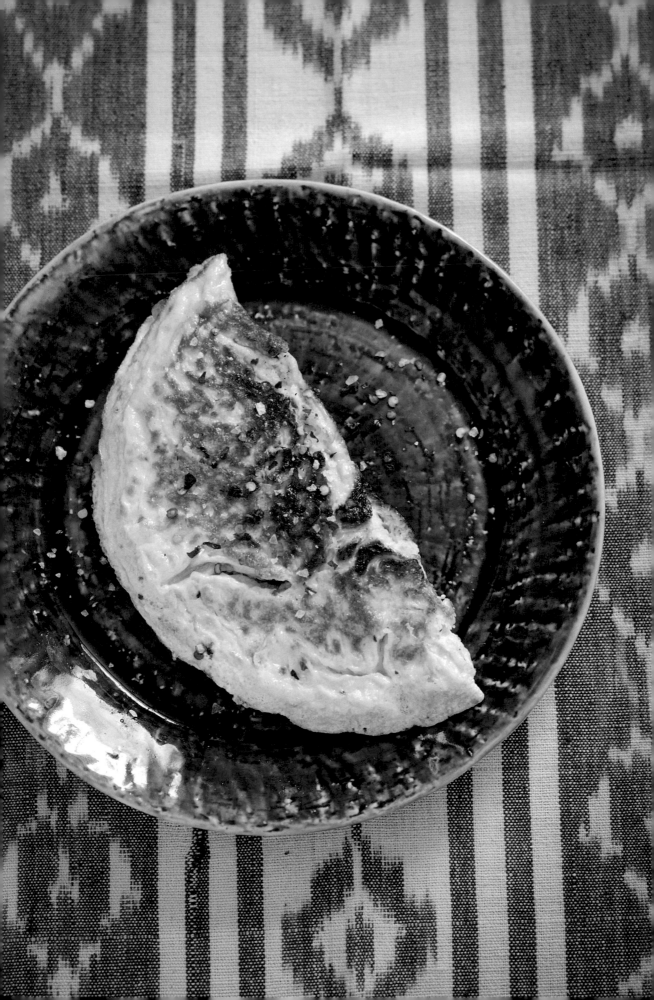

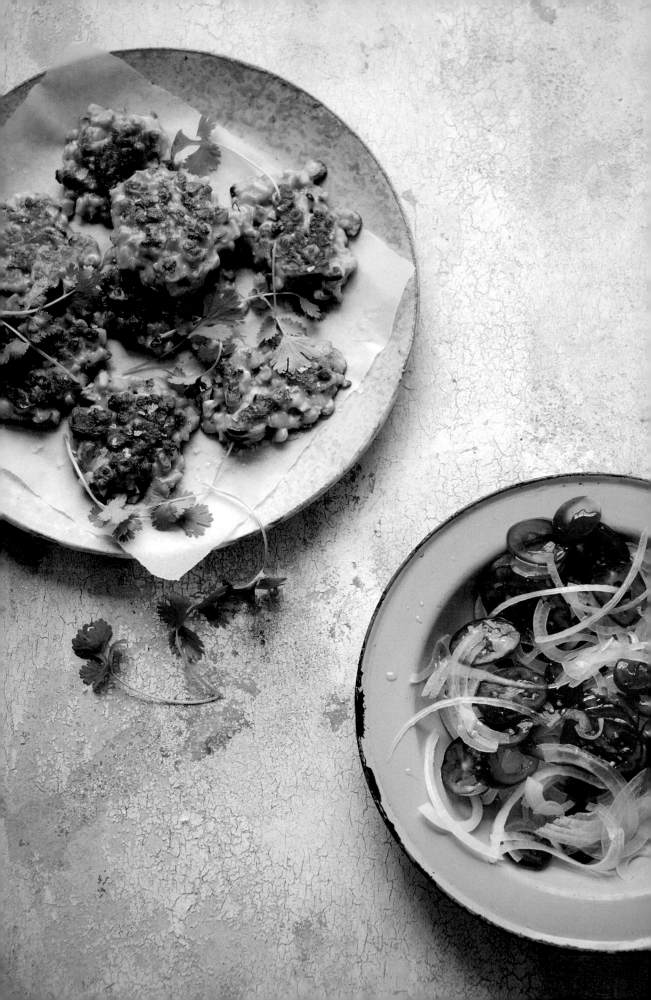

SWEETCORN FRITTERS WITH TOMATO & ONION SALAD

MAKES 8–10 FRITTERS TO SERVE 4 • 165 CALORIES PER SERVING

Once you have made these, you'll want to fritter everything in sight. It's so easy and tastes wonderful. Just make sure you use a non-stick frying pan and only a small drop of oil. This will ensure that your fritters are not soggy. For this recipe you need to use fresh corn on the cob. Tinned sweetcorn tastes very sweet, even if you buy the sugar-free version, and it has a softer texture than fresh kernels. The fritters are great for a starter or a sharing platter.

1 ear of sweetcorn (corn on the cob)

1 egg

50ml rice milk

A pinch of salt

A pinch of paprika

75g gluten- and wheat-free flour

2 spring onions, finely chopped

1 tsp olive oil, for frying

Fresh coriander, to garnish

FOR THE SALAD

3 ripe vine tomatoes, sliced

½ onion, finely sliced

Juice of ½ lemon

1 tsp runny honey

A pinch of salt

1 Preheat the grill to high. Remove the husks and silk from the sweetcorn, if necessary, then grill, turning occasionally, for 12 minutes until golden brown on all sides. Leave to cool.

2 Once cold, cut all the kernels off the cob. The easiest way to do this is to hold the cob at one end, upright at an angle, with the other end in the centre of a kitchen towel on your work surface, and to run a knife down the cob to remove the kernels. Do this all the way round. Discard the cob. Set the sweetcorn kernels aside.

3 Combine the egg, rice milk, salt and paprika in a large bowl and whisk together. Sift the flour into another bowl, then gently stir in the egg mixture to create a thick batter. Add the spring onions and sweetcorn. Leave to stand for about 10 minutes.

4 Meanwhile, combine all the salad ingredients in a bowl and mix together gently. Set aside.

5 Heat a large non-stick frying pan and add a drop of olive oil. Spoon the sweetcorn batter into the pan, using about a tablespoonful for each small

fritter (space them well apart to allow for spreading). Cook for 2–3 minutes on each side until golden. As each fritter is cooked, transfer it to a plate and keep warm, covered with foil. Add more oil to the pan as needed.

6 Serve the fritters warm, garnished with fresh coriander and with the tomato salad on the side.

RICH IN Vitamins B1 (thiamin), B6, B12 and C • Folate • Potassium

USEFUL FOR Heart ② • Immunity ① • Mind ① • Women ①

SWEET POTATO FRITTATA

MAKES 4 LARGE SLICES • 300 CALORIES EACH

This makes a substantial and filling lunch or dinner dish, and is great for a picnic too. We use sweet potato but you can also use butternut squash. The key is to caramelise the sweet potato in the oven, letting all the natural sugars work their magic. You'll need an ovenproof pan.

3 sweet potatoes, peeled and cut into 2.5cm cubes
1 tbsp olive oil, plus extra for drizzling
1 sprig of fresh rosemary
½ red onion, sliced
1 garlic clove, chopped
6 eggs
100ml rice milk
A handful of pumpkin seeds
Salt and pepper

1 Preheat your oven to 200°C/fan 180°C/gas 6. Line a baking tray with greaseproof paper.
2 Spread the sweet potato cubes on the baking tray and drizzle a little olive oil over them. Remove the leaves from the rosemary sprig (leave them whole or finely chop, as you like), then sprinkle over the sweet potatoes. Roast for 20 minutes.
3 Scatter the onion and garlic over the sweet potatoes and roast for a further 10 minutes until the potato cubes are soft and slightly golden.
4 Meanwhile, combine the eggs and rice milk in a bowl with some salt and pepper, and lightly whisk to mix.
5 Set a non-stick, ovenproof 24cm frying pan on high heat and add the tablespoon of olive oil. When hot, add the sweet potato and onion straight from the oven and spread out evenly in the pan. Cover with the egg mixture and turn the heat down to medium. Leave to cook until the egg mixture begins to set – you will see this happening round the edge.
6 Once the top of the frittata is almost set, sprinkle the pumpkin seeds over the surface and transfer the pan to the oven to cook for 10 minutes.
7 Leave the frittata to cool for a few minutes before turning it out on to a chopping board and cutting into slices.

RICH IN Vitamins B2 (riboflavin), B12 and D

USEFUL FOR Bones ① • Mind ① • Fatigue ⑤

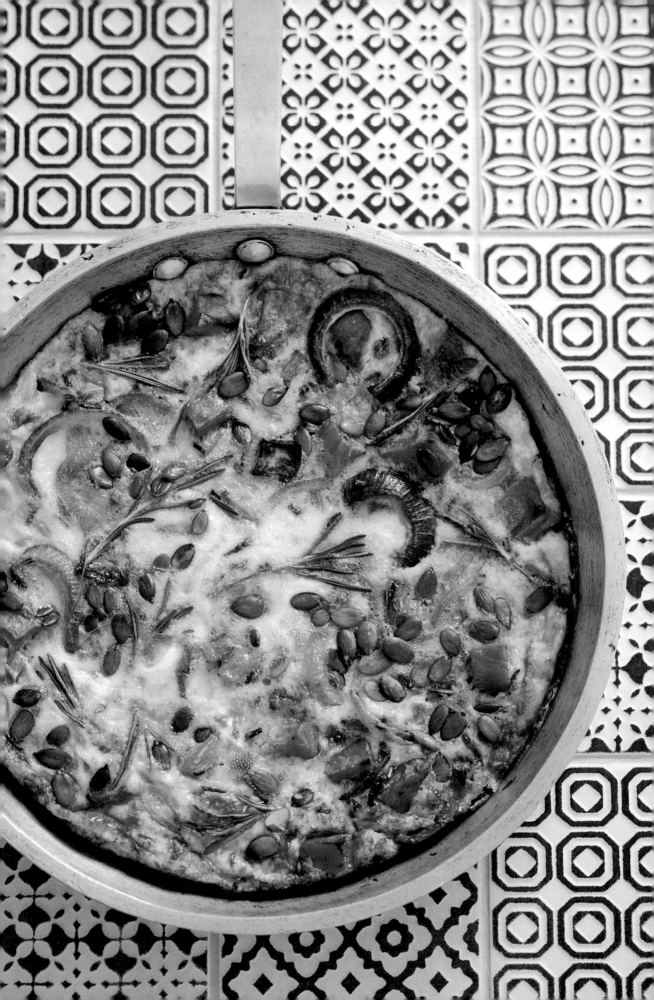

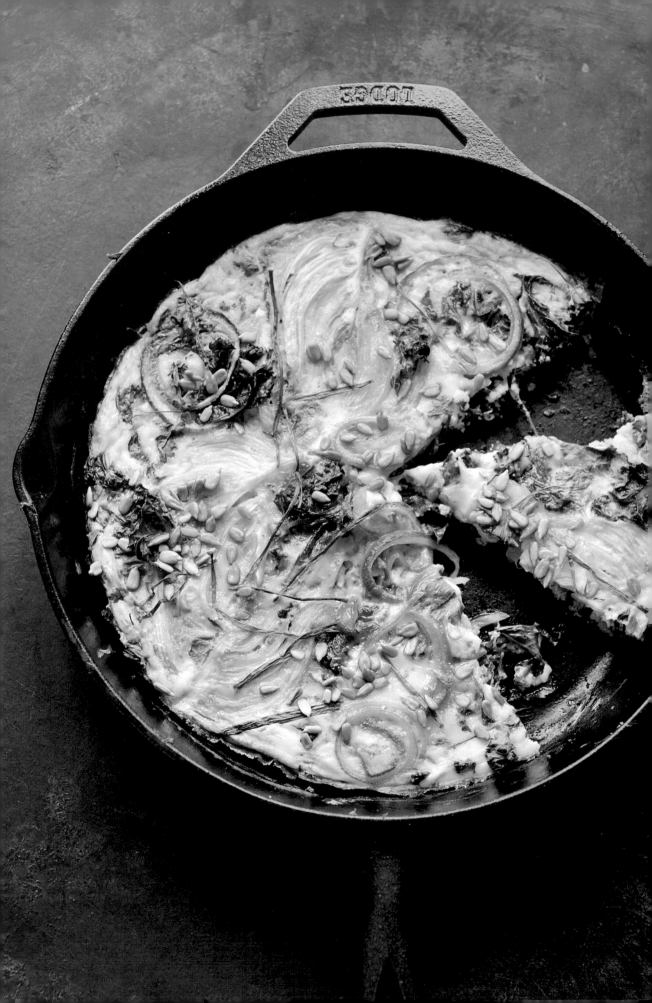

KALE, EDAMAME & FENNEL FRITTATA

SERVES 4 • 254 CALORIES PER SERVING

You can pretty much add any vegetable you like to a frittata and it will taste great. It's the perfect way to use up leftovers to create a really wholesome and filling dinner. Here we've used edamame beans, fennel and kale. Eating dark green vegetables such as kale provides non-meat-eaters a useful way to glean omega 3 from their diet. Kale is also a good source of copper, which helps with the absorption of iron. You need an ovenproof pan to make the frittata successfully.

1 fennel bulb, thinly sliced

2 red onions, thinly sliced

1 garlic clove, thinly sliced

1 tbsp olive oil, plus extra for drizzling

6 eggs

100ml rice milk

A handful of fresh chives, finely chopped

1 tbsp finely chopped fresh coriander

100g kale, shredded

A handful of edamame beans, thawed if frozen

A handful of sunflower seeds

Salt and pepper

RICH IN Vitamins B2 (riboflavin), B12 and D • Folate • Iron • Tryptophan

USEFUL FOR Bones ① • Mind ① • Fatigue ①③⑤ • Women ④

1 Preheat your oven to 200°C/fan 180°C/gas 6. Line a baking tray with greaseproof paper.

2 Spread out the fennel, onions and garlic on the baking tray. Drizzle some olive oil over the vegetables. Roast for 12 minutes.

3 Put the eggs and rice milk in a bowl with the chopped chives and coriander, season and lightly whisk to mix.

4 Set a non-stick, ovenproof frying pan, about 24cm diameter, on a high heat and add the tablespoon of olive oil. When the oil is hot, add the roasted vegetables, straight from the oven. Add the kale and edamame beans and sauté for a few minutes until the kale is slightly wilted.

5 Spread out the vegetables in the pan, then pour in the egg mixture. Turn the heat down to medium. Leave until the egg begins to cook (you will see this around the side of the pan). Once the top is almost set, sprinkle the sunflower seeds over the surface and transfer the pan to the oven to cook for 10 minutes.

6 Leave the frittata to cool for a few minutes before turning out on to a chopping board. Cut into slices and serve hot, or leave to cool – the frittata is delicious cold and will keep for a day in the fridge.

MEAT

Whether you choose to eat meat or not is a matter of personal preference, but in general, those who do eat meat tend to eat too much. Meat certainly doesn't need to be served up at every meal.

It is true that meat is highly nutritious. It provides a valuable source of protein and other key nutrients such as vitamin B12 and iron (these can help to protect against health conditions such as mild iron deficiency or anaemia, which can leave you feeling tired and fatigued). But adequate amounts of these key nutrients can be gained from eating just a small amount of meat in the diet, leaving room for other highly nutritious plant-based foods.

Whilst there is nothing wrong with eating small quantities of red meat, over-consumption has been linked to increased risk of certain diseases. At the Detox Kitchen we completely avoid red meat as well as processed meats, instead opting for lean white meats (chicken and turkey) and fish.

Most of our recipes use chicken or turkey breast. There are good reasons why breast is such a popular cut: not only is it robust enough to take on big, bold flavours, but it offers great versatility in cooking – from grilling and roasting, to pan-frying or stewing. Also, I find that breast goes really well with fruit, the combination offering a lovely balance of savoury and sweet. For me, nothing beats a chicken salad with quinoa and sweet peaches, nor a grilled chicken breast covered in a delicious cashew and basil pesto, a Thai-spiced chicken and noodle broth, or a comforting chicken and vegetable pie.

At the end of most of the recipes, you'll find a list of the main nutrients supplied in a serving as well as a list of health issues that may be benefited by including the recipe in your healthy diet. For more, see page 9.

TANDOORI CHICKEN WITH PINEAPPLE SALAD

SERVES 4 • 280 CALORIES PER SERVING

A good tandoori chicken should taste spicy and smoky. The smokiness comes from cooking in a tandoor – the smoked paprika in the recipe will give a similar flavour. Don't be shy with the chillies and spices, because the pineapple salad is very soothing and the sweetness will immediately reduce the heat in your mouth. The enzyme bromelain, found in the stem of pineapple, aids in the digestion of proteins.

2 thumb-sized pieces of fresh ginger, peeled and grated
4 garlic cloves, very finely chopped
2 fresh red chillies, seeded and finely chopped
Juice of 1 lemon
600g skinless, boneless chicken breasts, cut into bite-sized chunks
2 tbsp plain soya yogurt
1 tbsp smoked paprika
1 tsp ground turmeric
2 tbsp garam masala
1 tbsp olive oil
Lemon wedges, to serve

FOR THE SALAD
½ fresh pineapple, peeled, cored and diced
1 red pepper, seeded and finely diced
1 yellow pepper, seeded and finely diced
2 spring onions, finely diced
A handful of fresh coriander, finely chopped
Salt and pepper

RICH IN Vitamins B3 (niacin) and C • Potassium • Tryptophan • Beta-carotene • Bromelain

USEFUL FOR Heart ③ • Digestion ④ • Immunity ① • Skin, hair & nails ① • Mind ① • Fatigue ③

1 Combine the ginger, garlic, chillies and lemon juice in a large mixing bowl and mix well. Add the chicken and mix into the marinade so that all the pieces are coated. Cover and leave to marinate in the fridge for 20 minutes.

2 Add the yogurt, smoked paprika, turmeric, garam masala and olive oil and mix well. Cover again, return to the fridge and leave for 1 hour.

3 While the chicken is in the fridge, soak eight wooden skewers in water for an hour.

4 Preheat your grill to medium. Thread the chicken pieces on to the wooden skewers. Grill for about 20 minutes, turning occasionally.

5 Meanwhile, mix together the diced pineapple, peppers, spring onions and coriander in a bowl. Season to taste.

6 Serve two chicken skewers each, with a big helping of the salad and a wedge of lemon.

CAJUN CHICKEN WITH AVOCADO SALAD & MANGO SALSA

SERVES 4 • 415 CALORIES PER SERVING

This dish is all about the marinade. Rich spices and a punch of garlic create a smoky, aromatic flavour. By gently bashing out the breasts, the marinade can cover a greater area of the flesh. The chicken is perfectly balanced by the light, creamy avocado salad and sweet-spicy salsa made with mango. This fruit is a source of the antioxidant beta-carotene, which among its many other benefits may help delay the onset of cognitive decline in older people.

1 tbsp smoked paprika

2 tbsp ground cumin

1 tbsp ground coriander

1 tsp crushed dried chilli

1 garlic clove, crushed

1 tsp olive oil

4 skinless, boneless chicken breasts, about 150g each

FOR THE SALAD

150g spinach

A handful of fresh coriander

A handful of fresh mint

A handful of fresh flat-leaf parsley

¼ red onion, roughly diced

1 tsp rapeseed oil

2 avocados

FOR THE MANGO SALSA

1 mango, diced

4 cherry tomatoes, diced

A handful of fresh coriander, finely chopped

Juice of 1 lime

1 fresh red chilli, seeded and finely chopped

Salt and pepper

1 Mix together all the spices, garlic and oil with a pinch of salt in a large bowl. Add the chicken breasts and turn them so they are covered with the marinade.

2 Set a ridged griddle/grill pan on a medium heat and leave to heat up.

3 Meanwhile, one at a time, place the breasts on one half of a large sheet of clingfilm, fold the clingfilm over so that the spices are sealed in and gently bash the breasts with a rolling pin to flatten them to about 1cm thick; remove the clingfilm. Place the breasts on the griddle pan and cook for 6 minutes on each side.

4 Make the salad whilst the chicken is cooking. Finely chop the spinach, coriander, mint, parsley and red onion and mix together with the oil in a large bowl. Peel the avocados and remove the stone, then dice the flesh. Add to the bowl and fold in gently. Season with salt and pepper.

5 For the salsa, combine all the ingredients in another bowl. Use your hands to mix, squeezing the tomatoes to create a chunky, juicy salsa. Season to taste.

6 Serve each chicken breast with a big helping of the spinach salad and the mango salsa.

RICH IN Vitamins B2 (riboflavin), B3 (niacin), B6, C and E • Folate • Potassium • Beta-carotene • Tryptophan • Beta-sitosterol • Fibre

USEFUL FOR Heart ①②③ • Digestion ① • Immunity ① • Skin, hair & nails ① • Mind ① • Fatigue ③⑤ • Men ① • Women ①③

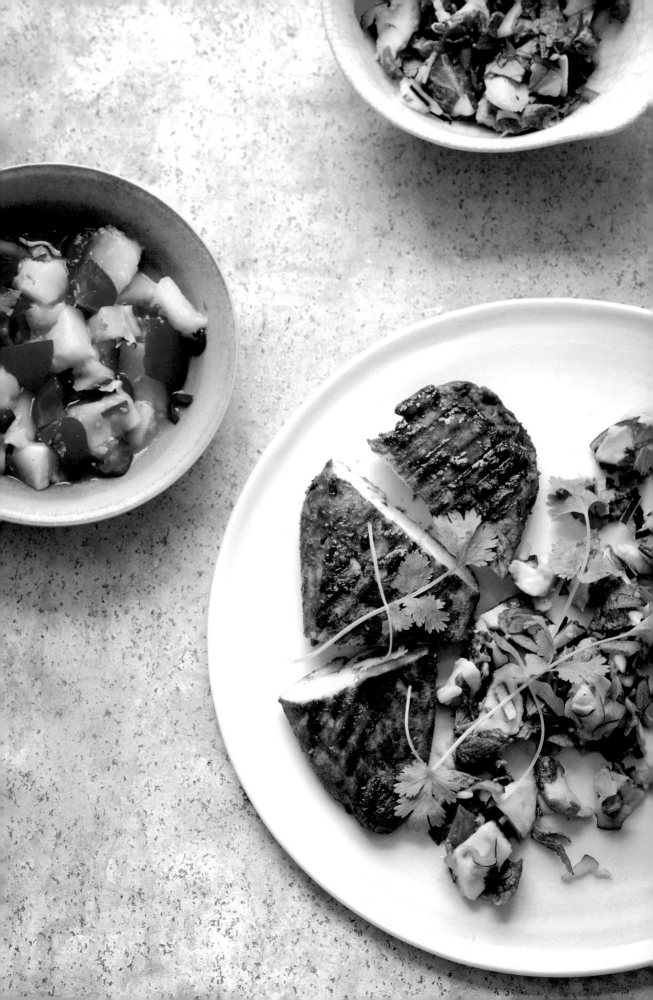

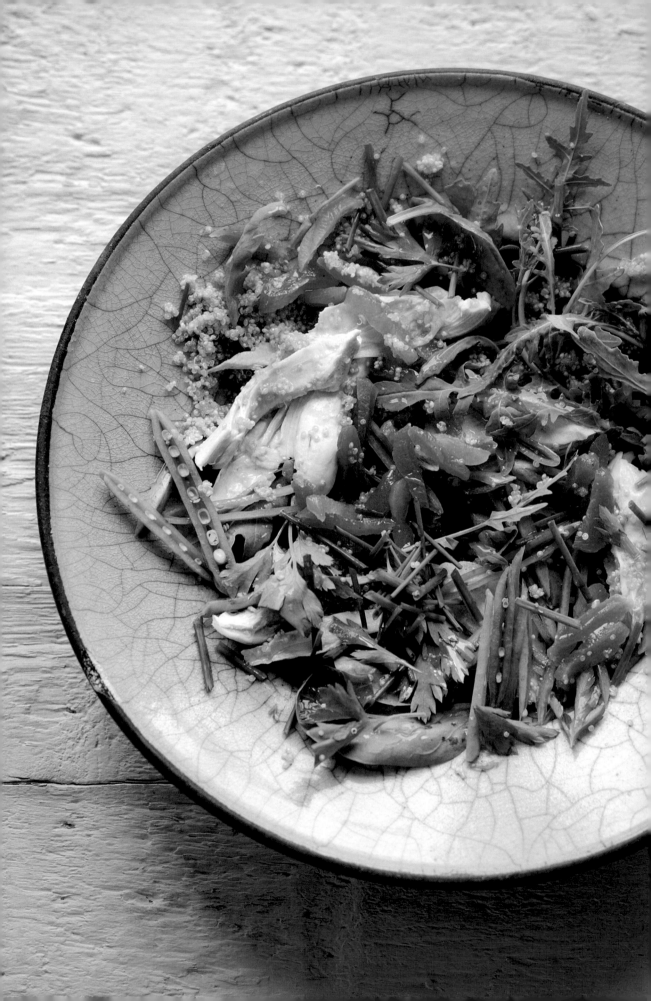

CHICKEN & QUINOA SALAD

SERVES 2 • 420 CALORIES PER SERVING

Two of our favourite ingredients sit happily together in this nutrient-dense salad. It is really delicious and filling. The very high protein content combined with complex carbohydrate in the quinoa make it the perfect lunch dish to help avoid mid-afternoon energy slumps.

2 skinless, boneless chicken breasts, about 150g each

2 sprigs of fresh thyme

2 lemon slices

2 garlic cloves, gently crushed with the skin on

100g quinoa

100g mange tout

150g rocket

100g baby spinach leaves

A handful of fresh chives, roughly chopped

A handful of fresh flat-leaf parsley

4 dried apricots, roughly cut into strips

Juice of 1 lemon

1 tbsp rapeseed oil

1 tsp flaked sea salt

A pinch of cracked black pepper

Salt

1 Preheat your oven to 200°C/fan 180°C/gas 6.

2 Place the chicken breasts on a baking tray and set a sprig of thyme, slice of lemon and garlic clove on each breast. Roast in the heated oven for about 20 minutes until thoroughly cooked. Allow to cool.

3 Put the quinoa in a medium-sized pan and cover with three times its volume of cold water. Set on a high heat and bring to the boil. Once boiling, season the water with salt and continue to boil for 6–8 minutes until just tender. Drain in a sieve and rinse under cold water until cool. Leave to one side to drain completely.

4 Bring a small pan of water to the boil. Drop in the mange tout and cook for no longer than 2 minutes; drain and rinse under cold water until cool.

5 Mix together the remaining ingredients in a bowl, then fold in the quinoa and mange tout.

6 Cut the chicken into strips and mix through the salad. Serve in a large sharing bowl.

RICH IN Vitamins B2 (riboflavin), B6, C and E • Folate • Potassium • Magnesium • Iron • Calcium • Selenium • Beta-carotene • Tryptophan • Fibre

USEFUL FOR Heart ①②③ • Bones ① • Digestion ① • Immunity ① • Skin, hair & nails ① • Mind ①② • Fatigue ①③⑤ • Men ① • Women ①③

PESTO CHICKEN WITH QUINOA & PEACH SALAD

SERVES 4 • 600 CALORIES PER SERVING

This pesto chicken is my foolproof dish when I have friends over. It pleases everyone – the basil gives the pesto a classic taste; the combination of nuts and seeds adds a rich depth of flavour; and the spinach enhances the vibrant green colour. When peaches are deliciously ripe and sweet in summer, they make a wonderful addition to the dish, perfectly complementing the bold flavours and adding a lovely texture.

4 skinless, boneless chicken breasts, about 150g each

1 tsp olive oil

300g quinoa

4 celery sticks, finely diced

Juice of 1 lemon

1 tsp rapeseed oil

2 ripe flat peaches

FOR THE PESTO

70g cashew nuts

50g sunflower seeds

2 handfuls of spinach

5 sprigs of fresh basil, leaves picked

1 tbsp rapeseed oil

Flaked sea salt and cracked black pepper

RICH IN B vitamins • Potassium • Magnesium • Zinc • Selenium • Iron

USEFUL FOR Heart ② • Immunity ① • Skin, hair & nails ① • Mind ①② • Fatigue ①⑤ • Men ①② • Women ①③

1 Preheat your oven to 200°C/fan 180°C/gas 6.

2 Place the chicken breasts on a baking tray. Drizzle the olive oil over them and season with a pinch each of sea salt and pepper. Roast in the heated oven for 20 minutes until cooked through.

3 Meanwhile, put the quinoa in a saucepan and cover with three times its volume of cold water. Bring to the boil, then reduce the heat and simmer for 6–8 minutes until just tender. Drain in a sieve and rinse, then tip into a mixing bowl. Add the celery, lemon juice, rapeseed oil and 1 teaspoon each of sea salt and pepper. Mix well, then set aside.

4 To make the pesto, place all the ingredients in a food processor and add 1 teaspoon sea salt and a pinch of pepper. Blitz to a rough paste.

5 To prepare the peaches, cut each in half around the stone, then pull the two halves apart. Slice each half into small bite-sized wedges. Sprinkle with salt and pepper.

6 Once the chicken is cooked, remove from the oven and cut into strips. Serve with the quinoa salad, peaches and pesto.

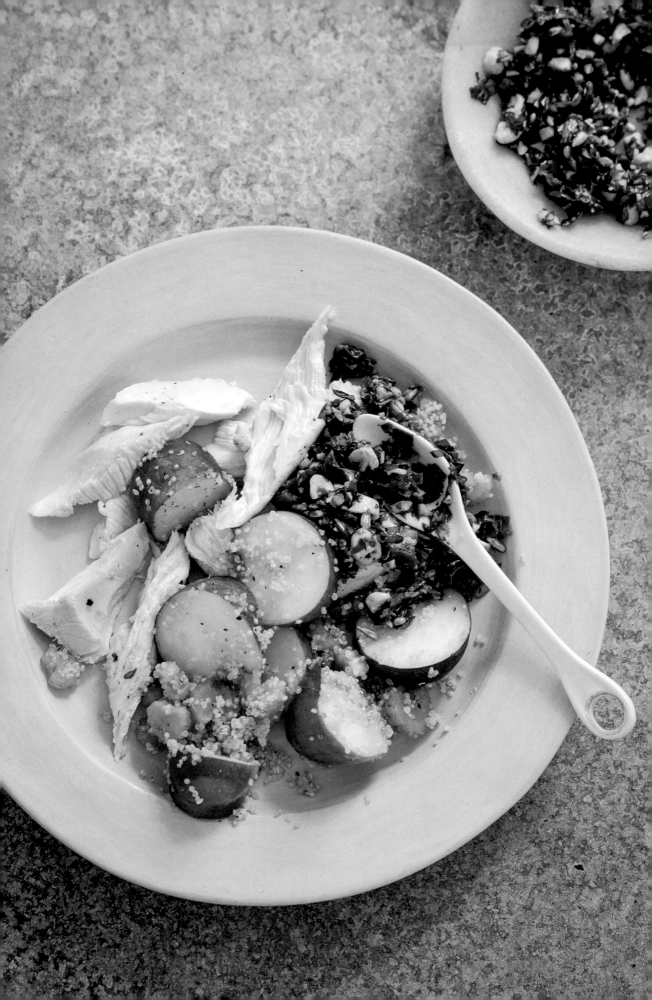

CABBAGE STUFFED WITH CHICKEN

MAKES 8 ROLLS TO SERVE 2 • 277 CALORIES PER SERVING

These cabbage rolls can be served as a starter for eight, but they are so delicious you'll want four each for a main dish. They can be made ahead, meaning all you have to do is pop them in the steamer. Overcooking vegetables can lead to a loss of vitamin C as it leaches into the cooking water. The cabbage leaves here are blanched for a very short time, just to make them pliable enough to roll up, so they retain their goodness. If you cannot buy minced chicken breast, ask your butcher to mince some for you.

1 Savoy cabbage
150g brown rice
1 tsp olive oil
1 onion, diced
1 garlic clove, chopped
1 sprig of fresh thyme
A handful of fresh marjoram, finely chopped
1 tsp ground cumin
1 tsp paprika
400g minced chicken breast
1 tsp salt
1 tsp pepper

1 Pull off the eight biggest outer leaves from the cabbage. Place them in a pan of boiling water and blanch for 3 minutes. Lift out and plunge into ice-cold water, then drain and set aside.
2 Put the brown rice in a saucepan and cover with twice its volume of water. Bring to the boil, then simmer for 20 minutes. Drain and set aside.
3 Set a non-stick frying pan on a medium heat. Add the olive oil and then the onion and garlic. Cook for 10 minutes until the onion is lightly browned. Add the thyme, marjoram, cumin, paprika and minced chicken and cook, stirring, for 5 minutes until the chicken has lost its raw look and is broken up. Remove from the heat and mix with the rice. Season with the salt and pepper.
4 To make each roll, put a small handful of the chicken and rice mixture in the middle of a cabbage leaf. Fold up the bottom end to cover the chicken, then tuck in the sides and roll over to seal. Place the rolls on a large plate with the cabbage flap underneath to ensure they stay compact. Chill for 30 minutes to firm up.
5 Bring water to the boil in the bottom of a steamer or saucepan. Set your steamer on top. Place the cabbage parcels in the steamer and steam for 10 minutes. Serve hot.

RICH IN Vitamins B1 (thiamin), B3 (niacin), B6 and C • Folate • Potassium • Selenium • Tryptophan

USEFUL FOR Heart ③ • Immunity ① • Mind ① • Fatigue ③ • Men ① • Women ①

PAD THAI WITH BROWN RICE NOODLES

SERVES 2 • 690 CALORIES PER SERVING

One of our all-time favourite dishes, this Thai staple has the perfect balance of sweet and spicy. We have used a tamarind paste to add acidity but do check that you buy a sugar-free version. Alternatively, lime juice will do the trick. The dish is bursting with B vitamins, including B12, low levels of which have been associated with depression.

RICH IN B vitamins • Vitamin C • Selenium • Magnesium • Potassium • Zinc • Iron • Tryptophan

USEFUL FOR Heart ③ • Bones ① • Immunity ① • Skin, hair & nails ①④ • Mind ①② • Fatigue ①③⑤ • Men ①② • Women ①③

120g brown rice noodles
4 tsp fish sauce
½ tsp tamarind paste mixed with 50ml water
30g runny honey
½ tsp crushed dried chillies, plus extra to serve
40ml (2 tbsp plus 2 tsp) groundnut oil
1 skinless, boneless chicken breast, about 150g, finely sliced
8 raw king prawns, peeled
2 spring onions, sliced
2 garlic cloves, finely chopped
2 large eggs
1 tbsp small dried shrimps
100g ready-to-eat beansprouts
A large handful of fresh coriander
50g roasted cashew nuts, roughly chopped
Lime wedges, to serve

1 Bring a pan of water to the boil. Add the noodles and leave for no more than 1 minute before draining in a colander. Cool under cold running water, then set aside.

2 To make the sauce, combine the fish sauce, tamarind, honey and chilli flakes in a small pan and heat gently for 3 minutes. Set aside.

3 Set a large wok on a high heat and add 2 tablespoons of the oil. Add the chicken and fry, stirring, for 5–7 minutes until it no longer looks raw. Add the prawns and stir-fry for a further 3 minutes. Add the spring onions and garlic and stir-fry for 3–4 minutes.

4 Add the noodles and stir-fry for 30 seconds, then add the sauce and mix into the noodles.

5 Push all the ingredients to the side of the wok and add the remaining 2 teaspoons oil. Crack the eggs into the wok and break the yolks. Cook, stirring, until the eggs begin to scramble, then mix with the other ingredients in the wok, plus the dried shrimps, beansprouts and coriander.

6 Serve the Pad Thai hot, with the cashew nuts, extra chilli flakes and lime wedges on the side.

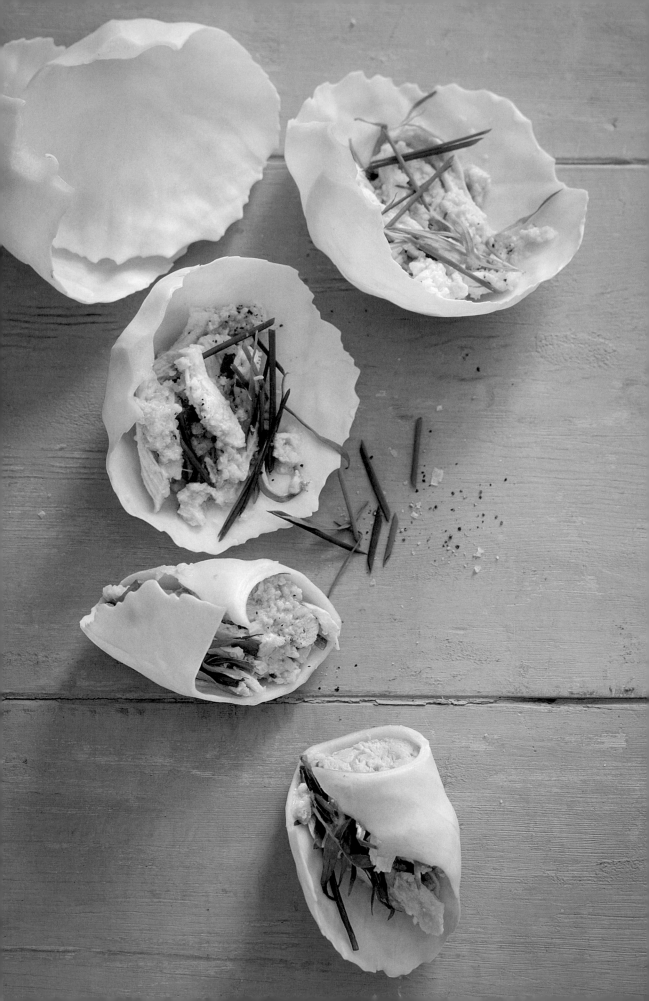

CHICKEN, CASHEW & TARRAGON WRAPS

SERVES 2 • 380 CALORIES PER SERVING

This is our version of chicken mayo, with cashew cream in place of mayonnaise. It's just as creamy and satisfying, and the cashew cream gives the wraps a much healthier fat profile. The chicken filling is wrapped in crunchy cabbage leaves, which are a great gluten-free alternative to traditional wraps.

30g cashew nuts
1 skinless, boneless chicken breast, about 150g
1 tsp olive oil, plus extra for drizzling
Grated zest of ½ lemon
1 tsp finely chopped fresh chives, plus extra to serve
1 tsp finely chopped fresh tarragon
4 white cabbage leaves
2 handfuls of rocket
Salt and pepper
Lemon wedges, to serve

1 Preheat your oven to 200°C/fan 180°C/gas 6. Put the cashew nuts to soak in water for about 20 minutes.
2 Meanwhile, place the chicken breast on a small baking tray and drizzle a little olive oil over it. Season with salt and pepper. Roast in the heated oven for 20 minutes until thoroughly cooked (slice the chicken through the centre to check). Leave to cool.
3 Drain the cashew nuts and put them in a mortar. Add the teaspoon of olive oil, the lemon zest and 1 tablespoon water and lightly bash with the pestle until smooth. Alternatively, for a very smooth cashew cream, use a mini blender/food processor.
4 Once the chicken is cool, cut it into small pieces and place in a bowl with the chives, tarragon and cashew cream. Mix thoroughly.
5 Wrap the chicken in the cabbage leaves with some rocket and chives. Add a squeeze of lemon juice too.

RICH IN Vitamins B1 (thiamin), B3 (niacin) and B6 • Selenium • Tryptophan

USEFUL FOR Heart ③ • Mind ① • Fatigue ③⑤ • Men ① • Women ①

MINCED CHICKEN IN LETTUCE WRAPS

SERVES 2 • 285 CALORIES PER SERVING

Based on a traditional Chinese dish, this recipe uses a staple Chinese vegetable: the water chestnut. It has a unique crisp texture that is hard to find in any other vegetable. Fresh water chestnuts are best as they are very crunchy, but they are rather difficult to get hold of, so we've used tinned, which are sold in most supermarkets. A serving of this dish provides 35 per cent of the RDA for selenium, a nutrient that offers protection against infection. Many people in the UK don't get adequate selenium in their diet.

300g skinless, boneless chicken breasts, minced or very finely diced
140g tin water chestnuts, drained and finely diced
2 tbsp tamari
1 spring onion, finely diced
1 garlic clove, finely diced
A handful of fresh chives, finely chopped
1 iceberg lettuce
2 tbsp puffed brown rice

1 Put the chicken in a bowl with the water chestnuts, tamari, spring onion, garlic and chives. Mix together, then leave to marinate for a few minutes.
2 Set a non-stick frying pan on medium heat and add the chicken mixture. Cook, stirring, for about 12 minutes until the chicken is cooked through. Remove from the heat.
3 Carefully take off four to six outer lettuce leaves, keeping them whole – these will be used for serving. Remove the core from the lettuce, then very finely shred it. Add to the chicken mixture along with the puffed brown rice. Stir thoroughly. The heat from the cooked chicken will make the lettuce wilt slightly.
4 Put a spoonful of the chicken mixture in each lettuce leaf, then fold in the bottom and sides and roll up.

RICH IN Vitamins B1 (thiamin), B3 (niacin) and B6 • Folate • Potassium • Selenium • Tryptophan

USEFUL FOR Heart ②③ • Mind ① • Fatigue ③ • Men ① • Women ①

TURKEY & CASHEW CURRY

SERVES 4 • 450 CALORIES PER SERVING

Cashew nuts are a great addition to any dish, offering a creamy texture and rich nutty flavour. Here they're used to create a curry paste. This acts as a binder in the dish and marries all of the ingredients together whilst also making a roux-like base to thicken the curry during the cooking process. This dish contains all of your daily requirement for vitamin B6, which you need to convert food into energy in the body.

RICH IN B vitamins • Vitamin C • Potassium • Zinc • Iron • Magnesium • Selenium • Curcuminoids • Tryptophan • Fibre

USEFUL FOR Heart ② ③ • Bones ① ② • Digestion ① • Immunity ① • Mind ① ② • Fatigue ① ③ ⑤ • Men ① ② • Women ①

100g cashew nuts
2 ripe vine tomatoes, roughly chopped
½ fresh green chilli, seeded and finely diced
2 garlic cloves, chopped
A thumb-sized piece of fresh ginger, peeled and roughly chopped
Juice of 1 lemon
400g skinless, boneless turkey breast, diced
2 tbsp ground almonds
1 tbsp ground cumin
1 tbsp ground coriander
1 tbsp ground turmeric
1 tbsp coconut oil
1 onion, diced
1 cauliflower, separated into florets
100ml coconut milk
100g podded fresh or thawed frozen peas

1 Soak the cashew nuts in warm water for about 20 minutes, then drain. Put them in a blender with the tomatoes, chilli, garlic, ginger and lemon juice and blitz to a paste. Transfer this to a large mixing bowl.

2 Add the turkey to the bowl and mix with the paste. Sprinkle the ground almonds, cumin, coriander and turmeric over the turkey and mix well. Cover and leave to marinate in the fridge for 20 minutes.

3 Meanwhile, set a large saucepan on a high heat and add the oil, then add the onion and cook for 5 minutes. Add the marinated turkey and cook for 5–7 minutes until it has lost its raw look.

4 Add the cauliflower, coconut milk and 100ml water and bring to a simmer. Keep the heat low and cook for 15 minutes, stirring occasionally. Add the peas, stir and simmer for a further 5 minutes.

5 Serve with a cucumber salad or brown rice.

SWEET POTATO & TURKEY MASSAMAN CURRY

SERVES 4 • 600 CALORIES PER SERVING (WITH RICE)

This is our take on a Thai Massaman curry, a deliciously fragrant dish traditionally made with beef and peanuts. We have swapped these with turkey and cashew nuts, which works really well. Cashew nuts are rich in magnesium, a deficiency of which may contribute to the onset of migraines. Don't be put off by the long list of ingredients – the curry is not difficult to make. It is served with an okra and ginger rice.

2 large onions, finely diced
1½ tbsp rapeseed oil
250g skinless, boneless turkey breast, diced
2 heaped tbsp grated fresh ginger
2 garlic cloves, finely chopped
1 tsp ground coriander
1 tsp ground cumin
A pinch of ground cinnamon
A pinch of ground cloves
1 fresh red chilli, seeded and chopped
1 stick of lemongrass, finely chopped
1 tsp fish sauce
400ml coconut milk
50g cashew nuts
4 cardamom pods
1 star anise
2 medium-sized sweet potatoes
Lime wedges, to serve

FOR THE RICE
200g brown rice
1 tsp coconut oil
150g okra
1 tbsp grated fresh ginger
A handful of fresh coriander, finely chopped
Salt and pepper

1 Set a large saucepan on a medium heat and fry the onions in a little of the rapeseed oil for about 10 minutes until lightly browned. Add the turkey breast and cook, stirring, until it has lost its raw look.

2 Put the ginger, garlic, ground spices, chilli, lemongrass and fish sauce in a small blender and blitz to a paste. Stir in the remaining 1 tablespoon of rapeseed oil to loosen.

3 Add the paste to the turkey and cook, stirring, on a low heat for 2 minutes, making sure that the spices don't burn.

4 Pour in the coconut milk and 100ml water and add the cashew nuts, cardamom pods and star anise. Bring to the boil, stirring occasionally, then simmer for 20 minutes.

5 Meanwhile, peel and dice the sweet potatoes. Stir into the curry and simmer for another 20 minutes until soft.

6 While the curry is simmering, prepare the rice. Put the brown rice in a large saucepan and cover with three times its volume of cold water. Set the pan on a high heat and bring to the boil, then cook for 20 minutes until the rice is tender.

7 Meanwhile, heat the coconut oil in a frying pan and lightly sauté the okra with the ginger for 6 minutes. Once the rice is cooked, drain it well and mix with the okra. Season with salt and pepper, and add the coriander.

8 Serve the curry with the okra rice and wedges of lime for squeezing over.

RICH IN Vitamins B1 (thiamin), B3 (niacin) and C • Folate • Potassium • Magnesium • Tryptophan • Beta-carotene • Fibre

USEFUL FOR Bones ① • Digestion ① • Immunity ① • Skin, hair & nails ① • Mind ①② • Fatigue ③⑤ • Women ①

TURKEY BURGERS
WITH CABBAGE SLAW

**MAKES 4 BURGERS TO SERVE 2 • 350 CALORIES
PER SERVING**

This will change the way you look at the classic Christmas bird, which has long been criticised for being dry and tasteless. Different methods of roasting have changed things, of course, and now turkey is readily available in supermarkets all year round. It's well worth eating more turkey because it contains the amino acid tryptophan, which is converted to serotonin – the 'feel-good' hormone – in the brain. So move away from the comfort of chicken and try these deliciously herby burgers.

300g skinless, boneless turkey breast
1 egg
1 tsp dried thyme
A pinch of dried tarragon
A handful of fresh flat-leaf parsley, finely chopped
A handful of fresh chives, finely chopped
Grated zest of 1 lemon
100g sweetcorn kernels (fresh or thawed frozen)
1 tbsp gluten- and wheat-free flour

FOR THE CABBAGE SLAW
½ small red cabbage, finely sliced
¼ small white cabbage, finely sliced
½ red onion, finely sliced
1 garlic clove, finely chopped
Juice of 1 lemon
A handful of fresh coriander, finely chopped, plus extra to garnish
A handful of fresh chives, finely chopped
A handful of fresh flat-leaf parsley, finely chopped
2 tbsp plain soya yogurt

1 Preheat your grill to medium.
2 Finely dice half of the turkey breast and place it in a large mixing bowl. Put the rest of the turkey breast in a food processor and pulse to create a minced consistency (not a paste). Add to the mixing bowl.
3 Add the egg, thyme, tarragon, parsley, chives, lemon zest, sweetcorn and flour. Mix together thoroughly with your hands. Shape into four medium-sized burgers.
4 Place the burgers on a baking tray, slide under the grill and cook for 8 minutes on each side until golden brown.

5 While the burgers are cooking, combine all the slaw ingredients in a bowl and mix together.
6 Serve two burgers each with a big bowl of slaw.

RICH IN B vitamins • Vitamin C • Folate • Potassium • Iron • Selenium • Tryptophan • Fibre

USEFUL FOR Heart ①②③ • Digestion ① • Immunity ① • Mind ① • Fatigue ①③ • Men ① • Women ①

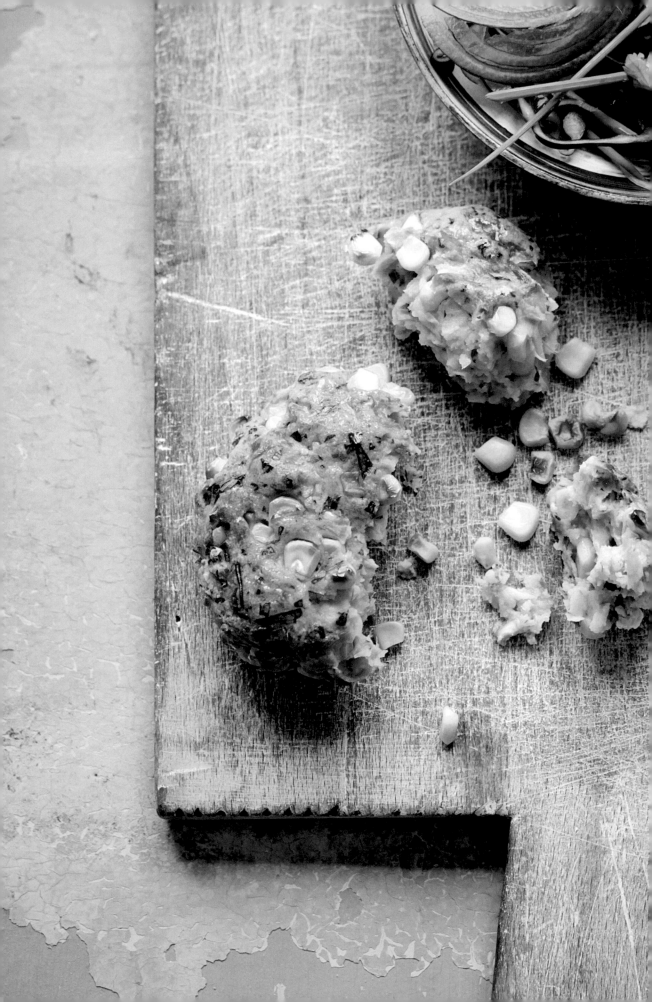

CHICKEN BURGERS WITH BEETROOT RELISH

SERVES 4 • 165 CALORIES PER SERVING

A chicken burger has featured on our menus since the very beginning. Made with good-quality meat and served with a punchy relish, it has always been popular. The minced chicken in most supermarkets tends to be made up from all parts of the bird, so if you want to stick to lean meat, ask a butcher to mince just the breast for you.

300g minced chicken breast
1 egg
1 tbsp rapeseed oil
A handful of fresh coriander, finely chopped
1 tsp dried thyme
A handful of fresh chives, finely chopped
Grated zest of 1 lemon
1 tsp salt
1 tsp cracked black pepper

FOR THE BEETROOT RELISH
4 large raw beetroots, peeled and cut into 2.5cm cubes
1 tbsp rapeseed oil
1 tsp capers
3 ripe vine tomatoes, diced
1 fresh green chilli, seeded and finely diced
½ red onion, finely diced
1 garlic clove, finely chopped

RICH IN Vitamins B3 (niacin) and C • Folate • Potassium

USEFUL FOR Heart ②③ • Immunity ①

1 Preheat your oven to 200°C/fan 180°C/gas 6.
2 To make the relish, pile the beetroot cubes in the centre of a piece of foil and drizzle the oil over them. Gather up the foil to form a parcel. Set it on a baking tray and bake for 30 minutes until the beetroot is softened but still has a crunch. Allow to cool. Leave the oven on for the burgers.
3 Once cooled, tip the beetroot into a blender and add the capers, tomatoes, chilli, onion and garlic. Pulse to create a coarse consistency. Transfer the relish to a bowl and set aside.
4 To make the burgers, combine the minced chicken with the rest of the ingredients in a large bowl, mixing with your hands. Take care not to mash the meat too much, which would make the burgers too dense. Shape into four good-sized patties and place them on a baking tray.
5 Cook the burgers in the oven for 25 minutes, turning once. Serve each topped with a dollop of the beetroot relish and a green salad alongside.

ROASTED POUSSIN WITH BRUSSELS SPROUTS

SERVES 2 • 450 CALORIES PER SERVING

A poussin is the perfect bird for two people. It is super-easy to cook and takes half the time a chicken does – and you can use the carcass afterwards to make a delicious stock. Poussins are also great for a dinner party because you can cook more birds and serve each couple a platter of poussin with leeks and Brussels sprouts to share. Brussels sprouts are from the same family as broccoli, cauliflower, kale and pak choi; all contain substances that may offer protection against certain types of cancer.

RICH IN Vitamins B2 (riboflavin), B3 (niacin), B6, C and E • Folate • Potassium • Iron • Zinc • Selenium • Beta-sitosterol • Tryptophan • Prebiotics • Fibre

USEFUL FOR Digestion ② • Immunity ① • Mind ① • Fatigue ①③⑤ • Men ①② • Women ①③

1 poussin
1 lemon, sliced
3 sprigs of fresh thyme
A pinch of flaked sea salt
A pinch of cracked black pepper
600ml chicken stock (see page 283)
2 leeks, finely diced
200g Brussels sprouts, cut in half
1 tbsp pumpkin seeds
1 tbsp sunflower seeds
1 tbsp home-shelled pistachios
A handful of fresh flat-leaf parsley, finely chopped
A handful of fresh coriander, finely chopped

1 Preheat your oven to 200°C/fan 180°C/gas 6. Line a small baking tray with greaseproof paper.

2 Place the poussin on the baking tray and top with a few lemon slices, the thyme sprigs, sea salt and cracked black pepper. Roast in the oven for 25 minutes.

3 While the poussin is roasting, set a saucepan on a medium heat and add the chicken stock. Bring to the boil, then add the leeks. Simmer for about 5 minutes until they have softened. Add the Brussels sprouts and simmer form a further 4 minutes until they are tender but still a little crunchy. Drain off excess stock, then keep the vegetables warm in the pan.

4 Remove the poussin from the oven and set aside to rest for a few minutes before carving into pieces or cutting in half.

5 Meanwhile, spread the seeds and nuts on another small baking tray and toast in the oven for 6 minutes until golden. Add these to the Brussels sprouts and leeks, then mix through the fresh herbs. Serve with the poussin.

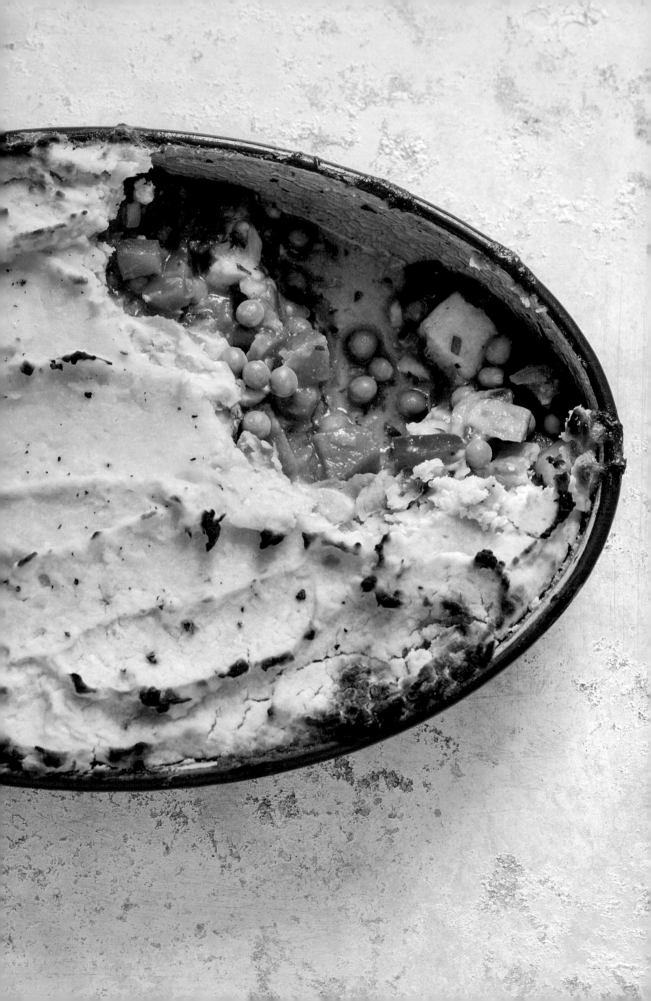

CHICKEN & VEGETABLE PIE

SERVES 6 • 320 CALORIES PER SERVING

Blended butter beans are the perfect substitute for mashed potatoes – they're the same colour and texture, and when baked as the topping on a pie, they form a lovely golden cover. Butternut squash, peas and peppers are used in the filling for this pie, but it is also a great way to use up any leftover vegetables you might have in your fridge, so feel free to experiment. It also makes a great vegetarian dish if you leave out the chicken and bump up the vegetables.

1 tbsp rapeseed oil

2 shallots, sliced

1 leek, finely diced

2 garlic cloves, chopped

4 skinless, boneless chicken breasts, about 150g each, diced

1 tbsp gluten- and wheat-free flour

400ml vegetable stock (see page 283)

A handful of fresh flat-leaf parsley, finely chopped

2 sprigs of fresh tarragon, finely chopped

1 bay leaf

2 carrots, diced

½ butternut squash, peeled, seeded and diced

1 red pepper, seeded and sliced

100g button mushrooms, cut in half

100g podded fresh or thawed frozen peas

FOR THE TOPPING

1 cauliflower, broken into florets

2 x 400g tins butter beans, drained

1 garlic clove, very finely chopped

200ml rice milk

Salt and pepper

1 Set a large saucepan on the heat and add the oil. When it is hot, add the shallots, leek and garlic and cook for 5 minutes. Add the chicken and cook, stirring occasionally, for 5–6 minutes until slightly golden. Sprinkle the flour over the mixture and stir well, then pour in half of the vegetable stock, stirring constantly to ensure there are no floury lumps.

2 Add the remaining stock along with the parsley, tarragon, bay leaf, carrots, squash, red pepper and mushrooms. Cook for a further 15 minutes, stirring occasionally, until the vegetables are tender. Transfer the mixture to a pie dish and top with the peas.

3 Preheat your oven to 200°C/fan 180°C/gas 6.

4 To make the topping, bring a medium-sized pan of water to the boil, add the cauliflower florets and cook for 10 minutes. Drain and tip into a food processor. Add the beans, garlic and rice milk to the processor and blitz for 2 minutes until smooth. Season to taste.

5 Spoon the bean mixture on top of the chicken and vegetable mixture to cover completely. Bake in the heated oven for 25 minutes. Serve hot.

RICH IN Vitamins B3 (niacin), B6 and C • Folate • Potassium • Selenium • Beta-carotene • Tryptophan • Fibre

USEFUL FOR Heart ①②③ • Digestion ① • Immunity ① • Skin, hair & nails ① • Mind ① • Fatigue ③ • Men ① • Women ①

LEMON CHICKEN

SERVES 4 • 340 CALORIES PER SERVING

This Moroccan-inspired dish is the result of my mum's ceaseless quest to find the ultimate lemon chicken recipe. She says she will continue to develop it until it's the best lemon chicken in the world. To my mind it already is. We serve the chicken with a steamed cauliflower 'cous cous', which does a wonderful job of soaking up all the delicious lemony sauce. This is the perfect winter meal, packed with vitamin C and selenium to keep your immune system healthy and B vitamins to ward off fatigue. You can find an alternative baked method for cauliflower cous cous on page 132.

3 large onions, finely diced
2 tbsp olive oil
4 skinless, boneless chicken breasts, about 150g each, cut across into 3 pieces
2 handfuls of fresh flat-leaf parsley, finely chopped
1 tbsp finely grated fresh ginger
A large pinch of saffron threads
10 large green olives, pitted
3 preserved lemons, finely chopped, plus a few extra slices to garnish
1.2 litres chicken stock (see page 283)
Fresh coriander, to garnish

FOR THE CAULIFLOWER COUS COUS
1 cauliflower, outer leaves removed
1 tbsp rapeseed oil
A pinch of saffron threads
Salt and pepper

1 In a deep, flameproof casserole, fry the onions in the olive oil for 10 minutes. Add the chicken and sauté for 6–8 minutes until lightly golden on both sides, turning the pieces occasionally. Add the parsley, ginger, saffron, green olives and chopped preserved lemon. Pour in the stock. Bring to the boil, then simmer for 10 minutes.

2 Meanwhile, preheat your grill to medium.

3 Remove the chicken and place it in a heatproof dish. Place under the grill and cook for about 10 minutes until golden brown on both sides; set aside and keep warm.

4 While the chicken is under the grill, turn the heat under the casserole to low and reduce the sauce for at least 40 minutes. It will end up thick and rich, bursting with flavour. Once reduced, add the chicken back in and season with salt and pepper to taste.

5 Whilst the sauce is reducing, make the cauliflower cous cous. Preheat the oven to 180°C/fan 160°C/gas 4. Remove the cauliflower florets from their stalks. Add the stalks and core to a food processor and blitz to create a fluffy cous-cous-like texture. Tip into a mixing bowl. Add the florets to the processor and blitz for a few seconds to create the same light texture (you may have to do this in a few batches). Add to the bowl along with the oil, saffron, and seasoning to taste. Mix together.

6 Lay a large square of foil on a baking tray (the foil should be at least three times the size of the tray). Pile the cauliflower cous cous in the middle and wrap it up in the foil so that there are no gaps. Steam in the oven for 20 minutes until soft.

7 Serve the lemon chicken garnished with fresh coriander and extra preserved lemon slices, and with the cauliflower cous cous alongside.

RICH IN Vitamins B1 (thiamin), B3 (niacin), B6 and C • Folate • Potassium • Selenium • Tryptophan

USEFUL FOR Heart ②③ • Immunity ① • Mind ① • Fatigue ③ • Men ① • Women ①

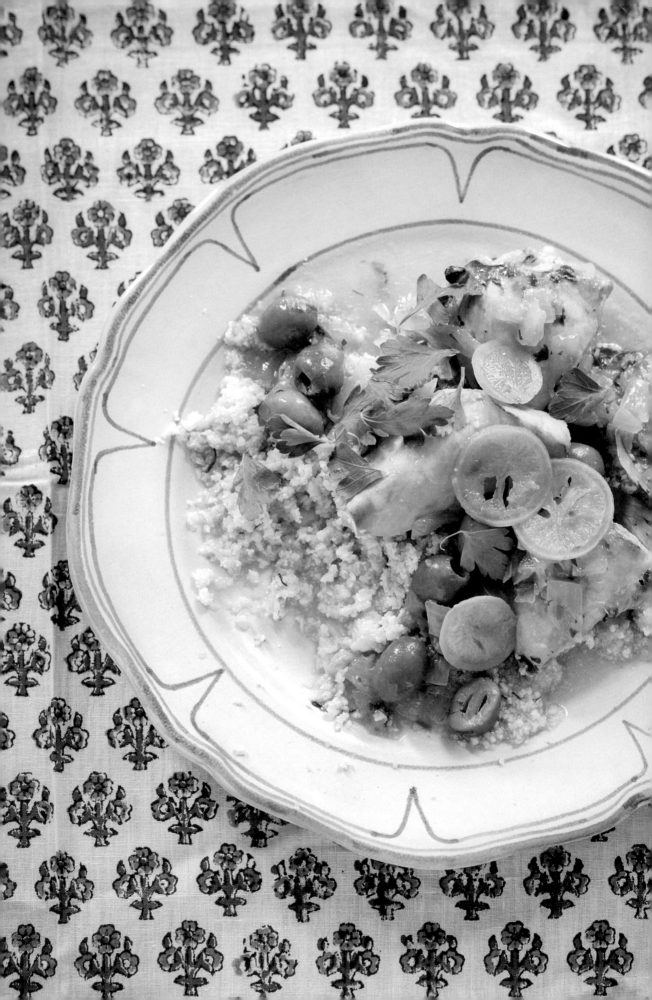

FISH

A perfectly cooked piece of fish with a huge helping of vegetables on the side makes a deeply appetising and nutritious meal. This is fish cookery at its simplest. In the recipes that follow we have used many different cooking techniques, from steaming to grilling, baking to barbecuing, with different flavourings, spices and herbs and great accompaniments. You'll find much inspiration here to expand your fish repertoire.

A healthy diet should include fish – current guidance is that we should eat at least a couple of servings per week, one of which should be oily fish, such as salmon, trout, tuna, sardines or herring, to ensure adequate amounts of heart-protective omega 3. (Oily fish contain substances that may be harmful in large amounts, so limit your intake to no more than four servings per week, or two if you are pregnant.) Fish and shellfish are also great sources of some key vitamins and minerals, including zinc and vitamins B6, B12 and D, as well as selenium, which is in short supply in the British diet.

Eating a variety of different fish is also important, not only to ensure a wider consumption of nutrients but also to preserve fish stocks. None of the fish that we have used in these recipes is endangered. When you are buying fish, check the label to ensure the fish is from sustainable sources (look for the Marine Stewardship Council symbol) or ask your fishmonger.

At the end of most of the recipes, you'll find a list of the main nutrients supplied in a serving as well as a list of health issues that may be benefited by including the recipe in your healthy diet. For more, see page 9.

CRAB & CHILLI WITH CUCUMBER SALAD

SERVES 2 | 185 CALORIES PER SERVING

In Goa, fresh crab is simply served with some lettuce leaves, fresh coriander and a wedge of lemon. The sweet flesh of the crab with the aromatic herb and zingy citrus is a perfect combination. It is the inspiration for this salad, which makes a substantial lunch or dinner. The salad contains more than 100 per cent of the RDA for selenium, an antioxidant mineral that is essential for a strong immune system to support good health.

200g fresh white crab meat
½ fresh red chilli, seeded and finely diced
Juice of 1 lime
A handful of fresh coriander, finely chopped
1 iceberg lettuce
Lime wedges, to serve

FOR THE CUCUMBER SALAD
1 cucumber
A handful of fresh mint leaves, finely chopped
2 spring onions, finely chopped
A handful of green beans, cut into 5mm pieces
Juice of ½ lemon
1 tsp rapeseed oil
1 tbsp plain soya yogurt

1 Mix the crab with the chilli, lime juice and coriander and set aside.
2 Peel the cucumber, cut in half lengthways and scoop out the seeds with a teaspoon. Finely dice the cucumber and place in a bowl. Add the mint, spring onions, green beans, lemon juice, oil and yogurt and mix thoroughly.
3 Peel off two large outer leaves from the lettuce; wash them and pat dry with kitchen paper. Spoon half of the cucumber salad into each one. Top with the crab and serve with wedges of lime.

RICH IN Vitamins B2 (riboflavin) and C • Folate • Selenium • Potassium • Tryptophan

USEFUL FOR Heart ② • Mind ① • Fatigue ③⑤ • Men ①

KING PRAWN, KOHLRABI & PEAR SALAD

SERVES 2 • 265 CALORIES PER SERVING

Kolrabi has leapt into the limelight over the last few years. A member of the cabbage family, it is a funny-looking vegetable, resembling an alien's head with leafy antennae. Don't let this put you off – it's very easy to prepare and will be a great addition to your diet. Finely sliced or diced, the pale, almost translucent green-white flesh is delicious served raw with just a squeeze of lemon juice and some seasoning. Kohlrabi is high in compounds called bioflavonoids, which work with other nutrients to prevent cell damage that promotes cancer.

30g walnuts
1 tsp groundnut oil
1 tsp finely grated fresh ginger
200g peeled raw king prawns (tails left on)
1 small kohlrabi
Grated zest and juice of 1 lemon
1 Conference pear
½ tsp black sesame seeds
Salt and pepper

1 Preheat your oven to 200°C/fan 180°C/gas 6. Spread the walnuts in a small baking tray and toast in the oven for 8 minutes. Tip into a mortar and lightly crush with the pestle. Set aside.
2 Heat the groundnut oil in a frying pan for 1 minute, then add the ginger and king prawns and cook, stirring, for about 4 minutes until the prawns are completely pink. Set aside to cool.
3 Meanwhile, peel the thick skin from the kohlrabi, then slice very thinly. It's best to use a mandoline but if you don't have one, you can slice the kohlrabi carefully by hand. Place the slices in a large bowl and add the lemon juice, a pinch of salt and some pepper.
4 Core the pear, then slice thinly. Add the pear to the bowl and mix gently with the kohlrabi. Divide between two plates.
5 Combine the king prawns, walnuts, lemon zest and black sesame seeds in a bowl and mix together. Place on top of the kohlrabi and pear salad to serve.

RICH IN Vitamins B12 and C • Folate • Potassium • Selenium • Tryptophan

USEFUL FOR Heart ② • Immunity ① • Mind ① • Fatigue ③ • Men ①

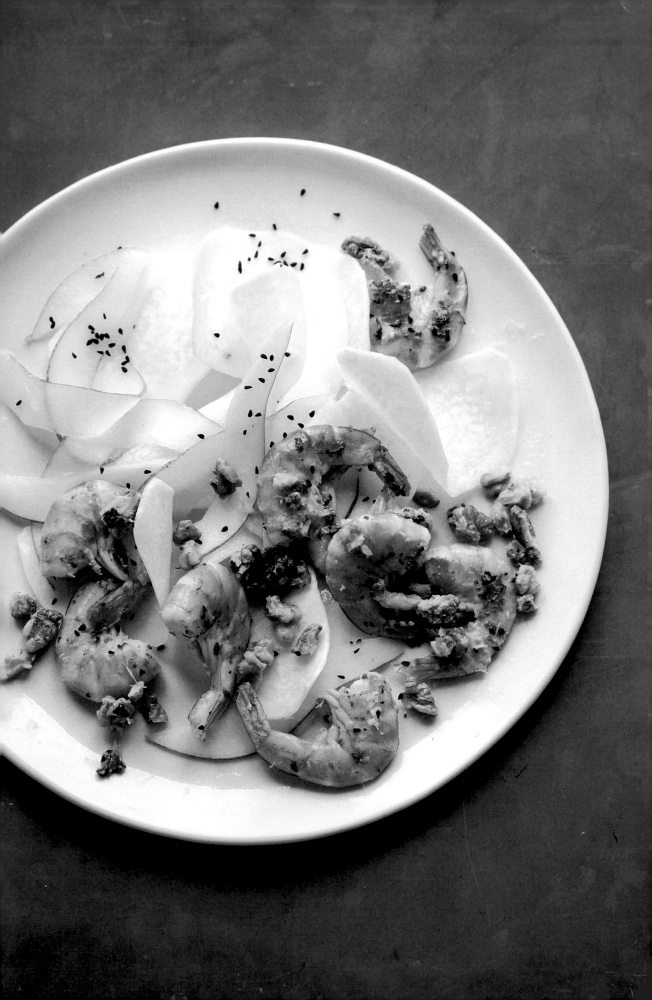

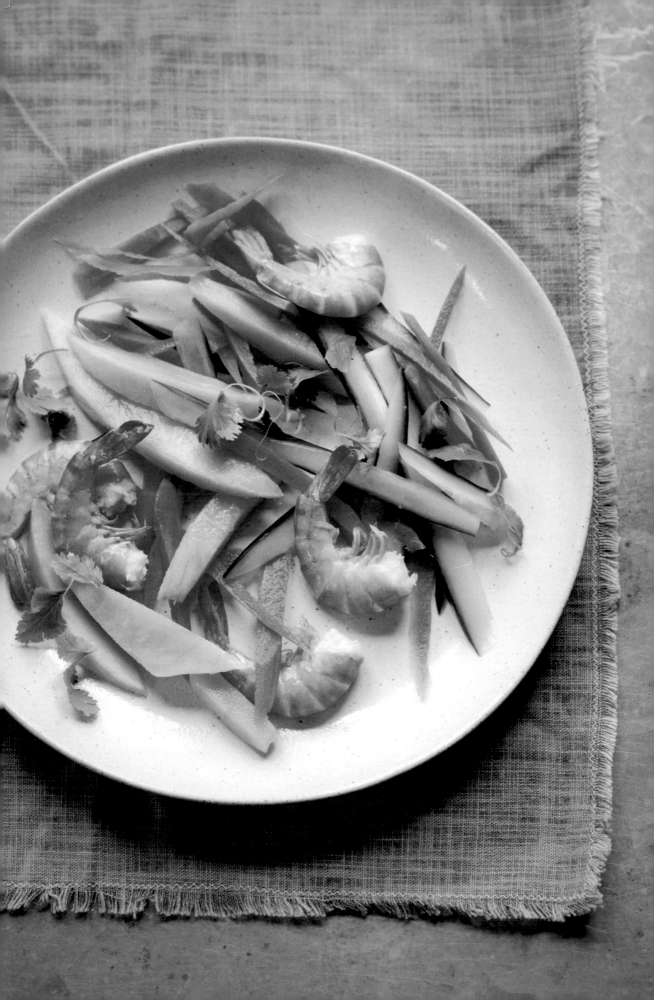

KING PRAWN & MANGO SALAD

SERVES 2 • 325 CALORIES PER SERVING

Putting a sweet, soft fruit into a seafood salad may seem odd, but it is very common in Asian cuisine. Mango certainly changes the whole dimension of this dish, adding a zingy sweetness and smooth texture that works perfectly with the juicy seafood. Prawns and other shellfish are a major source of zinc, a mineral that is essential for men's health.

1 mango
1 carrot, thinly sliced
½ cucumber, thinly sliced
150g peeled raw king prawns (tails left on)
A handful of fresh coriander

FOR THE DRESSING
Juice of 1 lime
1 tsp olive oil
½ tsp tamari
A thumb-sized piece of fresh ginger, roughly chopped with the skin on
½ fresh red chilli, roughly chopped
Salt and pepper

1 Cut the mango in half, around the flat stone; discard the stone. Set one half aside for the dressing. Score the flesh in the other half into long strips, then turn the half inside out and cut the slices away from the skin. Place them in a bowl and add the carrot and cucumber.
2 Bring a pan of water to the boil. Once boiling, turn the heat down to a simmer and add the prawns. Simmer for about 3 minutes until the prawns are completely pink. Drain. Add the prawns to the mango salad along with the coriander and season with salt and pepper.
3 To make the dressing, put the flesh from the reserved mango half in a blender with all the other ingredients and blitz to a smooth, runny consistency. Drizzle over the salad.

RICH IN Vitamins B2 (riboflavin), B6, B12 and C • Zinc • Selenium • Calcium • Magnesium • Beta-carotene • Tryptophan • Fibre

USEFUL FOR Heart ①②③ • Bones ① • Digestion ① • Immunity ① • Skin, hair & nails ①③ • Mind ①② • Fatigue ③⑤ • Men ① • Women ①

GRIDDLED SQUID WITH MUSHROOM SALAD

SERVES 4 • 225 CALORIES PER SERVING

If you haven't cooked squid before, it is definitely worth a go. It's a great lean source of protein. You can ask your fishmonger to prepare the squid, so that all you have to do is griddle it and serve. It is really easy to cook. Just be quick because it will continue to cook after you take it off the heat and can become chewy if overdone.

8 squid, prepared, with tentacles
1 tsp rapeseed oil
Juice of ½ lime

FOR THE SALAD
10 cherry tomatoes, cut into quarters
1 cucumber, diced
100g button mushrooms, thinly sliced
100g tinned sweetcorn, drained
2 spring onions, thinly sliced
A few sprigs of fresh coriander
A few fresh mint leaves

FOR THE DRESSING
A handful of fresh coriander, finely chopped
A handful of fresh mint, finely chopped
Juice of 1 lime
1 tsp rapeseed oil
Salt and pepper

1 First, make the salad by mixing together all the ingredients in a bowl. Cover with clingfilm and set aside in the fridge.
2 Mix the dressing ingredients together in a small bowl.
3 Slit the squid bodies open, then cut each in half lengthways so it lies flat, inner side up. Score the flesh in a diamond pattern.
4 Set a ridged griddle/grill pan on a high heat.
5 Once hot, add the oil, then place the squid, scored side down (with the tentacles), on the griddle. Hold the pieces down so that they don't curl up. Cook for 2 minutes on each side.
6 Transfer the squid to a plate and cut into slices. Sprinkle with the lime juice, then mix through the salad. Drizzle over the dressing and serve.

RICH IN Vitamins B6 and B12 • Folate • Selenium • Potassium • Tryptophan

USEFUL FOR Heart ② • Mind ① • Fatigue ③ • Men ① • Women ①

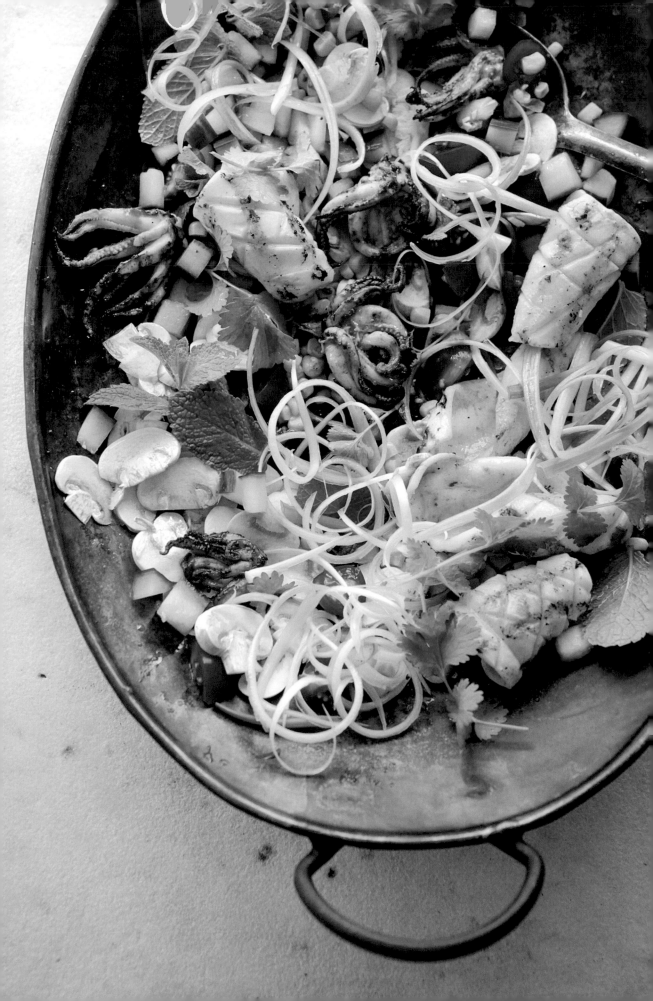

KING PRAWN STIR-FRY

SERVES 2 • 335 CALORIES PER SERVING

This easy, nutritious stir-fry makes a really quick dinner – after the ingredients are prepared, it takes only five minutes to cook. Containing three of your five-a-day, the dish is slightly sweet and slightly spicy to satisfy all of your tastebuds. You'll be surprised by how filling it is.

1 tsp olive oil
150g peeled raw king prawns
30g cashew nuts
4 spring onions, finely sliced on the diagonal
A thumb-sized piece of fresh ginger, grated with the skin on
2 garlic cloves, finely chopped
1 tbsp tamari
1 fresh red chilli, seeded and finely chopped
Juice of 1 lime
1 tsp runny honey
½ red pepper, seeded and finely diced
100g mange tout, finely sliced
100g Tenderstem broccoli
A handful of spinach, roughly chopped
2 pak choi, cut lengthways in half
A handful of fresh coriander, finely chopped
Lime wedges, to serve

1 Set a wok on a medium heat and add the olive oil. Once hot, add the prawns, cashew nuts, spring onions, ginger and garlic and stir-fry for 1 minute. Add the tamari, chilli, lime juice, honey and 2 tablespoons water and stir-fry for a further 2 minutes.
2 Add the red pepper and all the green vegetables and toss to coat with the sauce. Cook, tossing, for 2 minutes until the vegetables are slightly soft. Garnish with the coriander and serve with lime wedges for squeezing over.

RICH IN B vitamins • Vitamin C • Potassium • Calcium • Magnesium • Selenium • Zinc • Beta-carotene • Tryptophan • Fibre

USEFUL FOR Heart ①②③ • Bones ① • Digestion ① • Immunity ① • Skin, hair & nails ①③ • Mind ①② • Fatigue ⑤ • Men ①② • Women ①

PRAWN, CASHEW & BLACK RICE SALAD

SERVES 2 • 520 CALORIES PER SERVING

This combination of cauliflower, toasted cashew nuts and juicy king prawns is so good. The colour of black rice is due to a type of antioxidant in the flavonoid family called anthocyanins, which are thought to benefit heart health.

100g black or wild rice
50g cashew nuts
½ cauliflower, separated into small florets
1 spring onion, finely sliced
Juice of ½ lime
1 tsp groundnut oil
A handful of fresh coriander, finely chopped, plus extra to garnish
1 sprig of fresh mint, leaves picked and finely chopped
150g peeled raw king prawns
Lemon wedges, to serve

1 Preheat your oven to 200°C/fan 180°C/gas 6.
2 Put the black rice in a pan of cold water and bring to the boil, then cook for 20–25 minutes until tender. Drain and leave to one side.
3 While the rice is cooking, spread the cashew nuts in a small baking tray and toast in the oven for 8 minutes until golden. Set aside.
4 Put the cauliflower florets in a heatproof bowl. Cover with boiling water and leave for 3 minutes, then drain in a colander and refresh with cold running water. Put them back in the bowl and add the spring onion, cashew nuts, lime juice, oil, coriander and mint. Mix together.
5 Bring a pan of water to the boil. Drop in the prawns and poach for 4 minutes until they turn pink. Drain the prawns and add them to the cauliflower mixture. Toss to coat with the oil and herbs.
6 Serve the prawn and cauliflower salad on top of the black rice. Garnish with coriander and serve with lemon wedges.

RICH IN B vitamins • Vitamin C • Folate • Iron • Potassium • Zinc • Selenium • Tryptophan • Fibre

USEFUL FOR Heart ①②③ • Digestion ① • Immunity ① • Skin, hair & nails ①④ • Mind ① • Fatigue ①③ • Men ①② • Women ①

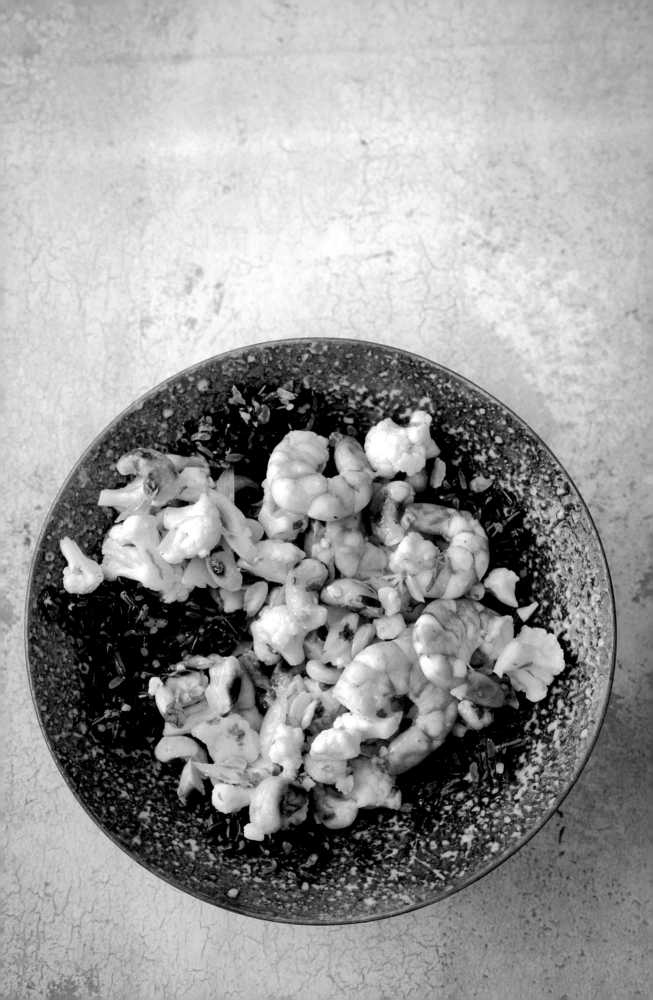

COURGETTE SPAGHETTI WITH KING PRAWNS

SERVES 2 • 285 CALORIES PER SERVING

Here, courgette spaghetti ingeniously tricks you into thinking you are tucking into a large bowl of pasta. Tossed with a sweet, delicious sauce and juicy king prawns, this is Italian-inspired comfort food at its best. It is a good dish for bone health because it contains a rich source of calcium, magnesium and phosphorus, all of which support strong bones.

5 courgettes
1 tsp flaked sea salt
1 tsp olive oil
1 red onion, finely chopped
1 fresh red chilli, seeded and finely sliced
200g cherry tomatoes, cut in half
1 garlic clove, finely sliced
150g peeled raw king prawns
A handful of fresh coriander, finely chopped

1 First make the courgette spaghetti using a julienne peeler/cutter (stop when you get to the soft seeded centre). If you don't have a julienne peeler, you can grate the courgettes. It won't give the same effect, but it will still taste great. Place the courgette spaghetti in a bowl and sprinkle with the sea salt. Set aside.
2 Heat the olive oil in a non-stick frying pan, add the onion and cook for 5 minutes. Add the chilli, cherry tomatoes and garlic and cook, stirring occasionally, for another 5 minutes until the tomatoes are soft. Stir in 50ml water and the prawns and cook for 5 more minutes until the prawns turn pink.
3 Pat the courgette spaghetti dry with kitchen paper, then add to the pan and mix through the sauce to heat. Serve immediately, sprinkled with coriander.

RICH IN Vitamins B1 (thiamin), B6, B12 and C • Potassium • Magnesium • Calcium • Iron • Zinc • Phosphorus • Beta-carotene • Lycopene • Tryptophan • Fibre

USEFUL FOR Heart ①②③ • Bones ① • Digestion ① • Immunity ① • Skin, hair & nails ①③ • Mind ①② • Fatigue ①③⑤ • Men ①② • Women ①③

SPICY PRAWN & TOMATO PASTA

SERVES 4 • 200 CALORIES PER SERVING

Blending curry flavours with a rich tomato sauce fuses Asian and Italian cooking, two of the cuisines that have heavily influenced the Detox Kitchen. This is a perfect dish for a family gathering, served from a big bowl in the middle of the table. Men in particular should enjoy it because the dish contains a rich source of zinc and the antioxidant lycopene, both of which can help to support men's health and fertility.

1 tbsp olive oil
4 shallots, finely sliced
1 tsp ground coriander
1 tsp garam masala
2 garlic cloves, chopped
100g cherry tomatoes, cut into quarters
150g gluten-free spaghetti
300g peeled raw king prawns
1 tbsp finely chopped fresh coriander
A pinch of crushed dried chilli

1 Set a medium-sized non-stick frying pan on a high heat and add the oil. Add the shallots and cook for 5 minutes until slightly browned. Turn the heat down to medium and add the ground coriander and garam masala. Cook for 1 minute, stirring, then add the garlic, tomatoes and 50ml water. Cook, stirring occasionally, for 10 minutes until the tomatoes are completely soft.
2 Meanwhile, bring a large pan of water to the boil. Add the pasta with 1 teaspoon salt and boil for 7–8 minutes until cooked. Scoop out half a cupful of the cooking water, then drain the pasta. Tip it back into the empty pan and add the reserved cooking water.
3 Add the prawns to the tomato sauce and cook for 4–5 minutes until they are completely pink.
4 Add the prawns and tomato sauce to the pasta along with the fresh coriander and chilli. Toss over a low heat for 2–3 minutes before serving.

RICH IN Vitamins B6, B12 and C • Magnesium • Potassium • Zinc • Lycopene • Fibre

USEFUL FOR Heart ②③ • Bones ① • Digestion ① • Immunity ① • Skin, hair & nails ①④ • Mind ①② • Fatigue ③⑤ • Men ①② • Women ①

BRAISED LETTUCE, MUSHROOMS & PRAWNS

SERVES 2 • 210 CALORIES PER SERVING

In this recipe, lettuce isn't a member of the supporting cast, it's the star of the show. Lightly braised, the lettuce becomes slightly soft whilst embracing all the flavours from the shallots, oyster mushrooms, garlic and ginger. Mushrooms are a concentrated source of glutamic acid, which is a naturally occurring form of monosodium glutamate, so act as a great flavour-enhancer in recipes, as well as providing a good source of B vitamins, which the body uses to convert food to energy in cells.

1 tbsp rapeseed oil

3 banana shallots, finely diced

150g oyster mushrooms, sliced

1 tbsp finely grated fresh ginger

1 garlic clove, finely chopped

150g peeled raw king prawns

300ml hot vegetable stock (see page 283)

1 tsp fish sauce

4 baby Gem lettuces, cut lengthways in half through the root

Salt and pepper

Chopped fresh coriander, to garnish

Lemon wedges, to serve

1 Heat the oil in a wok, then add the shallots and cook for a few minutes until softened. Add the mushrooms and cook for 5 minutes until lightly golden, stirring occasionally. Stir in the ginger, garlic and prawns. Cook for a further 2 minutes.

2 Pour in the hot stock and fish sauce and bring to a simmer. Add the lettuce halves and cook for 2 minutes until they are slightly softened but not sludgy. Season with salt and pepper.

3 Serve immediately with a sprinkle of coriander and wedges of lemon for squeezing over.

RICH IN Vitamins B1 (thiamin), B12 and E • Folate • Potassium • Selenium • Iron • Tryptophan

USEFUL FOR Immunity ① • Mind ① • Fatigue ①③ • Men ① • Women ③

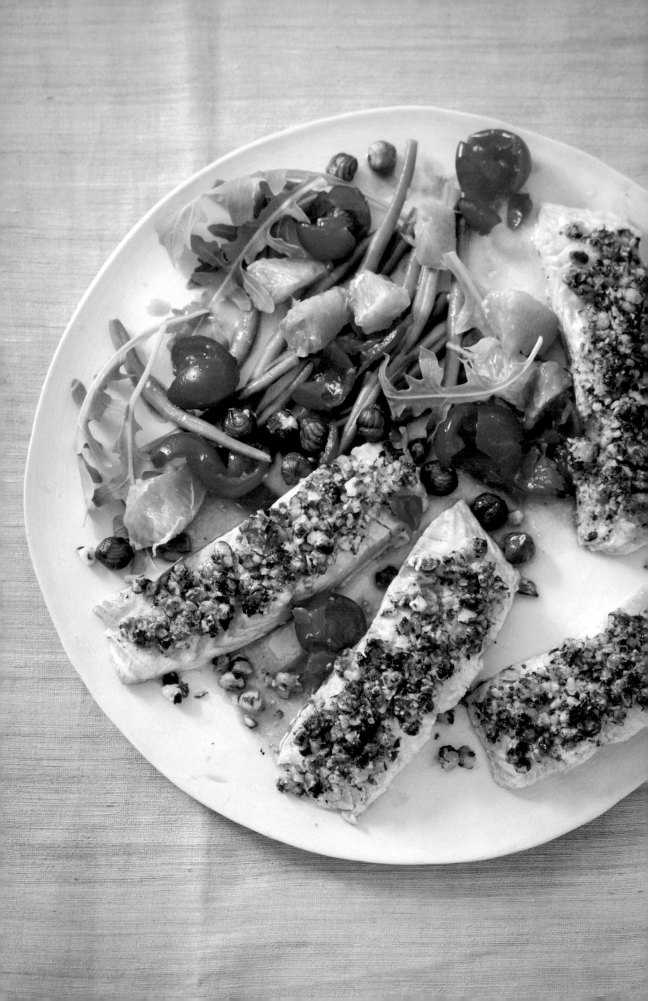

SALMON, GREEN BEANS, ORANGE & HAZELNUT SALAD

SERVES 4 • 410 CALORIES PER SERVING

This salad offers one of our favourite flavour combinations: hazelnuts and orange. It is a wonderfully colourful dish, and the salmon with the hazelnut dressing becomes crispy and extra rich under the grill. Salmon provides one of the few dietary sources of vitamin D, which is essential for strong bones.

60g hazelnuts
2 tsp rapeseed oil
Grated zest and juice of 1 orange
4 pieces of salmon fillet, 110–130g each
300g green beans
200g rocket leaves
150g cherry tomatoes
1 orange, peeled and segmented
Salt and pepper

1 Preheat your grill to medium. Line a baking tray with greaseproof paper.
2 Crush half the hazelnuts using a pestle and mortar, then tip into a small mixing bowl. Add the rapeseed oil and orange zest and stir to mix.
3 Remove the skin from your salmon fillets and place them on the baking tray. Grill them for 6 minutes. Turn the fillets over and cover with the crushed hazelnut mixture, then grill for a further 4 minutes. Remove the salmon from the grill and leave to cool slightly.
4 Meanwhile, bring a medium-sized saucepan of water to the boil. Drop in the green beans and blanch for no more than 1 minute. Drain in a colander and rinse under cold water to stop the cooking process and keep them bright green. Place the beans in a bowl and add the rocket leaves, orange juice and some salt and pepper.
5 Next add the tomatoes to the salad, one at a time: place between your thumb and forefinger and squeeze the tomato so that it rips apart and the juice oozes out. Add the halved orange segments and toss everything gently together.
6 Set a frying pan on a medium heat and add the rest of the hazelnuts. Toast for 3–4 minutes until lightly browned; keep swirling the nuts in the pan to ensure they brown evenly and don't burn. Add these to the salad and mix through.
7 Serve the salmon fillets with the salad on the side.

RICH IN B vitamins • Vitamins C, D and E • Potassium • Selenium • Omega 3 • Tryptophan

USEFUL FOR Heart ①② • Bones ①② • Digestion ③④ • Immunity ① • Skin, hair & nails ①②③ • Mind ① • Fatigue ②③ • Men ①② • Women ①③④

STEAMED SALMON WITH PESTO VEGETABLES

SERVES 2 • 465 CALORIES PER SERVING

This is a fail-safe weekday dish: healthy, fresh, filling and satisfying – everything you need to fuel your week. Steaming the salmon in a foil parcel retains all the rich, sweet flavour and keeps the nutrients packed in. The salmon is served with pesto-dressed roasted aubergine, courgette and sweet potato. Sweet potato is a highly nutritious starchy food with a low glycaemic load (GL) – a great food to include in your diet if you're trying to lose weight.

2 pieces of salmon fillet, 110–130g each
2 slices of lemon
2 sprigs of fresh thyme
Flaked sea salt
1 aubergine, cut into 1cm dice
2 courgettes, cut into 2.5cm dice
1 small sweet potato, cut into 2.5cm pieces with the skin on
1 tsp olive oil, for drizzling

FOR THE PESTO
A handful of fresh basil leaves
A handful of fresh chives
A handful of cashew nuts
1 garlic clove
2 tbsp olive oil
Grated zest of 1 lemon
Salt and cracked black pepper

1 Preheat your oven to 200°C/fan 180°C/gas 6. Line a baking tray with greaseproof paper.
2 Cut out two large squares of foil and place a salmon fillet in the centre of each. Top each fillet with a slice of lemon, a sprig of thyme, and a pinch each of sea salt and cracked black pepper. Wrap the salmon in the foil to seal and place the parcels on a baking tray. Bake in the heated oven for 20 minutes.
3 Meanwhile, spread out all the vegetables on the lined baking tray. Drizzle the olive oil over them and season with salt and pepper. Roast in the oven for 20 minutes.
4 While the salmon and vegetables are in the oven, put all the pesto ingredients in a blender (keep back a few basil leaves for the garnish) and blitz to a coarse paste. Season with a pinch each of salt and pepper. Transfer the pesto to a saucepan and set on a medium heat to warm through.

5 Remove the vegetables from the oven and mix gently with the pesto. Serve the salmon fillet with the pesto vegetables, garnished with a few basil leaves.

RICH IN Vitamins B6, B12, C and D • Folate • Potassium • Iron • Selenium • Beta-carotene • Omega 3 • Tryptophan • Fibre

USEFUL FOR Heart ①②③ • Bones ①② • Digestion ① • Immunity ① • Skin, hair & nails ①②③ • Mind ① • Fatigue ①③ • Men ① • Women ①③④

SALMON & BROWN RICE NOODLES

SERVES 2 • 460 CALORIES PER SERVING

Eating a big bowl of noodles is truly comforting, and this Asian-inspired salmon dish does the trick. The sharp lime juice with the nuttiness of the sesame, the salty tamari with the sweet salmon – these will all awaken your tastebuds. To make it more fiery, you could add a finely diced fresh red chilli. The dish contains over 200 per cent of your RDA for vitamin B12, which is involved in the production of healthy red blood cells.

2 pieces of salmon fillet, 110–130g each

A thumb-sized piece of fresh ginger, grated with the skin on

Juice of ½ lime

1 tbsp tamari

1 tsp toasted sesame oil

100g brown rice noodles

2 handfuls of small broccoli florets

Salt

Lime wedges, to serve

1 Preheat your oven to 200°C/fan 180°C/gas 6.

2 Place the salmon on a baking tray and cover with the grated ginger. Bake in the heated oven for 12 minutes until cooked. Remove from the oven and leave to cool.

3 Pull the skin off the salmon. You can leave the fillets whole, and let each person flake off pieces with their fork, or flake the salmon now using your fingers: going with the grain of the flesh, push off small pieces. Put the salmon and ginger in a bowl and add the lime juice, tamari and sesame oil.

4 To cook the noodles, bring a large pan of water to the boil. Add some salt, then drop in the noodles and broccoli and cook for 1 minute. Drain.

5 Divide the noodles and broccoli between two plates and top with the salmon. Pour over the tamari sauce and serve with lime wedges.

RICH IN Vitamins B3 (niacin), B6, B12, C and D • Potassium • Chromium • Selenium • Omega 3 • Tryptophan • Fibre

USEFUL FOR Heart ①②③ • Bones ①② • Digestion ①④ • Immunity ① • Skin, hair & nails ①②③ • Mind ① • Fatigue ②③ • Men ② • Women ①③④

SALMON & DILL FISHCAKES

SERVES 2 • 250 CALORIES PER SERVING

Salmon with dill is one of those classic flavour combinations that never fails to excite the tastebuds. The distinctive mild aniseed flavour brings out the delicate sweetness of salmon, and the feathery, soft leaves add a lovely texture and colour. The omega 3 in oily fish such as salmon may help with a number of inflammatory health conditions, including psoriasis and rheumatoid arthritis. Try to include up to four pieces of oily fish in your diet each week to help with such conditions.

1 tbsp capers, finely chopped
A handful of fresh chives, finely chopped
A handful of fresh dill, finely chopped
Grated zest of 1 lemon
A pinch of salt
A pinch of cracked black pepper
1 egg
200–220g salmon fillet, skin removed
1 tbsp gluten- and wheat-free flour
1 tbsp rapeseed oil

1 Preheat your grill to medium. Line a baking tray with greaseproof paper.
2 Mix together the capers, chives, dill, lemon zest, salt and pepper in a large bowl. Add the egg and mix well.
3 Finely dice the salmon – it is important to cut it into very small pieces, otherwise the fishcakes won't hold together. Add to the bowl along with the flour. Mix together with your hands to ensure everything is thoroughly amalgamated. Shape into two fishcakes.
4 Set a frying pan on a high heat and add the oil. Fry the fishcakes for 2–3 minutes on each side, then transfer them to the lined baking tray. Grill for 8 minutes on each side. Serve the fishcakes hot, with a green salad.

RICH IN B vitamins • Vitamin D • Selenium • Tryptophan • Omega 3

USEFUL FOR Heart ①②③ • Bones ①② • Digestion ③④ • Skin, hair & nails ①② • Mind ① • Fatigue ②③ • Men ①② • Women ①③④

GRILLED SALMON WITH GINGER

SERVES 2 • 240 CALORIES PER SERVING

This simple, easy dish is a staple in the Detox Kitchen. It was created when I was cooking with our friend Archie, and we still argue over who came up with the recipe. It is the perfect heart-healthy dish as it's high in omega 3 fatty acids, and also offers anticoagulant properties from the ginger and garlic that may help to improve blood flow.

2 pieces of salmon fillet, 110–130g each
1 fresh red chilli, seeded and finely chopped
1 garlic clove, finely chopped
2 tbsp tamari
A thumb-sized piece of fresh ginger, grated with the skin on
1 tbsp toasted sesame oil

1 Preheat your grill to medium.
2 Place the salmon skin-side down on a baking tray. Mix the rest of the ingredients in a bowl and pour equally over the fillets.
3 Grill for 12 minutes (no need to turn over). Once cooked, remove the skin and discard. Serve with spring greens and brown rice.

RICH IN Vitamins B3 (niacin), B6, B12 and D • Tryptophan • Omega 3

USEFUL FOR Heart ①②③ • Bones ①② • Digestion ③④ • Skin, hair & nails ①②③ • Mind ① • Fatigue ②③ • Men ①② • Women ①③④

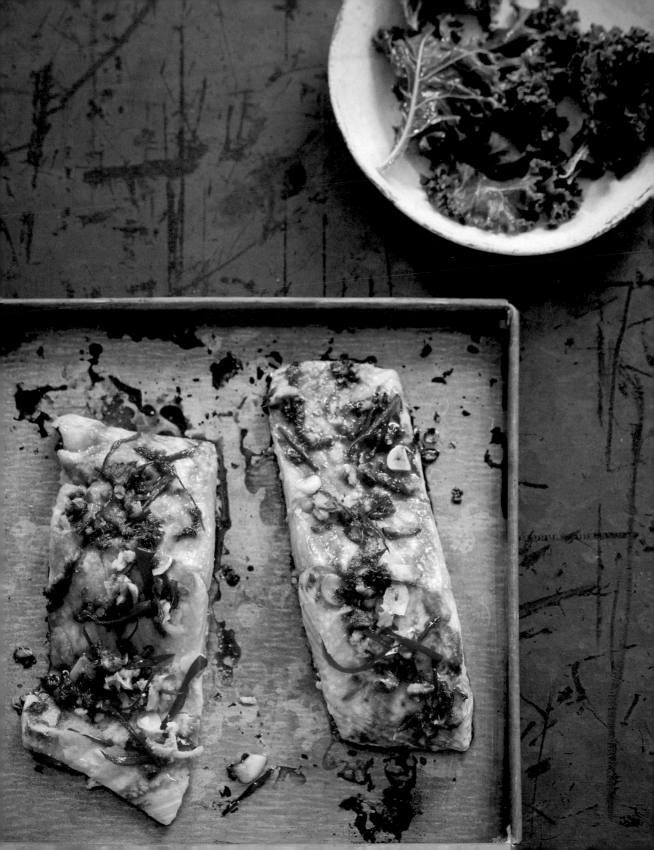

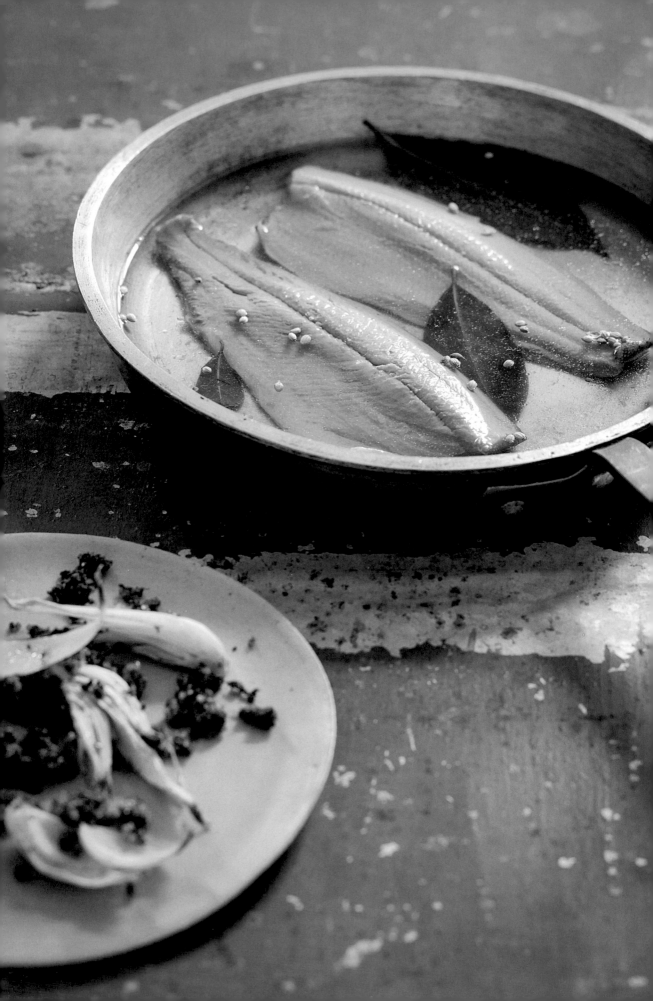

POACHED TROUT WITH FENNEL GRATIN

SERVES 2 • 420 CALORIES PER SERVING

Trout, with its rich flesh, is particularly delicious when poached. The soft texture that this cooking method lends complements the bold flavour of the fish. Omega 3 fatty acids found in trout and other oily fish may help to relieve the symptoms of rheumatoid arthritis, including joint pain and morning stiffness. A crisp, light fennel gratin works well with this fish dish as an alternative to new potatoes.

1.2 litres vegetable stock (see page 283)
2–3 bay leaves
2 trout fillets

FOR THE GRATIN
1 large fennel bulb (about 200g)
1 tsp fennel seeds
1 tsp coriander seeds
3 slices of gluten-free bread
Grated zest of 1 lemon
A handful of fresh chives, chopped
A handful of fresh coriander, chopped
1 tbsp olive oil
1 tsp flaked sea salt
½ tsp cracked black pepper

1 Preheat your oven to 200°C/fan 180°C/gas 6.
2 Trim the fennel bulb, then cut it lengthways, through the root, into slices about 1.5cm thick. Bring a pan of water to the boil on a high heat. Add the fennel and blanch for 4 minutes. Drain and spread out in a deep baking tray.
3 Place the rest of the gratin ingredients in a blender and blitz to rough crumbs. Sprinkle evenly over the fennel. Bake for 25 minutes.
4 While the gratin is baking, pour the stock into a shallow, wide pan and add the bay leaves. Bring to the boil, then reduce to a simmer. Gently place the fish in the stock and poach for about 8 minutes until cooked through.
5 Carefully lift the trout out of the stock and serve with the fennel gratin.

RICH IN Vitamins B6, B12, C and D • Folate • Potassium • Magnesium • Calcium • Selenium • Omega 3 • Beta-carotene • Tryptophan • Fibre

USEFUL FOR Heart ③ • Bones ①② • Digestion ① • Immunity ① • Skin, hair & nails ①③ • Mind ①② • Fatigue ③⑤ • Men ① • Women ①③④

HALIBUT WITH CHICKPEA STEW & PESTO

SERVES 4 • 340 CALORIES PER SERVING

This rustic, Italian-influenced stew makes a warming and filling dinner. Each serving is topped with a piece of fresh halibut that lightly flakes off and soaks up the sauce. The rapeseed oil and sunflower seeds in the dish make it very rich in vitamin E. Our bodies need this antioxidant to help keep the immune system strong to fight off harmful viruses.

1 tbsp rapeseed oil
4 pieces of halibut fillet, 110–130g each

FOR THE STEW
1 tbsp rapeseed oil
1 onion, chopped
1 fennel bulb, finely chopped
2 celery sticks, thinly sliced
2 small carrots, thinly sliced
1 yellow pepper, seeded and thinly sliced
400g tin cherry tomatoes
A handful of fresh flat-leaf parsley, finely chopped
1 tsp dried oregano
1 tsp dried thyme
300ml vegetable stock (see page 283)
400g tin chickpeas, drained and rinsed

FOR THE PESTO
A bunch of fresh basil
A handful of fresh flat-leaf parsley, leaves picked
1 garlic clove
A handful of toasted sunflower seeds
1 tbsp olive oil
Grated zest of ½ lemon
Salt and pepper

1 First make the stew. Heat the oil in a saucepan over a medium heat and cook the onion and fennel for a few minutes until the onion is slightly translucent. Add the celery, carrots and yellow pepper and cook for a further 5 minutes, stirring occasionally.

2 Add the tinned tomatoes, herbs and stock and stir well. Bring to the boil. Boil for 2 minutes, then reduce the heat, cover the pan and simmer for 40 minutes.

3 Meanwhile, make the pesto (keep a few basil leaves for the garnish). You can do this either by very finely chopping the herbs and garlic, then crushing the seeds in a mortar and pestle and pounding with the other ingredients, or by putting everything in a blender and blitzing for a few seconds to make a coarse paste. Set the pesto to one side.

4 Once the stew has been cooking for 40 minutes, stir in the chickpeas and cook for a further 7 minutes to heat them through. Add salt and pepper to taste.

5 While the chickpeas are heating through, set a large frying pan on a high heat and add the rapeseed oil. Once hot, place the halibut fillets, skin-side down, in the pan. When you put in each fillet, gently hold it down with your fingers for a few seconds so that it lies flat and will cook evenly. Then leave the fillets to cook for about 4 minutes. Gently flip them over and cook for a further 2 minutes.

6 Ladle the stew into four pasta bowls and place a halibut fillet on top of each. Garnish with the pesto and a few basil leaves.

RICH IN Vitamins B6, B12, C and E • Folate • Potassium • Iron • Magnesium • Calcium • Lycopene • Beta-carotene • Tryptophan • Fibre

USEFUL FOR Heart ①②③ • Bones ① • Digestion ① • Immunity ① • Skin, hair & nails ①③ • Mind ①② • Fatigue ①③⑤ • Men ① • Women ①③

KERALAN FISH CURRY

SERVES 4 • 205 CALORIES PER SERVING

This delicious dish is typically very tangy. In Kerala it is made with a fruit called kocum (*Garcinia indica*), which provides a sharpness similar to tamarind. Kocum isn't available in the UK, so we have used lime juice to achieve the same sour taste. This is a beautifully light curry, perfect for a weekday dinner.

1 tsp coconut oil
½ tsp fenugreek seeds
½ tsp mustard seeds
1 red onion, finely sliced
A thumb-sized piece of fresh ginger, grated with the skin on
1 garlic clove, finely chopped
1 fresh green chilli, finely chopped
5 curry leaves
1 tsp chilli powder
1 tsp ground coriander
½ tsp ground turmeric
4 vine tomatoes, finely diced
Juice of 1 lime
400g skinless white fish fillet, diced
1 tsp salt
200ml coconut milk

1 Heat the coconut oil in a medium-sized pan over a medium heat. Add the fenugreek and mustard seeds and cook for 1–2 minutes. Add the onion, ginger, garlic, green chilli and curry leaves and cook, stirring, for about 5 minutes until the onion is soft.
2 Stir in the chilli powder, coriander and turmeric, then add the tomatoes, 100ml water and the lime juice. Mix well. Bring to the boil, then reduce to a simmer. Add the fish and salt and simmer gently for 10 minutes.
3 Pour in the coconut milk and stir, then leave to simmer for a further 3 minutes to heat through. Serve with brown rice or quinoa.

RICH IN Vitamins B6, B12 and C • Selenium • Potassium

USEFUL FOR Heart ② • Mind ① • Men ① • Women ①

BAKED SEA BREAM WITH BRAISED LEEKS

SERVES 2 • 380 CALORIES PER SERVING

So delicious is fresh sea bream that it doesn't need to be served with anything flashy. Braised leeks are perfect – simple and flavoursome, with a good crunchy texture to accompany the soft fish. Leeks are rich in prebiotics that help to keep your gut healthy because they enable good bacteria to flourish.

2 sea bream fillets
Grated zest of 1 lemon
1 garlic clove, finely sliced
1 tbsp olive oil
A pinch of flaked sea salt

FOR THE LEEKS

3 leeks
1 tbsp olive oil
1 garlic clove, finely sliced
1 tbsp sunflower seeds
300ml vegetable stock (see page 283)
Salt and pepper

1 Preheat your grill to medium.
2 Place the bream on a chopping board and gently score the skin, making sure not to cut through into the flesh, then transfer the fillets, skin-side up, to a small baking tray.
3 Mix together the lemon zest, garlic and olive oil in a little bowl. Pour over the fish and sprinkle with the sea salt. Grill for 12 minutes (no need to turn the fillets).
4 Meanwhile, cut the leeks in half lengthways, then cut each half into three long strips. Set a non-stick frying pan on a high heat and add the oil. Once hot, add the leeks, garlic and sunflower seeds and shake the pan so everything is mixed with the oil and heats evenly. Cook for 2 minutes, shaking the pan, then add the stock and a pinch each of salt and pepper. Simmer for 10 minutes.
5 Serve the bream on top of the leeks.

RICH IN Vitamins B1 (thiamin), B6, B12, C and E • Folate • Potassium • Iron • Tryptophan • Prebiotics • Fibre

USEFUL FOR Heart ① • Digestion ② • Immunity ① • Mind ① • Fatigue ①③ • Women ①③

STEAMED SEA BASS WITH GINGER & GREEN CHILLI, WITH PAK CHOI

SERVES 2 • 230 CALORIES PER SERVING

The soft, sweet flesh of sea bass is the perfect backdrop for hot ginger and chilli. The fish is cooked by wrapping it in foil and steaming. This allows all the intense flavours to permeate the flesh and it becomes beautifully moist. It's served with the tastiest of Asian vegetables, pak choi, a slightly sweet, leafy Chinese cabbage, which is briefly cooked with garlic and tamari (this is a great gluten-free alternative to soy sauce).

2 sea bass fillets
A thumb-sized piece of fresh ginger, peeled and cut in julienne
1 fresh green chilli, seeded and finely sliced
1 spring onion, finely sliced
2 slices of lemon
1 tsp rapeseed oil
1 garlic clove, finely sliced
1 tbsp tamari
200g pak choi, cut lengthways into eighths
Lime wedges, to serve

1 Preheat your oven to 200°C/fan 180°C/gas 6 (or bring water to the boil in the bottom of a steamer).
2 Lay out two pieces of foil about 20cm square. Place a sea bass fillet in the centre of each piece and add half of the ginger, chilli and spring onion to each. Top each fillet with a slice of lemon. Fold the foil over the fish and fold in the edges to seal.
3 Place the parcels on a baking tray and bake in the heated oven for 15 minutes (or set the parcels on the rack in the steamer to cook for 10 minutes).
4 Meanwhile, set a large frying pan on medium heat and add the oil, then add the garlic and cook for 1 minute until golden. Add the tamari along with 1 tablespoon water, then put the pak choi in the pan. Cook for 1 minute.
5 Serve the fish with the pak choi and with lime wedges for squeezing over.

RICH IN Vitamins B6, B12 and C • Calcium • Iron • Tryptophan

USEFUL FOR Bones ① • Immunity ① • Mind ① • Fatigue ① • Women ①

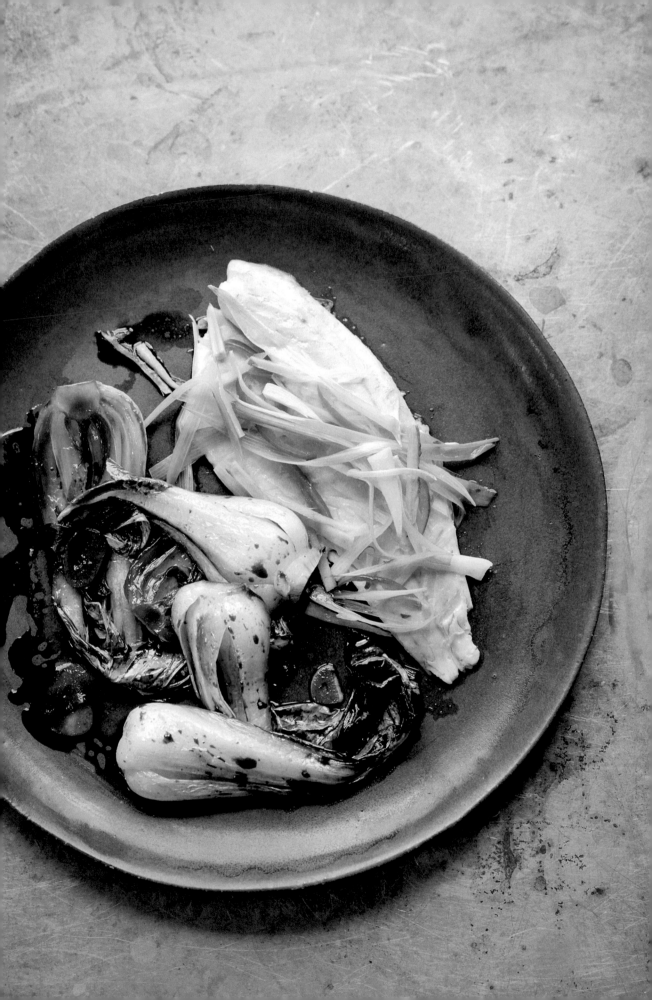

POLLOCK WITH TEMPURA GREEN BEAN CHIPS

SERVES 2 • 415 CALORIES PER SERVING

This dish is a lighter take on the classic British fish and chips. Pollock is succulent, meaty and flaky, perfect for roasting. Green beans deep-fried in a light tempura batter are gorgeous with it. These 'chips' may not be the healthiest side we've ever created, but they are certainly better than those made with potatoes.

200ml rapeseed oil

2 pieces of pollock fillet, 100–120g each

125g gluten- and wheat-free flour

A pinch of salt

1 egg

200ml sparkling water

250g green beans

Lemon wedges, to serve

1 Preheat your oven to 200°C/fan 180°C/gas 6.

2 Set a frying pan on the hob and add a drop or two of the rapeseed oil. Place the pollock fillets skin-side down in the pan and hold them down with your fingertips for a few seconds. Then continue to fry for 5 minutes. Transfer the fish to a baking tray and roast in the heated oven for 8 minutes.

3 While the fish is cooking, heat the remaining rapeseed oil in a saucepan to 160°C. (You can test if the oil is ready by dropping in a bread cube: it should turn golden in about 30 seconds.) Mix together the flour, salt, egg and sparkling water in a bowl to make a batter. Drop in the green beans and turn to coat thinly.

4 You'll need to fry the green beans in batches of about six at a time, to ensure they don't stick together. Lift a batch of beans out of the batter, shaking off the excess, then gently drop into the hot oil. Fry for 45–60 seconds until lightly golden on both sides. As each batch is cooked, remove and wrap it in kitchen paper to drain off the excess oil. Keep warm while you cook the other batches.

5 Serve the pollock with the green bean chips and lemon wedges.

RICH IN B vitamins • Vitamin C • Selenium • Potassium • Magnesium

USEFUL FOR Bones ① • Immunity ① • Mind ①② • Fatigue ③⑤ • Men ① • Women ①

POLLOCK & PRAWN FISHCAKES WITH COURGETTE SPAGHETTI

SERVES 2 • 460 CALORIES PER SERVING

Fishcakes are our friend Ed's speciality, so we nabbed his recipe and created this wheat-free version. The key is to take time preparing the fish, cutting it into tiny pieces rather than blitzing it in a blender. It offers a much more interesting texture. Courgette spaghetti adds freshness to the dish and is a lower calorie substitute for traditional pasta. For a more substantial dinner you could also serve some brown rice.

150g piece of skinless pollock fillet

6 raw king prawns, peeled

1 garlic clove, finely chopped

1 tsp capers, roughly chopped

Grated zest of 1 lemon

A pinch of crushed dried chilli

1 heaped tbsp gluten- and wheat-free flour

½ tsp bicarbonate of soda

1 tbsp olive oil

2 courgettes

Lemon wedges, to serve

FOR THE PESTO

30g sunflower seeds

1 tbsp finely chopped fresh coriander

4 fresh mint leaves

3 fresh chives, chopped

30g cashew nuts

Juice of ½ lemon

2 tbsp rapeseed oil

Salt and pepper

1 Finely dice the pollock fillet and prawns – you want tiny cubes that are about 5mm thick. Place the diced fish and prawns in a large mixing bowl. Add the garlic, capers, lemon zest, chilli, flour, bicarbonate of soda, a drizzle of the olive oil and a pinch each of salt and pepper. Mix together with your hands. Divide equally in half and shape each portion into a fishcake. Set aside.

2 To make the pesto, combine all the ingredients in a blender and blitz to a rough paste.

3 Set a non-stick frying pan on a medium heat. Add the rest of the olive oil and heat for about 30 seconds, then add the fishcakes. Cook for 6 minutes on each side, turning occasionally.

4 While the fishcakes are cooking, prepare the courgette spaghetti using a julienne peeler/cutter (stop when you get to the soft seeded centre). If you don't have a julienne peeler, you can grate the courgettes. It won't give the same effect, but it will still taste great.

5 Set a small pan on a medium heat, put the pesto in it and heat for 3 minutes. Add the courgette spaghetti and heat for another 3 minutes, stirring occasionally.

6 Serve the fishcakes on top of the pesto-dressed courgette spaghetti, with wedges of lemon.

RICH IN Vitamins B1 (thiamin), B12, C and E • Folate • Potassium • Selenium • Magnesium • Iron

USEFUL FOR Heart ②③ • Bones ① • Immunity ① • Mind ①② • Fatigue ③⑤ • Men ① • Women ③

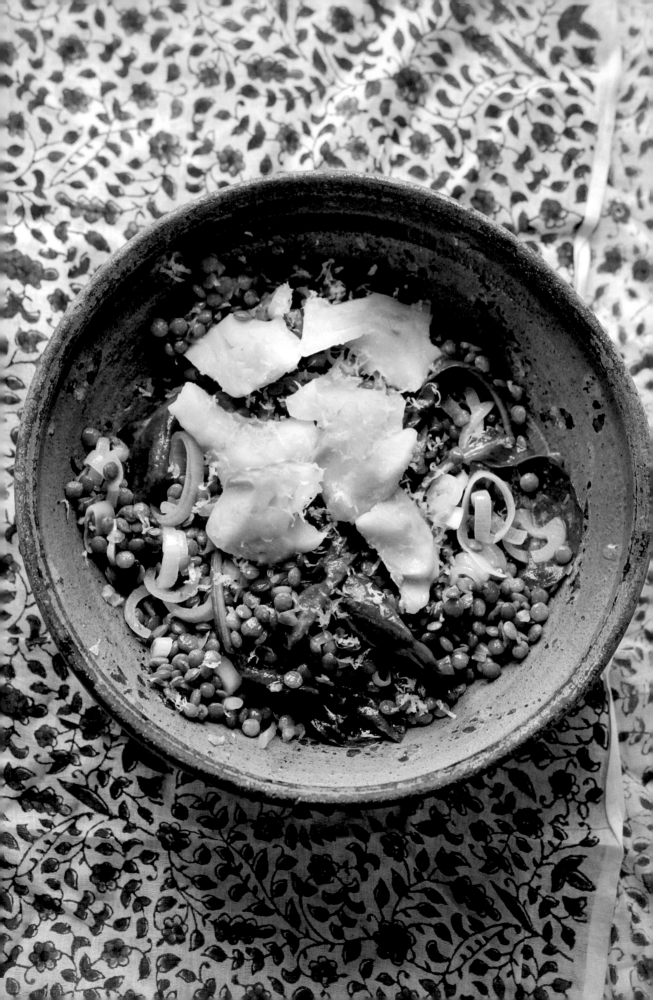

POLLOCK EN PAPILLOTE WITH BROWN LENTILS

SERVES 2 • 375 CALORIES PER SERVING

Cooking fish 'en papillote' (in paper) is a quick and easy technique that seals in lots of flavour. It also makes it less likely that you'll overcook the fish: 12–14 minutes of baking in a paper parcel results in flaky, succulent flesh. Here the pollock is served with some lemony lentils, but it also goes well with roasted vegetables.

RICH IN B vitamins • Selenium • Potassium • Iron • Magnesium • Zinc • Fibre

USEFUL FOR Heart ①②③ • Bones ① • Digestion ① • Skin, hair & nails ①④ • Mind ①② • Fatigue ①⑤ • Men ①② • Women ①

2 pieces of pollock fillet, 100–110g each
2 slices of lemon
2 garlic cloves, crushed with the skin on
2 sprigs of fresh thyme
1 tsp olive oil

FOR THE LENTILS
130g brown lentils
600ml vegetable stock (see page283)
1 bay leaf
1 tsp flaked sea salt
1 tbsp olive oil
3 shallots, sliced
1–2 garlic cloves, sliced
2 handfuls of spinach
Grated zest and juice of 1 lemon
1 tsp rapeseed oil
Salt and pepper

1 Preheat your oven to 200°C/fan 180°C/gas 6.
2 Lay out two 30cm squares of baking parchment and place a pollock fillet in the middle of each one. Set a lemon slice, garlic clove and sprig of thyme of top of each fillet. Add a drizzle of olive oil and seasoning of salt and pepper.
3 Gather up the edges of the paper and tie them together with string, ensuring there are no gaps. Place the parcels on a baking tray and bake in the heated oven for 12–14 minutes until the fish is just cooked.
4 Meanwhile, put the brown lentils in a saucepan with the vegetable stock, bay leaf, sea salt and a pinch of pepper. Bring to the boil and cook for 15 minutes until the lentils are tender. Drain in a sieve and tip into a large bowl.
5 Heat the olive oil in a non-stick frying pan, add the shallots and garlic, and cook for 5 minutes until translucent. Add the spinach with the lemon zest and cook for 1 minute until wilted.
6 Add the spinach to the lentils along with the lemon juice and rapeseed oil. Season well and toss to mix. Serve with the pollock.

MACKEREL & CUCUMBER GAZPACHO

SERVES 2 • 370 CALORIES PER SERVING

On a hot day, there is nothing quite like a chilled, refreshing cucumber gazpacho. On its own it is delicious but topped with a fresh mackerel fillet, it is transformed into a filling lunch. Mackerel is best between April and September, making this dish a top choice for a summer lunch. It will provide you with at least two of your five-a-day plus a healthy dose of omega 3 fatty acids.

1 tsp olive oil

2 mackerel fillets

1 tbsp plain soya yogurt

Shredded zest of ½ lemon

FOR THE GAZPACHO

1 cucumber

1 avocado

1 yellow pepper, seeded and roughly chopped

1 garlic clove

2 spring onions, roughly chopped

3 sprigs of fresh mint, leaves picked

Juice of 1 lemon

A handful of fresh chives

1 First make the gazpacho. Cut the cucumber in half lengthways and scoop out the seeds. Roughly chop the flesh, then place it in a blender. Cut the avocado in half and discard the stone; scoop the flesh into the blender. Add the yellow pepper, garlic, spring onions, mint leaves, lemon juice, chives and 75ml cold water to the blender. Blitz for about 2 minutes until smooth. Pour into a jug and leave to chill in the fridge.

2 Meanwhile, set a large frying pan on a high heat and drizzle in a little oil. Once hot, gently place the mackerel fillets, skin-side down, in the pan. Hold down with your fingers so that the fillets lie flat and cook for 3 minutes. Then gently turn them over and cook for a further 2 minutes.

3 Take the gazpacho out of the fridge and pour into two bowls. Top each with a warm mackerel fillet, a dollop of soya yogurt and sprinkle of lemon zest, then serve.

RICH IN B vitamins • Vitamins C, D and E • Potassium • Selenium • Omega 3 • Beta-sitosterol • Fibre

USEFUL FOR Heart ①②③ • Bones ①② • Digestion ① • Immunity ① • Skin, hair & nails ①②③ • Mind ① • Fatigue ②③ • Men ①② • Women ①③④

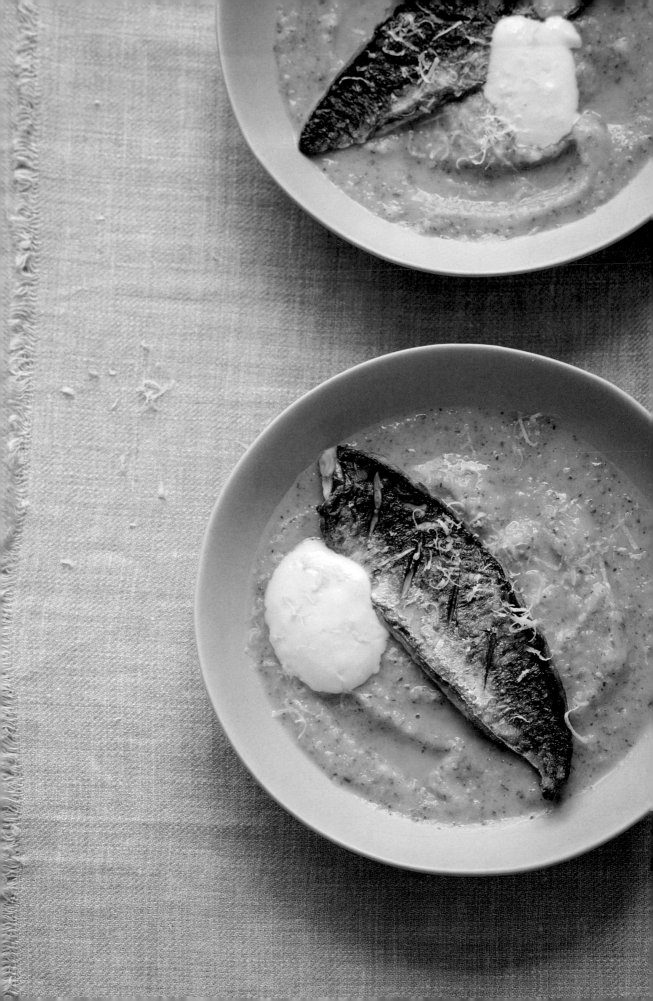

MACKEREL WITH WILD RICE, PEPPER & YOGURT SALAD

SERVES 2 • 600 CALORIES PER SERVING

There is something deeply appetising about freshly cooked fish topped with a creamy, tart dressing. Soya yogurt is a dairy-free option, and here we add some lemon zest to give it an extra punch. The lemon also works well with the smoky, salty flavour of the mackerel.

150g wild rice

1 tsp rapeseed oil

1 red onion, sliced

1 garlic clove, finely chopped

1 red pepper, seeded and finely sliced

1 green pepper, seeded and finely sliced

100g podded fresh peas

2 mackerel fillets

A handful of fresh coriander leaves, roughly chopped

A handful of fresh flat-leaf parsley, finely chopped

5 tbsp plain soya yogurt

½ cucumber, peeled, halved and sliced

Grated zest of 1 lemon

A handful of fresh mint leaves, finely chopped

A handful of fresh chives, finely chopped

Salt and pepper

1. Set a saucepan of water on a high heat and bring to the boil. Add the wild rice and cook for 20–25 minutes until tender.
2. Meanwhile, set a frying pan on a medium heat. Add a little of the rapeseed oil and then the onion, garlic and peppers. Cook for 10 minutes until soft. Add the peas and cook for a further 3 minutes. Tip into a large mixing bowl.
3. Wipe out the frying pan, then place it on a high heat and drizzle in a little more rapeseed oil. Once hot, gently place the mackerel fillets, skin-side down, in the pan. Hold the fillets down with your fingers so that they lie flat, and cook for 3 minutes. Then gently turn them over and cook for a further 2 minutes.
4. Once the wild rice is cooked, drain it and return to the pan. Stir the pepper mixture through the rice along with the coriander and parsley. Season with salt and pepper. Keep warm.
5. Mix the yogurt with the cucumber, lemon zest, mint and chives. Season to taste.
6. Spoon the wild rice salad into the centre of each plate and set a mackerel fillet on the rice. Top with a dollop of the cucumber yogurt. Serve with some steamed green beans.

RICH IN B vitamins • Vitamins C and D • Potassium • Selenium • Iron • Omega 3 • Beta-carotene • Phytoestrogens • Fibre

USEFUL FOR Heart ①②③ • Bones ② • Digestion ① • Immunity ① • Skin, hair & nails ①②③ • Mind ① • Fatigue ②③ • Men ①② • Women ①③④

GRILLED MACKEREL WITH GINGER & SAFFRON RICE

SERVES 2 • 585 CALORIES PER SERVING

It takes a rich, flavoursome fish like mackerel to stand up to bold flavours. Mackerel is packed full of heart-healthy omega 3 fatty acids, which have a powerful anti-inflammatory effect on the body.

200g brown rice
1 tsp salt
2 cloves
2 bay leaves
A small pinch of saffron threads
A handful of edamame beans, thawed if frozen
2 mackerel fillets
A thumb-sized pieces of fresh ginger, grated with the skin on
1 fresh green chilli, sliced
Juice of 1 lime
A pinch of flaked sea salt
1 tsp olive oil
2 handfuls of spinach, chopped
A handful of cherry tomatoes, finely chopped
Cracked black pepper

1 Preheat your grill to medium. Line a baking tray with greaseproof paper.
2 Put the rice in a saucepan and cover with three times its volume of water. Bring to the boil, then add the salt, cloves, bay leaves and saffron. Cook for 16 minutes. Add the edamame and cook for a further 2 minutes until the rice is tender. Drain in a sieve; discard the cloves and bay leaves.
3 While the rice is cooking, place the mackerel fillets, skin-side down, on the baking tray. Top each fillet with half of the ginger, chilli, lime juice and sea salt and add a drizzle of olive oil. Grill for 6 minutes until the mackerel is cooked.
4 Serve the mackerel on top of the rice with the chopped spinach and tomatoes, and a sprinkle of freshly cracked black pepper.

RICH IN B vitamins • Vitamin D • Selenium • Potassium • Magnesium • Phytoestrogens • Omega 3 • Tryptophan • Beta-carotene

USEFUL FOR Heart ①②③ • Bones ①② • Digestion ① • Immunity ① • Skin, hair & nails ①②③ • Mind ①② • Fatigue ②③⑤ • Men ①② • Women ①③④

SEARED TUNA & BEETROOT SALAD

SERVES 2 • 360 CALORIES PER SERVING

Fresh tuna steaks make a delicious and quick weekday dinner. Searing is the best way to cook this wonderfully meaty fish, retaining its rich strong flavour. When buying your tuna, make sure to pick steaks with dark red flesh, and avoid using bluefin tuna as this is an endangered species. Here the tuna is served with a chilli-spiked beetroot and raisin salad. The dish is very high in vitamin B12, which is essential for blood health, fighting off tiredness and fatigue.

2 raw beetroots
Juice of 1 lemon
½ fresh green chilli, seeded and finely diced
1 red onion, very finely sliced
A handful of raisins
A pinch of salt
A pinch of pepper
2 tsp olive oil
2 tuna steaks, patted dry
A handful of fresh coriander, roughly chopped
1 tsp black sesame seeds
Lime wedges, to serve

1 Peel and finely grate the beetroots. Tip into a bowl and cover with the lemon juice, green chilli, red onion, raisins, salt and pepper. Mix together, then set aside.
2 Set a frying pan on a high heat and add the oil, then gently place the tuna steaks in the pan. For medium rare tuna, cook the steaks for 3 minutes on each side. If you would prefer the tuna to be completely cooked through, cook for 5 minutes on each side, but turn the heat to medium/low after 2 minutes of cooking on each side.
3 Transfer the tuna to kitchen paper and pat off any excess oil. Place on the plates and sprinkle with the coriander and black sesame seeds. Cut each steak into four or five slices.
4 Serve with the beetroot salad on the side and wedges of lime.

RICH IN B vitamins • Vitamin C • Folate • Selenium • Potassium • Omega 3

USEFUL FOR Heart ①② • Bones ② • Digestion ③④ • Immunity ① • Skin, hair & nails ①②③ • Mind ① • Fatigue ② • Men ① • Women ①③④

SWEET TREATS

The recipes in this chapter truly are treats – delicious and indulgent. You might think it's impossible to make sweet treats without using refined sugar, but the recipes here will show you how achievable it is. Refined sugar has no place in the Detox Kitchen. We use only natural sugars – found in fruit (and some vegetables), honey and sweet spices – in moderation, plus raw cacao powder for a rich chocolate hit.

      Whilst our sweet treats may be high in calories (they are intended to be little 'treats' after all, to be enjoyed occasionally), they are still good for you. Natural sugars (from honey and fruit) and fat (from nuts and seeds) are indeed calorific, but they provide beneficial nutrients too, making the results healthier than biscuits, cakes and so on sweetened with refined sugar. You get much more bang for your buck by eating the right types of natural, whole foods.

      'Detox' baking can be a big challenge. You might expect to find yourself anxiously peering through the window of the oven door, praying that by some miracle your cake will rise. But don't worry. Although baking without wheat, dairy or refined sugar can be tricky at first, it is quickly mastered. You'll find that our recipes are very simple, and you'll soon be enjoying a truly guilt-free sweet treat.

At the end of most of the recipes, you'll find a list of the main nutrients supplied in a serving as well as a list of health issues that may be benefited by including the recipe in your healthy diet. For more, see page 9.

BANANA BREAD

CUTS INTO 8 SLICES • 335 CALORIES PER SLICE

If you ever have some overripe bananas lying around, use them for this recipe. The riper they are, the sweeter and lighter the bread will be. The addition of orange zest, cinnamon and nutmeg highlights the sweetness of the bananas and makes the loaf smell delicious. Bananas are a rich food source of potassium, and a slice of this bread will contribute 20 per cent of the RDA. You can make the mixture by hand or using a food processor.

350g bananas
50g runny honey
50g coconut oil
1 tsp ground cinnamon
A pinch of grated nutmeg
½ tsp bicarbonate of soda
Grated zest of ½ orange
½ vanilla pod, split open lengthways
4 eggs
200g ground almonds
2 tbsp flaked coconut
2 tbsp desiccated coconut

1 Preheat your oven to 200°C/fan 180°C/gas 6. Line a 10 x 24cm loaf tin with baking parchment.

2 Peel the bananas and cut a slice from one of them; keep for the decoration. Put the remaining banana flesh in a large bowl and, using a fork, mash to a chunky paste. Add the honey, coconut oil, cinnamon, nutmeg, bicarbonate of soda and orange zest. Scrape the seeds from the vanilla pod and add them. Mix everything together well. Add the eggs and beat in with a wooden spoon. Mix in the ground almonds until thoroughly amalgamated.

3 Tip the mixture into the lined loaf tin. Top with the flaked and desiccated coconut, and then with the reserved slice of banana. Bake in the heated oven for about 50 minutes until a wooden cocktail stick or skewer inserted into the centre of the loaf comes out dry.

4 Remove from the oven and allow to cool in the tin for 20 minutes, then turn out on to a wire rack and leave to cool completely. The bread can be kept in an airtight container in the fridge for up to 5 days.

RICH IN Vitamin E • Beta-sitosterol

USEFUL FOR Heart ① • Men ① • Women ③

ORANGE & CRANBERRY DROPS

MAKES 18 DROPS • 90 CALORIES EACH

We make these little biscuits to sell in our deli at Christmas – we wanted to create a little gift bag of spiced seasonal treats, and these perfectly sum up the holiday's flavour. Nuts and seeds provide a source of monounsaturated fats that are beneficial for heart health when eaten in place of saturated fats.

50g gluten- and wheat-free flour
½ tsp baking powder
100g ground almonds
25g flaked almonds, plus 1 tbsp to finish
25g pumpkin seeds
25g sunflower seeds
Grated zest of ½ orange
A pinch of ground cinnamon
A pinch of ground cloves
A pinch of grated nutmeg
1 tsp runny honey
50g dried cranberries
3 egg whites

1 Preheat your oven to 200°C/fan 180°C/gas 6. Line a baking tray with baking parchment.
2 Sift the flour and baking powder into a large mixing bowl and add the remaining ingredients, except for the egg whites. Mix together with your hands.
3 In another bowl, whisk the egg whites to stiff peaks. Gently fold them into the spicy mixture with a large metal spoon until completely combined.
4 Roll the mixture into small balls and place them on the baking tray. Place a flaked almond on top of each ball.
5 Bake in the heated oven for 12–14 minutes until lightly golden. Leave to cool on the tray for 5 minutes, then transfer to a wire rack to finish cooling. The drops can be kept in an airtight container for 5 days.

MINI CARROT & ORANGE MUFFINS

MAKES 12 MINI MUFFINS • 140 CALORIES EACH

These little muffins are just bursting with wonderful flavours. While they're baking, their sweet spiced scent fills the kitchen. Enjoy them as a pudding, with a fruit such as blueberries, or on their own as a snack. Carrots and other orange fruits and vegetables provide essential nutrients that support good eye health.

75g gluten- and wheat-free flour
¼ tsp baking powder
55g ground almonds
1 tbsp arrowroot powder
A pinch of salt
1 tsp ground cinnamon
1 tsp ground allspice
4 egg whites
110g runny honey
1½ tbsp rapeseed oil
2 carrots, grated
Grated zest of 1 orange

1 Preheat your oven to 200°C/fan 180°C/gas 6. Line a 12-hole mini muffin tin with mini paper cases.
2 Sift the flour and baking powder into a large mixing bowl. Add the almonds, arrowroot, salt and spices and stir with a wooden spoon.
3 Put the egg whites, honey and oil in a blender or food processor and blitz until smooth and thickened.
4 Gradually stir the egg white mixture into the dry ingredients in the bowl, then add the carrots and orange zest and mix thoroughly with a wooden spoon. Pour the mixture into a jug to make it easier to distribute among the muffin cases. Fill each case just over halfway.
5 Bake in the heated oven for 35 minutes. Transfer the muffins to a wire rack and leave to cool completely. They can be kept for 3 days in an airtight container.

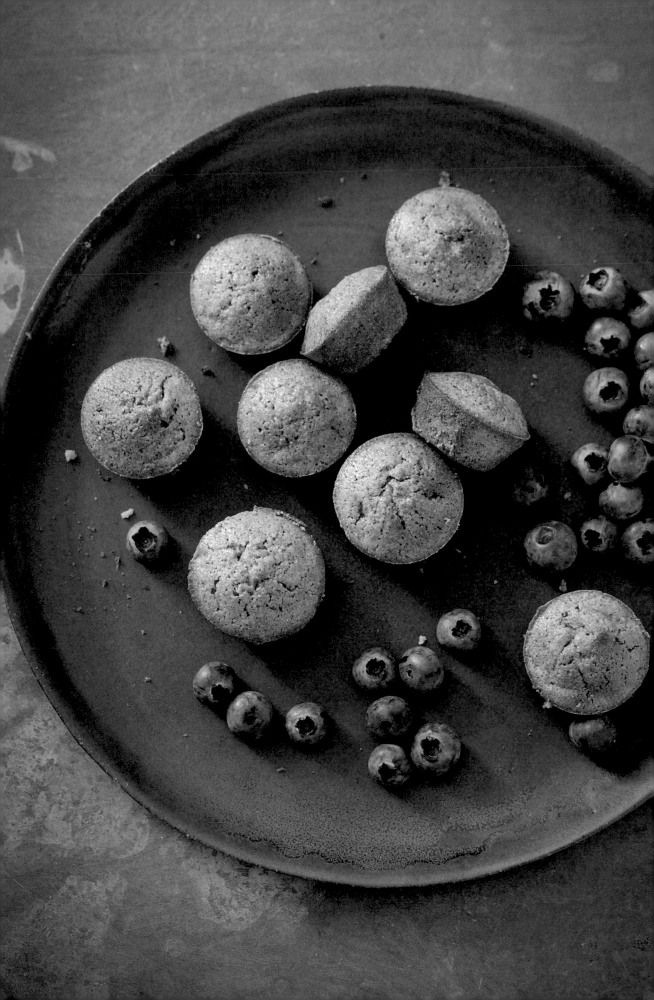

MINI MINCE PIES

MAKES 12 MINI PIES • 160 CALORIES EACH

These little beauties are crisp, golden and fat, as mince pies should be. Traditional shortcrust is replaced with an almond pastry, which is just as easy to make. If you want a decorative top pastry lid, it's worth investing in some little star cutters.

FOR THE FILLING

100g raisins

50g sultanas

50g dried goji berries

Grated zest and juice of 1 orange

1 tsp runny honey

1 tsp ground cinnamon

FOR THE PASTRY

250g ground almonds

2 tbsp runny honey

2 tbsp rapeseed oil

1 egg

½ vanilla pod, split open lengthways

1 tbsp gluten- and wheat-free flour, for dusting

1 To make the filling, put all the ingredients in a bowl and mix together well. Cover with clingfilm and leave to macerate in the fridge for at least 3 hours, or overnight if possible.

2 To make the pastry, combine the almonds, honey, oil and egg in a large bowl. Scrape the seeds from the vanilla pod and add to the bowl. Mix everything together with your hands to make a fairly dry mixture. Transfer to a board and add 50ml water. Work the mixture into a dough, then cover with clingfilm and leave to rest in the fridge for 1 hour.

3 Preheat your oven to 200°C/fan 180°C/gas 6. Flour a 12-hole mini muffin tin.

4 Remove the pastry from the fridge. Dust your work surface with a little flour and roll out the pastry to about 3mm thick. Cut out 3cm rounds and place them carefully into the holes in the muffin tin to line the bottom and side of each one. Gather the trimmings, roll out again and cut out a top for each pie (preferably star-shaped).

5 Fill each pastry case with the fruit mixture and cover with a pastry top. Bake for 25 minutes until golden and crisp. Allow to cool slightly in the tin, then remove carefully – the pastry can be crumbly whilst hot but will firm up once cool.

RICH IN Vitamin E

USEFUL FOR Women ③

OAT SCONES

MAKES 12 SCONES • 210 CALORIES EACH

These are perfect little treats for an afternoon tea. Made with a wheat-free dough, they tend to be more crumbly than classic scones, but topped with a little nut butter and some jam (see recipe for Apricot & Ginger Jam on page 71), they are an afternoon delight. They are very high in a mineral called manganese, which is essential for the proper functioning of the thyroid hormone that helps to control metabolism.

300g porridge oats, plus extra for topping
½ tsp bicarbonate of soda
100g runny honey
2 tbsp olive oil
A pinch of ground cinnamon
1 banana
150g sultanas

TO SERVE
Cashew Nut Butter (see page 63)
Jam

1 Preheat your oven to 200°C/fan 180°C/gas 6. Line a baking tray with greaseproof paper.
2 Put the oats, bicarbonate of soda, honey, oil, cinnamon and banana flesh in a blender and blitz until a soft dough forms. Add the sultanas and mix in by hand or with a spoon.
3 Turn out the dough on to a lightly floured surface and flatten to about 2.5cm. Using a 5cm round cutter, stamp out circles – you should get 12 (you'll need to gather up the trimmings and roll out again). Sprinkle extra oats on the top of each round.
4 Place them on the lined baking tray. Bake in the heated oven for 15–20 minutes until lightly golden. Allow to cool before serving.

RICH IN Fibre

USEFUL FOR Heart ① • Digestion ①

APPLE, BLACKBERRY & COCONUT CUPCAKES

MAKES 12 CUPCAKES • 150 CALORIES EACH

Here is a cupcake that, although free of wheat, dairy and refined sugar, still gives you a feeling of indulgence. The apple creates a lovely soft texture, and the plump blackberries add a touch of tartness, perfectly complemented by the sweet coconut. Blackberries, along with other purple and blue fruits, contain a plant chemical called ellagic acid, which acts as an antioxidant that helps to protect the body against cancer.

100g gluten- and wheat-free flour
100g ground almonds
1 tbsp arrowroot powder
1 tsp salt
¼ tsp baking powder
1 tsp ground cinnamon
2 eating apples, peeled, cored and finely diced
5 eggs
1 tbsp rapeseed oil
2 tbsp coconut milk
3 tbsp runny honey
24–36 blackberries (2–3 for each cupcake)
Desiccated coconut, to sprinkle

1 Preheat your oven to 200°C/fan 180°C/gas 6. Line a 12-hole cupcake tin with paper cases.
2 Sift the dry ingredients into a large bowl.
3 Put the diced apples in a small saucepan with a splash of water and cook on a low heat for 6–8 minutes until soft, adding more water if the apples begin to stick. Drain the apples and place in a blender. Add the eggs, oil, coconut milk and honey and blitz until smooth.
4 Add the apple mixture to the bowl and fold with the dry ingredients until completely combined. Pour the mixture into a jug, then fill each paper case to just over halfway. Place two to three blackberries on each cupcake and sprinkle with desiccated coconut.
5 Bake in the heated oven for 30 35 minutes until firm to the touch. Leave to cool in the tin for about 10 minutes, then transfer to a wire rack to finish cooling. These are best freshly baked but can be kept for a day.

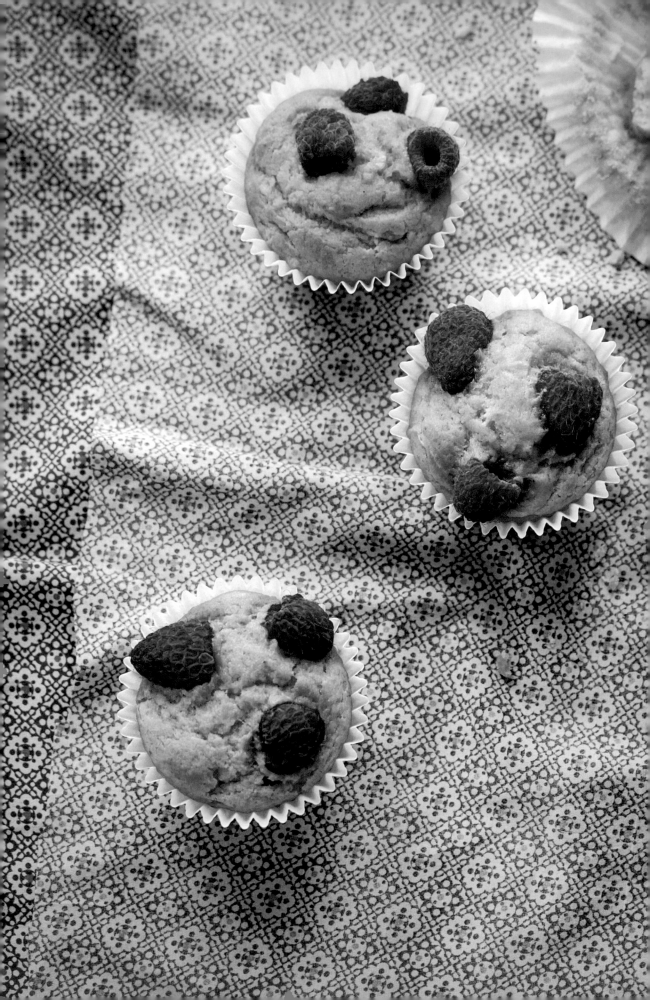

SPICED MUFFINS

MAKES 8 MUFFINS • 380 CALORIES EACH

These delicious muffins have a lovely sweet and aromatic flavour. At the Detox Kitchen we make pumpkin purée in large batches and freeze it – it is a great addition to cakes, giving them an earthy sweet flavour. The use of rapeseed oil in these muffins provides 30 per cent of the RDA for vitamin E, which acts as an antioxidant, helping maintain a good strong immune system.

FOR THE PUMPKIN PURÉE

200g peeled pumpkin flesh, diced
1 tbsp rapeseed oil
1 tsp ground cinnamon

FOR THE MUFFINS

300g gluten- and wheat-free flour
1½ tsp baking powder
½ tsp bicarbonate of soda
½ tsp salt
1 tsp ground cinnamon
1 tbsp grated fresh ginger
100ml rapeseed oil
300g runny honey
Raspberries, for topping

1 Preheat your oven to 190°C/fan 170°C/gas 5. Line an 8-hole muffin tin with paper cases.
2 To make the pumpkin purée, spread the pieces of pumpkin in a roasting tin. Drizzle the rapeseed oil over them and sprinkle with the cinnamon. Roast for 40 minutes until soft. Leave to cool, then transfer the pumpkin to a blender or food processor and blitz to a purée. You need 200g purée for the muffins.
3 In a bowl, whisk together the flour, baking powder, bicarbonate of soda, salt, cinnamon and ginger. Whisk the oil and honey together in a jug, then add to the dry ingredients and whisk to make a smooth mixture.
4 Gently fold in the pumpkin purée until well distributed throughout the mixture.
5 Pour into the muffin cases, filling them equally, and put a few raspberries on top of each. Bake in the heated oven for 15–20 minutes until the muffins bounce back when gently pressed in the centre. Leave them to cool in the tin and serve at room temperature.

RICH IN Vitamin E

USEFUL FOR Men ① • Women ③

BEETROOT, APPLE, CARROT & GINGER CAKE

CUTS INTO 12 PIECES • 305 CALORIES EACH

Moist and sweet, this cake is beautifully colourful. The fat used is sunflower oil, which is a very rich source of vitamin E – 1 tablespoon provides nearly 50 per cent of the RDA. It is not an oil we use on a daily basis but works well in cakes and is a useful way of gleaning this nutrient.

175g runny honey
175ml sunflower oil
3 eggs
2 small eating apples, peeled, cored and grated
100g grated carrots
100g grated raw beetroot
1 tbsp ground ginger
A thumb-sized piece of fresh ginger, peeled and finely grated
30g walnuts, roughly chopped
50g raisins
50g pitted dates, finely chopped
Grated zest of 1 orange
170g gluten- and wheat-free flour
1 tsp bicarbonate of soda
1 tsp baking powder
1 tsp ground cinnamon
½ tsp grated nutmeg
10g flaxseeds

1 Preheat your oven to 190°C/fan 170°C/gas 5. Grease an 18cm round, loose-based cake tin with olive oil (cover your fingertips with oil and run them over the bottom and side of the tin).
2 Combine the honey, sunflower oil and eggs in a bowl and whisk until slightly fluffy. Add the apples, carrots and beetroot and stir into the egg mixture. Add the ginger, walnuts, raisins, dates and orange zest and mix well. Now sift in the flour, bicarbonate of soda, baking powder, cinnamon and nutmeg and fold together.
3 Pour the mixture into the tin and sprinkle the flaxseeds over the top. Bake in the heated oven for about 40 minutes until a skewer inserted into the centre of the cake comes out clean. Leave to cool in the tin for 10 minutes, then turn out on to a wire rack to finish cooling. The cake can be kept for 3 days in an airtight container.

RICH IN Vitamin E

USEFUL FOR Women ③

APPLE & GINGER CAKE

CUTS INTO 8 PIECES • 205 CALORIES PER PIECE

The smell of a home-made apple cake baking is very comforting. This one has a slightly crumbly texture, wetter than your average sponge cake, and it's perfectly sweet. There are no strong binding ingredients, so it's really important to let the cake cool and set before slicing, otherwise it will crumble apart. Red-skinned apples are rich in an antioxidant called quercetin, which acts as a powerful anti-inflammatory in the body.

2 eggs
2 tbsp rapeseed oil
100g runny honey
6 large, juicy, red-skinned eating apples, cored and cut into 1cm cubes
200g ground almonds
100g flaked almonds
A thumb-sized piece of fresh ginger, peeled and finely grated
1 tsp ground ginger
1 tsp mixed spice
½ vanilla pod, split open lengthways
70g pecans

1 Preheat your oven to 180°C/160°C/gas 4. Line the bottom of an 18cm round loose-based cake tin with baking parchment.
2 Put the eggs, oil and honey into a large mixing bowl and whisk together for a few minutes to combine and create a smooth, light texture. Add the apples, ground and flaked almonds, fresh and ground ginger, and mixed spice. Scrape the seeds from the vanilla pod and add to the bowl. Mix everything together well.
3 Transfer the mixture to the prepared cake tin. Cover the top with the pecans. Bake in the heated oven for about 1 hour and 10 minutes until a skewer inserted into the centre comes out clean.
4 Remove from the oven and leave to cool for 30 minutes, then place the tin in the fridge to cool completely for at least 2 hours.
5 Remove the cake from the tin and serve, or place in an airtight container. The cake can be kept for up to 5 days.

RICH IN Vitamin E

USEFUL FOR Women ③

COCONUT MACAROONS

MAKES 18 MINI MACAROONS • 150 CALORIES EACH

The perfect coconut macaroon should be crunchy on the outside and chewy in the middle. We think shredded coconut makes for a wetter, chewier centre than desiccated, and like the macaroons to be slightly golden. If you would prefer a whiter finish, cook for slightly less time.

1 tbsp cacao butter
100g shredded coconut
100g ground almonds
1½ tbsp runny honey
A pinch of flaked sea salt
½ vanilla pod, split open lengthways
2 egg whites

1 Preheat your oven to 170°C/fan 150°C/gas 3. Line a baking tray with baking parchment.
2 Melt the cacao butter, either in the microwave or in a heatproof bowl set over a pan of boiling water. Pour the melted butter into a blender or food processor and add the shredded coconut, ground almonds, honey and salt. Scrape the seeds from the vanilla pod and add them to the blender. Blitz for a few seconds to combine, then transfer to a bowl.
3 In another bowl, whisk the egg whites to stiff peaks. Fold into the coconut mixture.
4 Form into little balls and place on the baking tray. Bake in the heated oven for 20–25 minutes until the macaroons are firm to the touch. Leave to cool on the tray for 5 minutes, then transfer to a wire rack to finish cooling. The macaroons can be kept in an airtight tin for up to 3 days.

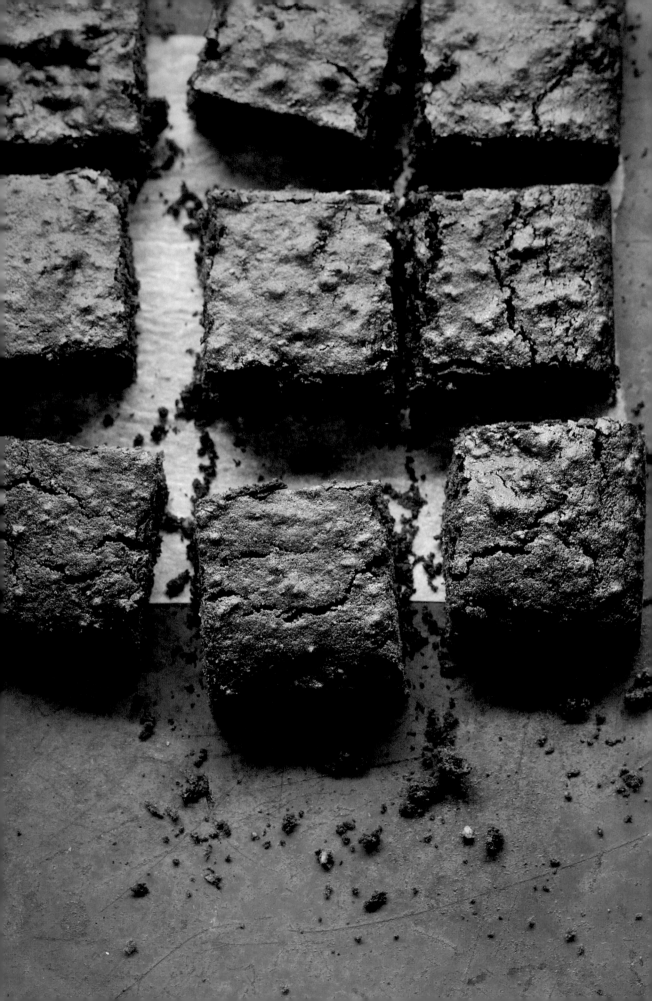

BEETROOT BROWNIES

MAKES 9 BROWNIES • 260 CALORIES EACH

Brownies can be far too sweet. These, though, are just right. The beetroot keeps them moist and gives them a lovely earthy flavour, whilst also giving them a brilliant deep red colour. Raw cacao powder contains no sugar and is much richer in nutrients than drinking chocolate.

150g peeled raw beetroot, cut into small cubes
50g hazelnuts
100g gluten- and wheat-free flour
1 tsp baking powder
60g raw cacao powder
150g runny honey
½ tsp salt
3 eggs
75ml rapeseed oil

1 Preheat your oven to 200°C/fan 180°C/gas 6. Line the bottom and sides of a 20cm square cake tin with greaseproof paper.

2 Put the beetroot in a microwave-safe bowl with 50ml water, cover with clingfilm and cook on a high heat for 7 minutes until soft. If you don't have a microwave, wrap the beetroot in foil and bake in the heated oven for about 40 minutes until soft.

3 Put the hazelnuts in a blender and blitz until they are roughly chopped. Transfer them to a large mixing bowl. Sift in the flour, baking powder and cacao powder.

4 Now blitz the cooked beetroot in the blender for 1–2 minutes until smooth. Add to the dry ingredients in the bowl but do not mix just yet.

5 Using the blender for the third time, put the honey, salt and eggs in it and blitz for 3 minutes. Pour into the bowl and mix with the rest of the ingredients using a wooden spoon. Be gentle, as you want to keep air in the mixture whilst combining it thoroughly.

6 Pour the mixture into the prepared cake tin and bake in the heated oven for about 30 minutes or until a skewer inserted into the centre comes out clean. Allow to cool completely before cutting into squares.

BAKED APPLES

SERVES 4 • 180 CALORIES PER SERVING

Low in refined sugar, fat and carbs, this is a great after-dinner midweek treat. The dish contains the insoluble fibre pectin, which is good for reducing cholesterol, so this is the perfect heart-healthy dessert. It is also very simple to make.

50g pecans
6 Braeburn apples
2 tbsp runny honey
A pinch of ground cinnamon
A pinch of salt

TO SERVE
4 tbsp plain soya yogurt
½ vanilla pod, split open lengthways

1 Preheat your oven to 200°C/fan 180°C/gas 6. Line a baking tray with greaseproof paper.
2 Crush the pecans by placing them in a plastic bag and using a rolling pin to gently break them up into pieces.
3 Peel the apples, slice them in half and cut out the core. Put the apples, cored side up, on the baking tray.
4 Mix together the honey, cinnamon and salt in a bowl. Drizzle this mixture over the apples, then sprinkle the pecans on top. Bake in the heated oven for 20–25 minutes until the apples are soft and slightly golden.
5 Put the soya yogurt in a bowl. Scrape the seeds from the vanilla pod and stir into the yogurt.
6 Serve the apples hot with a dollop of vanilla yogurt on top.

RICH IN Phytoestrogens • Fibre

USEFUL FOR Heart ① • Men ① • Women ①③④

APPLE & RASPBERRY CRUMBLE

SERVES 8 • 280 CALORIES PER SERVING

Here's a sugar-free version of the British favourite that gives as much pleasure as a traditional crumble. We've added spices to bring out the sweetness of the apples, whilst the raspberries add a welcome tart note and bright pink colour.

10 eating apples, peeled, cored and sliced
300g fresh raspberries
1 cinnamon stick
1 star anise
1 tbsp runny honey

FOR THE CRUMBLE
200g porridge oats
100g ground almonds
50g gluten- and wheat-free flour
1 tbsp rapeseed oil
3 tbsp runny honey
A pinch of ground cinnamon

1 Preheat your oven to 200°C/180°C/gas 6.
2 Put the sliced apples, half of the raspberries, the cinnamon stick, star anise, honey and 80ml water in a saucepan. Set on a medium heat and bring to a simmer. Simmer gently for 10 minutes, adding more water if necessary. Remove the cinnamon stick and star anise, and pour the fruit into an ovenproof dish about 20cm square. Scatter the rest of the raspberries over the top.
3 To make the crumble, combine all the ingredients in a large mixing bowl and mix together thoroughly, using your fingers.
4 Cover the fruit evenly with the crumble. Bake in the heated oven for 20–25 minutes until the crumble topping is golden brown and crisp.

RICH IN Vitamin E • Fibre

USEFUL FOR Heart ① • Digestion ① • Women ③

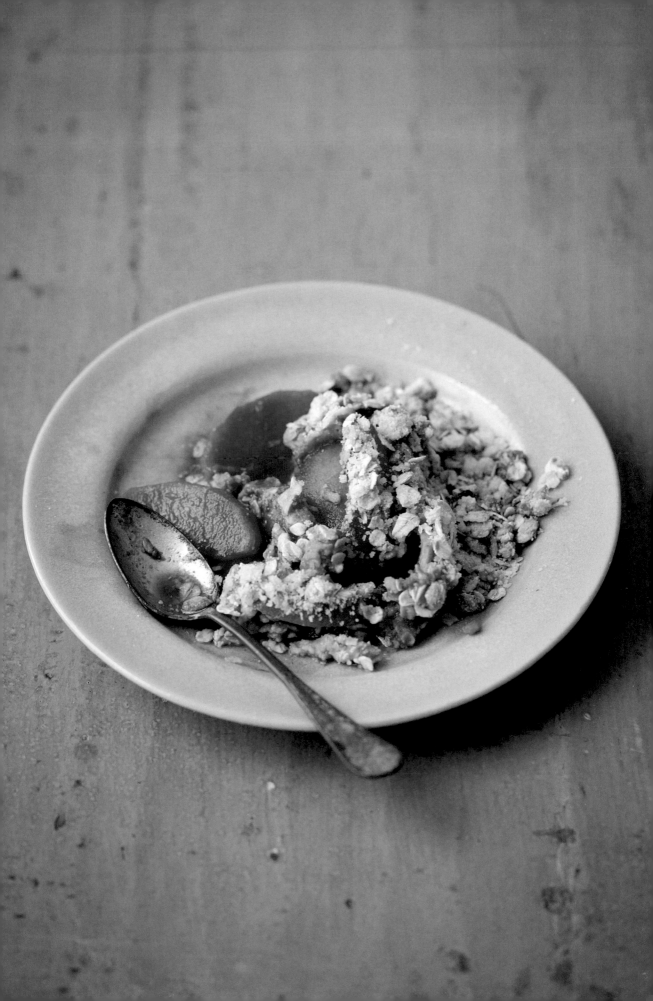

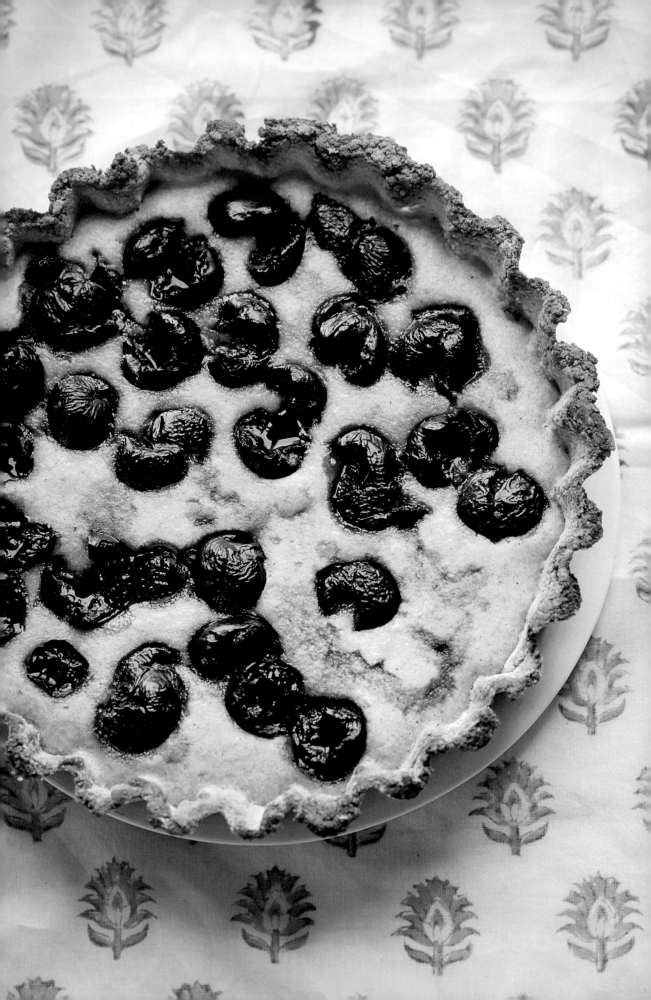

CHERRY & ALMOND TART

SERVES 8 • 290 CALORIES PER SERVING

Cherry and almond is a classic combination that works brilliantly in a pie. In this recipe lusciously sweet fresh cherries fill a crumbly nut pastry case, with cinnamon, orange and vanilla adding to the flavour. Cherries are a natural source of melatonin, the hormone that helps to regulate sleep, so a piece of this pie could be the perfect midnight snack!

FOR THE PASTRY

175g porridge oats
120g ground almonds
Grated zest of 1 orange
2 tbsp runny honey
½ vanilla pod, split open lengthways
1 egg
1 tbsp gluten- and wheat-free flour, for dusting

FOR THE FILLING

150g ground almonds
60ml rapeseed oil
2 tbsp runny honey
1 vanilla pod, split open lengthways
3 eggs
500g fresh cherries, stoned and halved

1 First make the pastry. Put the oats, ground almonds, orange zest and honey in a blender. Scrape the seeds from the vanilla pod and add to the blender along with the egg. Pulse until a dough starts to form. (If you don't have a blender, you can rub the ingredients together with your fingertips and then knead to form a dough.)

2 Dust your work surface with some of the flour and scoop out the dough on to it. Bring the dough together by hand to form a ball. Wrap in clingfilm and leave to rest in the fridge for 30 minutes.

3 Preheat your oven to 200°C/fan 180°C/gas 6. Dust a 20cm round, fluted, loose-based tart tin with some of the flour.

4 Remove the dough from the fridge and roll out on the floured surface to a circle about 3mm thick. Carefully place the pastry in the tart tin and line the bottom and sides evenly; trim off the excess pastry. Prick the pastry case with a fork, then cover with baking parchment and fill with rice or baking beans. Blind bake for 10 minutes. Remove the paper and rice, and leave the pastry case to cool while you make the filling. (Leave the oven on.)

5 Put the ground almonds, oil, honey, seeds from the vanilla pod and eggs in a large mixing bowl and whisk together until smooth.

6 Tip the mixture into the pastry case and cover with the cherries. Bake in the heated oven for 15–20 minutes until the egg mixture has just about set. Allow to cool before serving warm.

RICH IN Vitamin E • Magnesium • Melatonin

USEFUL FOR Heart ②③ • Bones ① • Fatigue ③⑤ • Women ①③

LAVENDER POACHED PEARS

SERVES 4 • 90 CALORIES PER SERVING

If you're looking for a sweet treat whilst trying to lose weight, try this delicious low-calorie and low-fat dessert. The distinct floral, slightly sweet flavour of lavender can be overpowering – the lightest dusting goes a long way – but the right balance with a sweet fruit like pears is delightful. It's a very sophisticated dish.

1 tbsp runny honey

1 cinnamon stick

Grated zest of 1 lemon

1 sprig of lavender, plus extra to garnish

4 Conference pears

1 Fill a saucepan with enough water to cover the pears, and add the honey, cinnamon stick, lemon and lavender. Bring to the boil.

2 Peel the pears, then place them in the pan. Cover with a lid and reduce the heat to low. Poach for about 20 minutes until the pears are tender but not soft.

3 Remove the pears and place them in a serving bowl. Return the pan to the heat and boil to reduce the poaching liquid to a runny sauce.

4 Pour the sauce over the pears. Allow to cool, then chill for 2 hours. Serve garnished with lavender.

RICH IN Fibre

USEFUL FOR Heart ① • Digestion ①

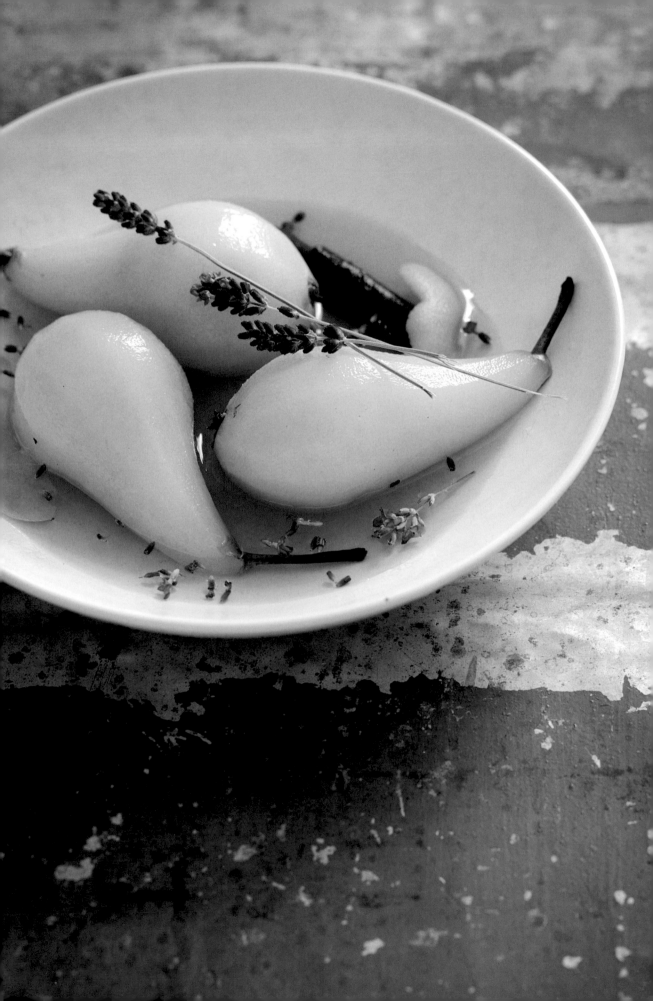

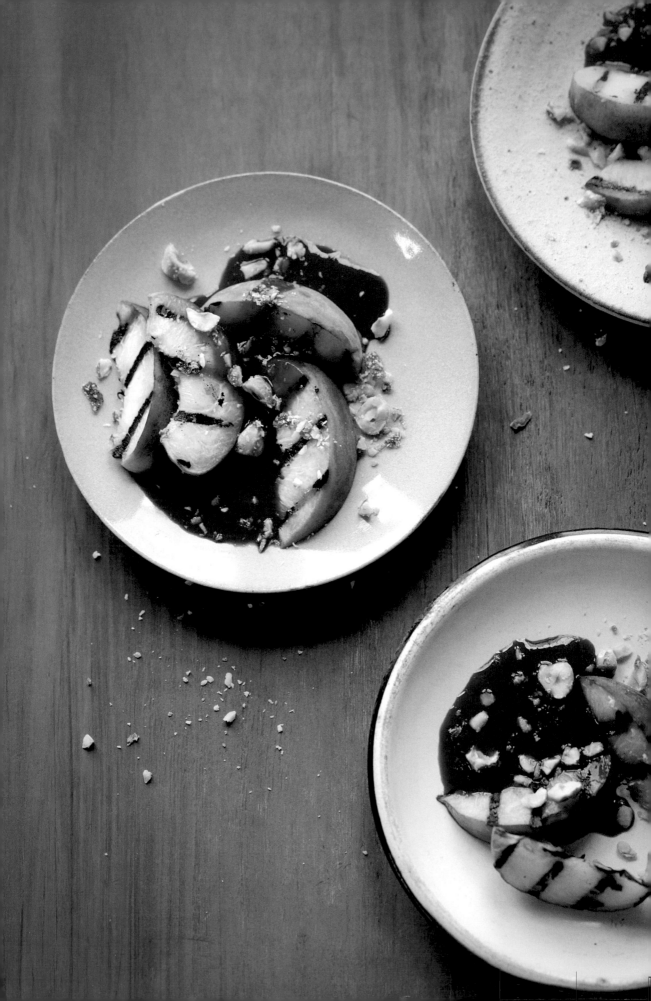

GRILLED PEACHES, HAZELNUTS & RASPBERRY

SERVES 4 • 150 CALORIES PER SERVING

At the height of summer, when you find a perfectly ripe peach, its flesh seems to want to burst out of its skin. That's when it's time to make this recipe for fragrant peaches with tart-sweet raspberries. It is the ultimate summer pudding. Fruit-based desserts like this offer a useful way to increase your fibre intake, which will help to maintain healthy digestion.

150g fresh raspberries
50g hazelnuts
1 tbsp runny honey
4 of the ripest peaches you can find

1 Preheat your oven to 180°C/fan 160°C/gas 4. Line a small baking tray with greaseproof paper.
2 First make the coulis. Put the raspberries in a blender and blitz for 2 minutes to make a purée. Pass through a sieve to remove the seeds and set aside.
3 Mix the hazelnuts with the honey and spread on the baking tray. Roast in the heated oven for 10 minutes. Allow to cool, then place in a plastic bag and gently bash the nuts to break them down into smaller pieces.
4 Set a ridged griddle/grill pan on a high heat. You want to get the griddle as hot as possible so that the peaches won't stick. Cut them into eighths (discard the stones). Place the peach wedges on the griddle and cook for 30 seconds on each side.
5 To assemble the dish, place the peaches on the plates and sprinkle with the hazelnuts. Pour the coulis over and around the peaches.

RICH IN Vitamin C

USEFUL FOR Immunity ①

PINEAPPLE CARPACCIO & COCONUT SHARDS

SERVES 4 • 285 CALORIES PER SERVING

Coconut shards add a delicious sweet crunch to any pudding and work perfectly with some slices of fresh fruit or berries. A bright yellow pineapple carpaccio is an ideal backdrop for the shards, and the dish looks very inviting on the plate. It is as refreshing as it is indulgent, and can aid digestion at the end of a meal due to the enzyme bromelain found in the pineapple.

2 egg whites
1 tbsp runny honey
150g desiccated coconut
1 ripe pineapple
A handful of fresh mint leaves, finely chopped

1 Preheat your oven to 180°C/fan 160°C/gas 4. Line a large baking tray, at least 1cm deep, with greaseproof paper.
2 Whisk the egg whites to stiff peaks, then gently fold in the honey and desiccated coconut using your hands. Tip the mixture on to the baking tray and pat gently with your hands to flatten the mixture to about 1cm. Bake in the heated oven for 15 minutes. Leave to cool, then break into rough shards.
3 Peel the pineapple and use a corer to remove the central core. (If you don't have a corer cut the pineapple in half lengthways, then carefully cut out the core.) Slice the pineapple into very thin rings (or half-moons).
4 Arrange the pineapple on a large plate. Place the coconut shards on top and sprinkle the mint around the plate.

RICH IN Bromelain • Fibre

USEFUL FOR Digestion ①④

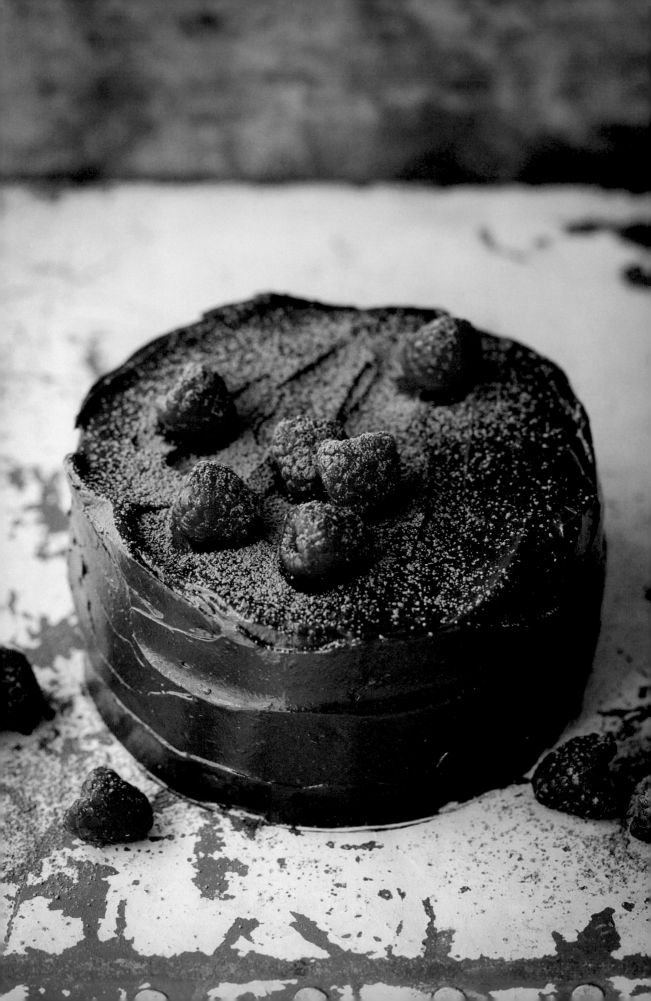

RAW CACAO, AVOCADO & RASPBERRY CAKE

SERVES 16 • 420 CALORIES PER SERVING

Created by one of our very talented chefs, Virginia, this is everything a chocolate cake should be: rich, creamy and intensely chocolatey. There is no baking involved, and the sweet avocado icing is a brilliant alternative to a cream cheese frosting. Just a small sliver of this cake is enough.

900g pitted dates
360g blanched (skinned) hazelnuts
120g raw cacao powder
300g raspberries
125g toasted and roughly blitzed hazelnuts

FOR THE ICING
4 avocados
4 tbsp runny honey
150g raw cacao powder

1 To make the cake mixture, put the dates and blanched hazelnuts in a bowl, cover with boiling water and leave to soak for 20–30 minutes.
2 Meanwhile, make the icing. Scoop the flesh from the avocados into a food processor and add the honey and cacao powder. Blitz until smooth. Taste and add more honey or cacao powder if the icing seems a bit bitter or tastes too much like avocado. Set aside in the fridge.
3 Drain the dates and hazelnuts. Blitz in the cleaned food processor, adding the cacao powder little by little until you get a smooth, thick consistency. Chill until cold.
4 Line the bottom of a 15cm round, loose-based tin with greaseproof paper.
5 Use about half of the cake mixture to smoothly line the bottom and sides of the tin, creating a well in the middle. Fill the well with 200g of the raspberries. Spread the rest of the cake mixture over the top, gently patting the mixture down to even the surface. Chill for 2 hours to set.
6 Before serving, remove the cake from the tin and cover with the icing. Decorate with the remaining raspberries and toasted hazelnuts. The cake will keep well overnight in the fridge.

RICH IN Vitamin E • Potassium • Magnesium • Iron • Fibre

USEFUL FOR Heart ①② • Bones ① • Digestion ① • Mind ② • Fatigue ①⑤ • Women ①③

CARAMEL SQUARES

MAKES 25 SQUARES • 112 CALORIES EACH

Because this indulgent treat contains lots of dates, a small square will be enough to satisfy anyone's sweet tooth. And it will provide 16 per cent of the RDA for vitamin E (this acts as an antioxidant in the body and helps to maintain healthy skin). We've used raw honey, which tends to be less sweet that everyday honey but is far more nutritious because it is unpasteurised and unprocessed. It is great for digestion and boosting energy levels. Try these squares with a cup of peppermint tea after dinner.

400g pitted dates
200g ground almonds
100g pecans, lightly toasted and finely chopped
1 heaped tbsp cacao butter, melted

FOR THE CARAMEL TOPPING
100g raw honey
1 tbsp coconut oil
1 tbsp raw cacao powder

1 Soak the dates in boiling water for 10 minutes. Drain, then divide equally in half and set aside one portion for the topping. Put the remaining dates into a blender and blitz until smooth. Transfer to a large mixing bowl.
2 Add the rest of the ingredients for the base to the bowl and mix well with the date purée. Line the bottom of a 15cm square cake tin with greaseproof paper. Spread the base mixture evenly in the tin and press flat. (If you don't have a tin this small, you can use a larger tin: just push the mixture into one of the corners and make a 15cm square base; the mixture should be thick enough to keep its shape.) Place in the freezer to set for 30 minutes.
3 Meanwhile, put the dates for the topping in the blender and blitz until smooth. Add the rest of the topping ingredients along with 50ml hot water and blitz for a few minutes until completely smooth.
4 Once the date base has set, remove it from the freezer and top with the caramel. Place in the fridge and leave to set for 2 hours.
5 To serve, cut into 3cm squares. They can be kept for up to 2 weeks in a sealed freezer bag in the freezer; thaw before serving.

RAW CACAO & CHILLI TRUFFLES

MAKES 12 TRUFFLES • 60 CALORIES EACH

These truffles look so delicate and pretty that people will think you have been slaving over them for hours, but they are actually very easy to make. Chilli adds a zing in this recipe but orange zest also works really well. The truffles are very rich, so make them small, then dust them with raw cacao powder, or nuts or seeds. Raw cacao contains a mild stimulant known as theobromine, which has less after-effect than the caffeine in coffee.

2 tbsp cashew nuts
5 pitted dates
2 heaped tbsp raw cacao powder
1 tbsp runny honey
½ tsp salt
½ tsp ground cinnamon
¼ fresh red chilli, seeded and very finely chopped
1 vanilla pod, split open lengthways
1 tbsp cacao butter
1 tbsp coconut oil

TO FINISH
Raw cacao powder, very finely chopped nuts, desiccated coconut or sesame seeds

1 Soak the cashew nuts in a bowl of hot water for 20 minutes, then drain.
2 Put the cashews in a blender or food processor and add the dates, cacao powder, honey, salt, cinnamon and chilli. Scrape the seeds from the vanilla pod and add to the blender. Blitz until smooth.
3 Melt the cacao butter and coconut oil – in the microwave for 1 minute or in a small pan on a low heat. With the blender running, gradually add the melted mixture to the other ingredients and blitz until completely combined.
4 Spread the mixture on a flat tray and leave to cool and firm up in the fridge for 1 hour.
5 Once the mixture is firm, break off small pieces and roll into balls about the diameter of a 10p coin. Dust with cacao powder or roll in chopped nuts, coconut or sesame seeds (if you give each batch of four truffles a different coating, they will look even more special). These can be kept in an airtight container for 5 days.

RICH IN Theobromine

RAW CACAO, GINGER & AVOCADO MOUSSE

SERVES 4 • 315 CALORIES PER SERVING

If you tell people the ingredients used to make this dish, they are likely to opt out of having any pudding. Yes, avocado in a sweet dish does seem strange but here it acts as a deliciously thick cream to bring the dark, bitter cacao and spicy ginger flavours together, resulting in a very sophisticated-tasting mousse. A compound in raw cacao can help to boost your mood with its effect on the brain – the same chemical is released when you're in love.

2 tbsp coconut oil
2 avocados
1 vanilla pod, split open lengthways
1 tsp finely grated fresh ginger
3 tbsp coconut water
3 tbsp raw cacao powder
3 tbsp runny honey

1 Put the coconut oil in a small pan and heat gently for 5 minutes until melted. Remove from the heat.
2 Whilst the coconut oil is melting, slice the avocados in half and remove the stones. Scrape all the flesh into a blender or food processor. Scrape the seeds from the vanilla pod and add to the blender.
3 Add the grated ginger and coconut water and blitz until smooth. Now add the coconut oil along with the raw cacao powder and honey. Blitz for 2 minutes until completely smooth. (If you don't have a blender you can mix everything together by hand although the texture may not be as smooth.)
4 Spoon the mixture into four small ramekins or dessert glasses and leave to set in the fridge for 1–2 hours before serving.

RICH IN Potassium • Magnesium • Beta-sitosterol • Phenylethylamine • Fibre

USEFUL FOR Heart ①② • Bones ① • Digestion ① • Mind ①② • Fatigue ⑤ • Men ① • Women ①

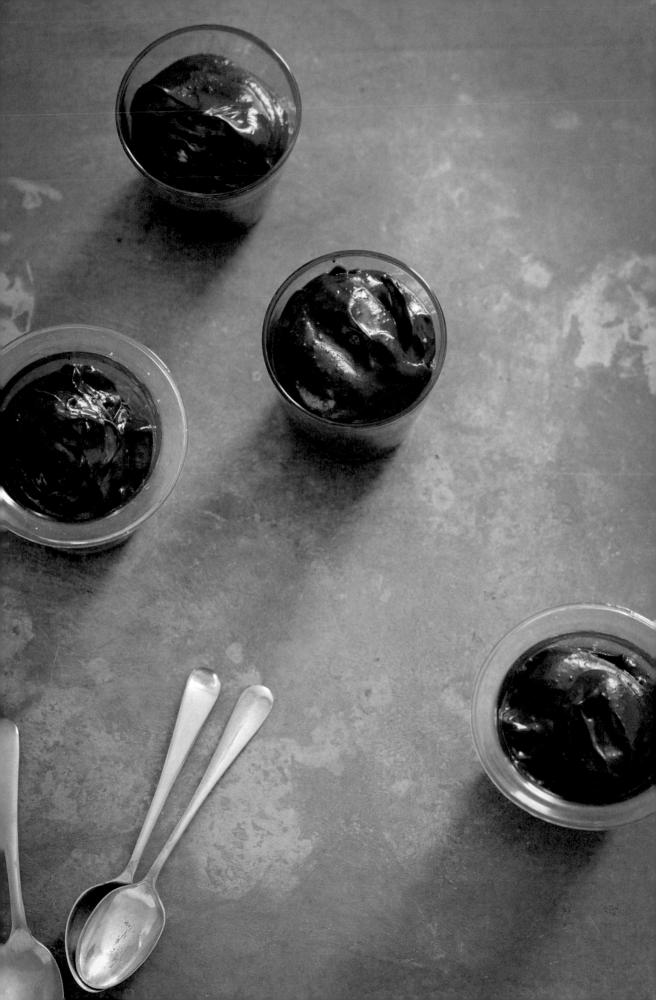

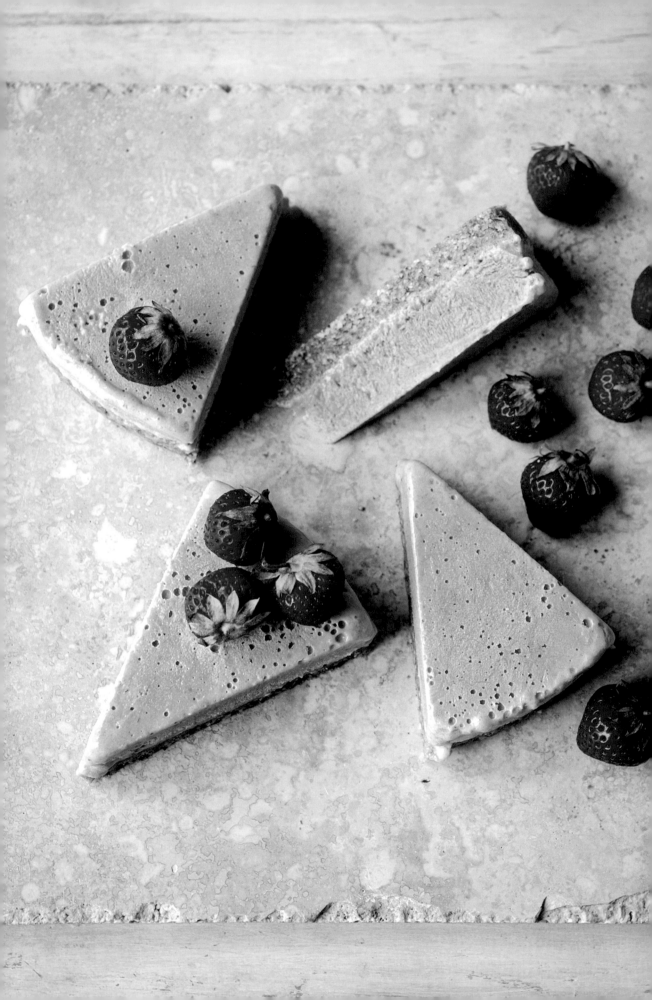

STRAWBERRY CHEESECAKE

CUTS INTO 10 PIECES • 285 CALORIES EACH

A cheese-free cheesecake might seem like an impossibility, but coconut and soya yogurts combined with ripe berries create the smooth, creamy texture that every cheesecake should possess. The base is made from dates, so it is suitably sweet, and nuts and seeds give it a lovely crunchy texture. The brazil nuts also make it that little bit more nutritious – they are one of the richest sources of selenium. You can use other fruit in the filling: raspberries, blackberries and mango are all delicious.

FOR THE BASE
100g brazil nuts
100g hazelnuts
100g sunflower seeds
20 dates, pitted and soaked in hot water
for 10 minutes
2 tbsp coconut oil
A pinch of salt

FOR THE FILLING
250g fresh strawberries, plus extra to decorate
50ml runny honey
100g plain soya yogurt
175g coconut yogurt

1 To make the base, toast all the nuts and seeds in a dry frying pan until they are golden brown. Tip into a blender or food processor and blitz to a chunky crumble. Add the drained dates, the coconut oil and salt to the blender and blitz just until everything is combined.
2 Spread the mixture evenly over the bottom of a 20cm round, loose-based cake tin. Chill in the freezer while you make the filling.
3 Put the strawberries and honey in the (cleaned) blender or food processor and blitz to a purée. Add the soya and coconut yogurts and blitz until smooth.
4 Pour the filling mixture over the base, then return to the freezer. Leave for 2 hours until set.
5 Remove from the freezer and top with extra strawberries. Serve immediately.

RICH IN Vitamins C and E • Selenium • Phytoestrogens

USEFUL FOR Immunity ① • Men ① • Women ①③④

STRAWBERRY & BANANA ICE CREAM

SERVES 4 • 156 CALORIES PER SERVING

In the height of summer, try keeping a few bananas in the freezer. They are great to throw into smoothies, and are delicious sliced up and mixed with some fresh berries and coconut yogurt. But the best way to use frozen bananas is to blend them into this brilliant low-fat ice cream, which is packed with vitamin C. So delicious is this simple recipe that you will have your freezer stocked with bananas in no time.

4 bananas
12 strawberries, stalks removed
200ml almond milk
½ vanilla pod, split open lengthways

1 Peel the bananas and place them in a freezer bag with the strawberries. Freeze overnight.
2 The next day, put the bananas and strawberries in a blender with the almond milk. Scrape the seeds from the vanilla pod and add them to the blender. Blitz briefly until smooth.
3 Transfer to a freezerproof container and freeze for 30 minutes before serving.

RICH IN Vitamin C

USEFUL FOR Immunity ①

MANGO & RASPBERRY SORBET

SERVES 4 • 170 CALORIES PER SERVING

Sorbet can take time to make, but the continual churning produces a creamy, refreshing result. If you don't have an ice-cream machine, you can achieve nearly the same texture by repeatedly blitzing in a food processor. Try this sorbet topped with fresh raspberries and a sprinkle of granola (see a recipe on page 30). As well as vitamin C, this sorbet contains a little beta-carotene, which helps to maintain a strong immune system.

200g raspberries
200g peeled mango flesh, chopped
Grated zest and juice of 1 lime
Juice of 1 lemon
180g runny honey

1 Put all the ingredients in a food processor with 200ml water and blitz until smooth. Transfer to an ice-cream machine and churn until frozen. For a very smooth sorbet, churn, then put the sorbet in the freezer for 1½ hours before churning it a second time.
2 If you don't have an ice-cream machine, pour the mixture into a freezerproof container and place it in the freezer. After 30–40 minutes the mixture should be frozen on top. Now put it back in the food processor and blitz until smooth. Repeat this process two or three times until a sorbet texture is achieved.
3 Transfer the sorbet to a freezerproof container, if necessary, then leave it in the freezer to 'ripen' for a few hours before serving. If it is very hard, let it soften a bit in the fridge before scooping.

RICH IN Vitamin C

USEFUL FOR Immunity ①

APPLE & LYCHEE GRANITA

SERVES 4 • 120 CALORIES PER SERVING

This refreshing, semi-frozen Sicilian dessert is perfect in the heat of summer or as an after-dinner palate-cleanser. The texture should be slightly slushy and more crystalline than that of a sorbet. A serving of the granita contains nearly all of your daily vitamin C requirements, which is good news if you're continually getting coughs and colds. This is also the perfect dessert to soothe a sore throat and rehydrate you if you've picked up something nasty.

4 eating apples
500g fresh lychees, peeled and stoned, plus extra for serving
Juice of ½ lime

1 Wash the apples, then juice them. Pour the juice into a blender. Add the lychees and lime juice, and blitz until smooth.
2 Transfer the mixture to a shallow freezerproof dish and place in the freezer. After 30 minutes the top will have frozen. Now, using a fork, crush and scrape the frozen part to break up the ice crystals and mix them with the rest of the mixture. Return to the freezer.
3 Repeat the crushing and scraping of the ice crystals three or four times until the mixture reaches the granita texture – like soft crushed ice without any ice crystals. Serve with extra lychees. The granita is best served on the day you make it, but can be kept in the freezer for a few days.

RICH IN Vitamin C

USEFUL FOR Immunity ①

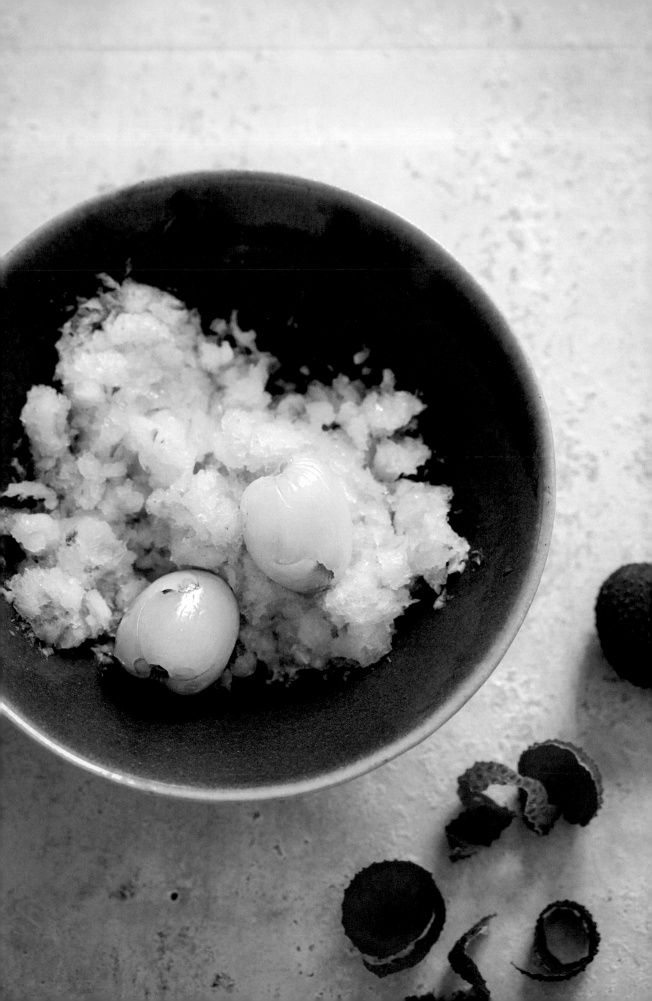

BASIC STOCKS

In the Detox Kitchen we always make our own stock, but at home there are times when you're in a hurry and want something quick and tasty. The brand of stock powder to turn to then is Marigold Organic Swiss Vegetable Bouillon. It has a rich, clean taste and is free of preservatives, artificial colourings and stabilisers.

VEGETABLE STOCK

MAKES ABOUT 1 LITRE

1 onion, cut in half
8 celery sticks, roughly chopped
2 carrots, roughly chopped
1 swede, roughly chopped
1 broccoli stalk, diced
A handful of fresh flat-leaf parsley, roughly chopped
2 bay leaves
4 white peppercorns

1 Put all the ingredients in a large pan and add 2.4 litres of water. Bring to the boil, then reduce the heat and leave to simmer for 1 hour.
2 Strain the liquid into a bowl (discard the solids), then return it to the pan. Simmer for a further 20 minutes to reduce. Allow to cool.
3 The best way to store the stock is in icecube trays in the freezer. Alternatively, it can be kept in the fridge in an airtight container for a week.

CHICKEN STOCK

MAKES ABOUT 1 LITRE

400g chicken bones (the backbone and neck are the best)
2 leeks, roughly chopped
4 celery sticks, roughly chopped
1 carrot, roughly chopped
1 onion, cut in half
½ fennel bulb, roughly chopped
4 white peppercorns
1 bay leaf
A sprig of fresh thyme
A handful of fresh flat-leaf parsley, roughly chopped

1 Put the chicken bones in a large pan and cover with 2.4 litres cold water. Bring to the boil, then reduce the heat and leave to simmer for about 20 minutes.
2 Skim all the foam from the surface before adding the rest of the ingredients. Simmer for a further 2 hours. Strain (discard the solids) and allow to cool.
3 The best way to store the stock is in ice-cube trays in the freezer. Alternatively, it can be kept in the fridge in an airtight container for 5 days.

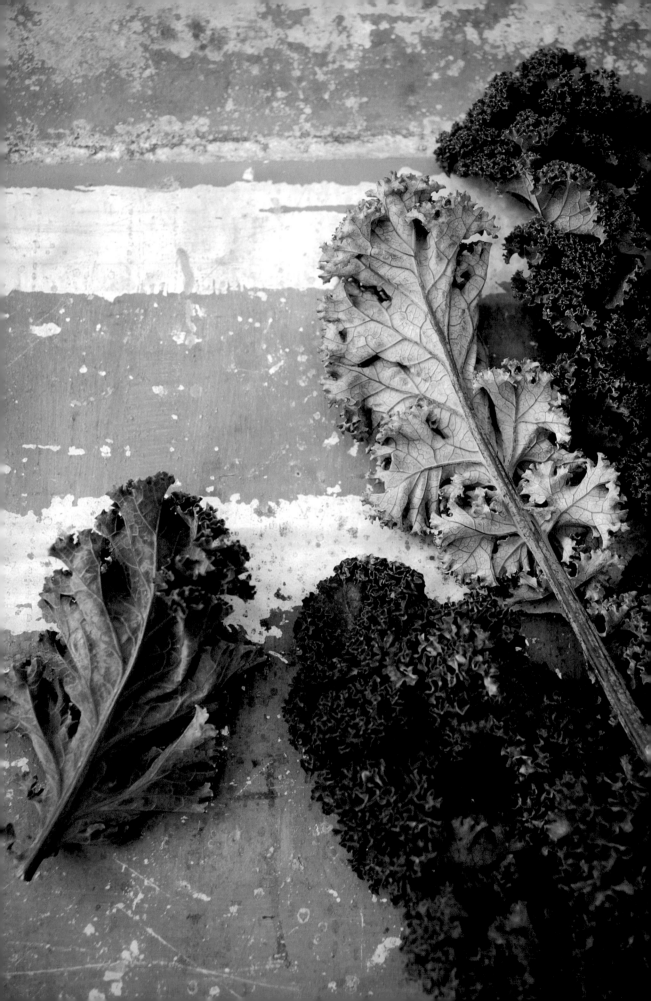

NUTRITION

NUTRITION BASICS

There's a lot of information out there about nutrition and healthy eating, some reliable and some less so. The latter usually focuses on specific nutrients or foods, often with a contradictory 'kill or cure' message, so explaining the basics of nutrition seems to be a good place to start this section of our book.

Nutrition science is still a relatively new and exciting area of research. New findings and theories about the best way to eat in order to maintain good health seem to make the headlines on a weekly basis. Unfortunately, the research is often misrepresented in the media and given too much importance, which leads to confusion and the assumption that a single food or nutrient can offer superior positive effects on our health if eaten in large amounts (these foods are often referred to as 'superfoods' – a buzzword with little scientific relevance).

As well as telling you about the current advice regarding nutrition and health, I want to introduce you to some new ideas and research that have gathered momentum in recent years, and show how these can be translated into the food choices you make. Some of these concepts are a little complicated, but I've done my best to simplify them into something that doesn't require a degree in science! What is particularly interesting is to see how our Detox Kitchen model fits both traditional and more modern ideas about eating well.

Balance & variety If you look at what's been reported over time, on the whole it always seems to revert back to the same old message: the key to good nutrition and health is eating a balance of foods with as much variety as possible. Quite how that balance should look is a matter of debate for some health experts, but in general it reflects the diagram in the Key Food Groups section (see opposite), with the majority of food coming from plants.

In some cases, including or excluding particular foods may be helpful in the management of specific health conditions or problems, but this should always be done within the boundaries of a balanced, varied diet.

Calories = energy What we do know about the basics hasn't really changed much over the years. The food we eat provides the energy needed to carry out our daily routine. This energy is measured in calories, which are gleaned from carbohydrate, fats and protein (the macronutrients). Other nutrients supplied by our diet that protect us from ill health and promote well-being are vitamins and minerals (micronutrients).

We give the calories for each recipe in our book because counting calories is still the simplest way of monitoring your daily energy intake. However, not all calories are created equal – opting for healthy, nutrient-dense foods from the key food groups (such as choosing wholegrain carbohydrates over refined) is most important.

THE KEY FOOD GROUPS

All foods can be split into the following five groups, which are illustrated in the diagram below. (We refer to wheat-free, dairy-free and sugar-free foods following the guiding principles of the Detox Kitchen.) Choosing mostly plant-based foods, some dairy alternatives, a little protein and healthy fats should provide you with everything you need to enjoy optimal health.

FRUIT & VEGETABLES Although you're probably bored with listening to nutritionists telling you to eat more fruit and vegetables, they really do have an important role to play by providing fibre, vitamins, minerals and antioxidants to support good health and protect us against disease. You should *aim to eat at least five servings daily* (new findings suggest that this number should be more like ten to receive the most benefit), with more vegetables than fruit. Try to keep fruit to a couple of portions per day, with juice only at breakfast – although fruit juices contain natural sugars, these are quickly digested because the fibre in the fruit has been removed, and this can impact on blood sugar (guzzling lots of juice can also notch up your calorie intake).

STARCHY FOODS Foods such as grains, corn, potatoes and wheat-free bread and pasta provide one of the most accessible forms of energy (starch is a carbohydrate found in plants), so *try to include a starchy food with most meals throughout the day*. Wholegrain varieties, such as brown rice, quinoa (actually the seed of a grain, although used in cooking as a grain), barley and oats, also offer valuable sources of fibre, which helps with digestion and regulates your blood sugar levels.

Modern diets contain too much wheat, which can cause digestive problems for some people. The highly refined varieties (found in white bread and pasta) that make up the majority of wheat consumption can lead to rapid spikes and troughs in blood sugar levels, which is not beneficial for health in the long term (research is beginning to associate excess consumption of refined carbohydrates, including sugar, to heart disease and other conditions).

At the Detox Kitchen we prefer to avoid using wheat in favour of the huge range of wheat-free carbohydrate alternatives, which includes rice, quinoa, barley, corn and buckwheat, as well as starchy vegetables such as sweet potatoes.

HEALTHY DIET

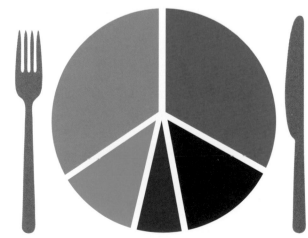

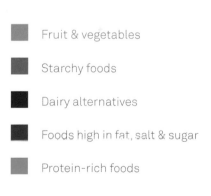

- Fruit & vegetables
- Starchy foods
- Dairy alternatives
- Foods high in fat, salt & sugar
- Protein-rich foods

This plate illustrates the proportion that each of the food groups should contribute to your diet over the course of a week. Most of these foods should come from plant-based origins, which includes vegetables, fruit, wholegrains, pulses, nuts and seeds.

DAIRY ALTERNATIVES The Detox Kitchen eating plan is dairy-free because some people experience a degree of digestive upset when eating dairy foods (the degree to which this affects them can vary depending on the amount eaten). In some cases this can aggravate certain existing health conditions.

Whilst dairy foods do provide a valuable source of calcium, you can obtain this bone-friendly mineral from plenty of other foods, including fortified plant milks such as rice milk, sesame seeds and tahini, dried fruit, tofu, dark green leafy vegetables such as kale, and certain nuts such as almonds (dried herbs provide an additional useful source). All offer many additional nutrients to the diet. You should *aim to include two to three servings of these foods daily* to acquire the necessary calcium in your diet.

PROTEIN-RICH FOODS Essential for the body's growth and repair, protein-rich foods (meat, fish, eggs and pulses) are also a useful way to control appetite for weight maintenance, so *aim to include a source of protein with every meal*. Try to avoid relying solely on animal proteins, instead exploring other protein-rich foods such as eggs, pulses, nuts and soya products.

Soya foods have been at the root of much controversy surrounding food production. One of the issues is genetic modification (representing over 90 per cent of the soya crop in the US), where the plant is changed at a DNA level, creating a species that would not normally occur in nature: GMO soya produces a higher yield of crop that is more resistant to pests and diseases. Some experts believe genetic modification may do more harm than good, but until scientifically proven the jury is still out. At the Detox Kitchen we prefer to use ingredients that have been left to grow the way nature intended, so we always opt for non-GMO foods, including soya.

Be sure to include oily fish in your diet each week for a source of omega 3 fats. The current guidance is that we should eat two portions of fish per week, with one of these an oily fish. It also recommends limiting oily fish intake to four portions per week (two for pregnant women) to avoid any risk of a toxic heavy metal build-up.

FOODS HIGH IN FAT, SALT & SUGAR Puddings and desserts and savoury snacks should make up the smallest part of your diet, although they can be useful for those wanting to increase their body weight (a group that is all too often forgotten about in today's obsession with losing weight; see page 346). In the Detox Kitchen recipes and eating plans, we opt for sweetening with natural alternatives to refined sugar, such as fruit and honey, and use healthy oils along with fats such as those obtained from avocados and nuts. We recommend extra virgin olive or rapeseed oils for their high monounsaturated and omega 3 fatty acid content, and use extra virgin coconut oil for sautéing and baking as it maintains its structure at high temperatures.

MACRONUTRIENTS

These major components of the diet provide energy (which is measured in calories). The body requires energy to carry out its normal day-to-day processes – over 1000 calories every day in most healthy adults (a number that is surprising to most people) – plus additional energy to fuel activities that can include anything from gardening to running a marathon.

Macronutrients include carbohydrate, fat and protein, each of which is composed of smaller units. Some of these units the body is able to make 'in house' whilst others need to be obtained from the diet. For example, the body can make some amino acids – the smaller units of proteins – but others have to come from the food we eat.

Whilst each of the macronutrients is processed using different mechanisms in the body, for them to be used as an energy source they need to be broken down to glucose, which is the simplest of sugars and the main energy source for cells in the body.

CARBOHYDRATE

Because little energy is required to break it down to glucose, carbohydrate is considered to be the most efficient source of energy compared to protein and fat. As a result, it has long been advised that carbohydrates should make up about 50 per cent of the calories we get from our diet (although modern thinking is that we should be eating a little less than this). Most of the carbohydrate-rich foods we eat come from plants in the form of starches and sugars, the only exception being the sugar found in milk (lactose).

COMPLEX CARBOHYDRATES Natural starches are found in carbohydrate foods that do not undergo any processing (such as removing the outer husk from brown rice to yield white rice). As such, these foods contain high amounts of fibre. Processed or refined starches such as wheat are found in foods such as white pasta, white bread, biscuits and cakes.

Natural starches are broken down slowly in the body as a result of their high fibre content, meaning that they have less of an effect on blood sugar and help to keep us feeling fuller for longer (as well as being more nutritious). These are commonly referred to as 'complex carbohydrates', and they should make up the majority of the carbohydrate we get from our diet. The foods rich in complex carbohydrates include oats, brown rice, barley, buckwheat (in soba noodles), quinoa and starchy vegetables such as sweet potato and butternut squash; beans and lentils also provide some complex carbohydrate.

I'm a big fan of including the 'right' type of carbohydrates – the complex carbs – in your diet. I'm not anti the protein-heavy diets, as it's often 'different strokes for different folks', but I haven't had a client yet who hasn't experienced improved energy levels and digestion as well as weight loss by eating plenty of fibre-rich wholegrains – something that is echoed by our customers at the Detox Kitchen. I also find this way of eating less restrictive and more sustainable long term.

Natural sugars (such as fructose), which are found in fruit and vegetables as well as honey, are not complex carbohydrates but often occur in foods in the presence of fibre (which is the case in fruit and vegetables), meaning they also have less of an effect on blood sugar when compared to their more refined counterparts. Refined sugars, used in confectionery, soft drinks, cakes and biscuits, and sweet snack foods, include all types of white and brown sugar, and also agave and maple syrups. The majority of sugar in the diet should come from natural sources.

As carbohydrates are broken down to glucose to be used as fuel, the body produces the hormone insulin, which helps to transport the available glucose into cells for energy. When the cells have taken all they need, most of the remaining glucose is stored in muscles and the liver (as glycogen) and excess is stored as fat (triglycerides) around the body (insulin also helps transport triglycerides into fat cells). Controlling the pace at which this process occurs helps to balance blood sugar levels, making you feel more centred, neither fizzing with energy nor slumped and lethargic.

The speed at which foods are broken down and the effect they have on your blood sugar (and as a result your energy levels) is measured by the glycaemic index (GI). As complex carbohydrates are broken down slowly in the body, they have a low GI (see page 290).

GLYCAEMIC INDEX VS GLYCAEMIC LOAD

The glycaemic index (GI) was developed as a method of rating foods according to the effect they have on blood sugar levels – in other words, how quickly they're digested and broken down by the body. Foods that have a high GI are digested and broken down quickly, which causes a rapid increase in blood sugar, whilst those with a low GI take longer to be digested and so have much less of an effect.

The problem with the GI rating is that it doesn't take into account the effect of portion size. So often seemingly healthy foods (such as certain fruit and vegetables, including melons and carrots) are given a high GI, implying that they may be 'unhealthy'.

The glycaemic load (GL) accounts for this and so gives a more accurate predictor of how a food may affect blood sugar levels. It's not practical to try to calculate the GL of every dish you eat and, quite frankly, life is just too short! But as a rule of thumb, foods that taste sweet will generally have a high GL, as will those made with refined white wheat flour, so these should be kept to a minimum in the diet.

Those foods with a higher fibre content, such as fruit (not fruit juice), vegetables, oats, wholegrains, pulses, nuts and seeds, will have a low GL and should make up the majority of the food we eat. By adding protein and fats to high GL foods you can reduce the spikes in blood sugar – for example, eating white rice (high GL) with vegetables and salmon.

Maintaining steady blood sugar can help to control energy and mood levels as well as hunger, which is helpful if you are trying to lose weight. Regulating blood sugar is also used as a strategy in the prevention and control of certain diseases, such as the reduction of insulin resistance, which is a key issue in a number of health conditions, including diabetes.

SIMPLE CARBOHYDRATES Simple carbohydrates are the refined starches and sugars mentioned on the previous page. They have usually had some or all of their fibre removed (many people still prefer white foods to brown), which reduces their nutritional content, and they are broken down quickly in the body, meaning they have a high glycaemic load (see left).

An excess of this type of carbohydrate in the diet can lead to a high level of the blood sugar-regulating hormone insulin, which will promote fat storage, raising the level of triglycerides that are associated with coronary heart disease, diabetes and fatty liver disease. Maintaining a healthy body weight and opting for complex carbohydrates (see page 289) will help to keep the body's fat levels in check, as will replacing some saturated fat with healthier versions found in oils such as extra virgin olive and rapeseed.

Refined sugar & fructose The amount of sugar in our diet has become a hot topic, and it's clear from food surveys that most of us eat too much of it, especially refined sugar, with the majority coming from soft drinks and table sugars. Cooking from fresh and avoiding processed foods is the best way to have more control over the amount of sugar in your diet, which will benefit your health. At the Detox Kitchen, for sweetening dishes we only advocate the use of sugar from natural sources such as fruit and honey (in relatively small quantities).

Much of the demonising of sugar relates to the overuse of high-fructose corn syrup (HFCS), a cheap sweetener that is often found in processed food products, including soft drinks. It also goes by names such as 'glucose-fructose sugar' and 'maize sugar' if you're looking at the ingredient list on a packet or tin.

Although fructose is found naturally in fruit and honey, the type used by the food industry is manufactured in a process that converts some of the glucose found in corn syrup into fructose, which increases its sweetness so it tastes like sucrose (table sugar). In the United States, HFCS is the preferred choice of food manufacturers because it's a cheaper option than sugar (due to sugar production quotas, import taxes on foreign sugar and subsidies on American corn). HFCS is not widely used in the UK but is still found in some processed foods.

Compared to other sugars, fructose behaves a little differently in the body: it can only be broken down by the liver, which assimilates it using a small amount for energy if there is not enough glucose present. The excess is converted into trigylcerides (main fat storage molecules in the body), which circulate in the bloodstream as well as producing free radicals (see right).

The excessive consumption of fructose via processed foods is thought to have played a big part in the rise of obesity and associated diseases in countries where processed foods are consumed in large amounts. The theory is that our bodies are not adept at dealing with fructose in large quantities because historically this type of sugar would only have been obtained from eating ripe fruit seasonally. This doesn't mean, though, that you shouldn't eat fruit, because the amount of fructose you'll get is comparatively low.

As with most of the new ideas and findings relating to nutrition, these concepts can get blown out of proportion in the media (causing a lot of confusion in the general public). Whilst obesity is an important health issue, simply avoiding processed foods will ensure that you radically cut down your sugar intake and give you more control over what you eat. If you do need to grab something on the go, then look for low-sugar foods with less than 5g per 100g.

It is also worth remembering that a little refined sugar in the diet is fine in moderation. You may not want to adopt the Detox Kitchen eating principles as a way of life, but instead will choose to dip in and out of our detox plans to give your body a healthy break. When you're not following a plan, it's good to take a sensible approach to how you eat. But try not to view particular foods as good or evil because this will only skew your attitude to and enjoyment of food.

FREE RADICALS

If you were to cut an apple, or your skin, a process called oxidation would occur as the cells react with oxygen. This process happens naturally to all cells in nature, including those in your body. When it occurs, cells undergo a change, such as the apple going brown or skin cells dying (they are then replaced with new cells, an ongoing process of regeneration).

These reactions occur between atoms (these make up cells). However, in some cases the atoms become unstable – they are then referred to as 'free radicals'. Problems arise when free radicals build up and react with other components of the cell, causing it to function poorly or die.

Not all free radicals are bad – some are used in a positive way by the immune system to kill off harmful bacteria or infections. The body is well equipped with antioxidants (obtained from the food we eat) to deal with the small amounts of free radicals produced during normal cell activities. But a build-up can occur as a result of environmental factors such as sun damage, stress, smoking or eating a poor diet (which, amongst other things, may result in inadequate intake of protective antioxidants).

It's worth noting that you would be wrong to assume that taking huge amounts of antioxidant supplements will protect against disease. Some studies have shown that this has had the opposite effect by encouraging certain diseases to develop (such as with the antioxidant beta-carotene, which in high quantities may increase the risk of cancer in smokers).

In some instances, where nutrient intake is compromised, supplements can help to bridge the nutrition gap, but the rule is 'food first, always'.

FIBRE

Fibre is composed of the indigestible parts of plants, meaning they pass through us relatively unchanged. Whilst in itself not a macronutrient, fibre is included here as it's largely carbohydrate and has long been considered a key component of a healthy diet (although we're only beginning to understand the important role it has to play in the prevention of disease and maintenance of good health). Current guidelines suggest a daily fibre intake of 24g, which can be achieved by eating foods such as wholegrains, fruit, vegetables, nuts and seeds. Many people fail to meet this guideline by opting for low-fibre foods that are typical of our Western diet.

All plant foods contain some form of fibre, of which there are two types: soluble and insoluble. Some plant foods tend to be richer in one type or the other. Soluble fibre, which can be found in foods such as lentils, oats, barley and pectin-rich fruit like apples and pears, absorbs water, swells and softens stools. Insoluble fibre, found in oat bran, nuts and seeds, isn't digested in the gut, so adds bulk and improves stool transit.

Each type of fibre offers its own range of health benefits. Soluble fibre has been shown to be effective in reducing cholesterol levels (you may have seen the soluble fibre beta-glucan mentioned on the packet of oats in your cupboard). It forms a thick, gel-like binding to excess cholesterol, preventing it from being absorbed back into the body, which in turn may help to reduce the risk of developing heart disease and stroke.

Insoluble fibre helps relieve constipation and prevents bowel disorders, such as diverticulosis and haemorrhoids, as stools become soft and bulky. The World Cancer Research Fund recommends intake of this type of fibre to help reduce your risk of developing bowel cancer.

A healthy digestive system is the bedrock of well-being, for which fibre in the diet is essential. Fibre is also helpful in controlling blood sugar levels in the case of diabetes, and in maintaining a healthy body weight. Most of the Detox Kitchen recipes offer a rich source of fibre (more than 30 per cent of the recommended intake), so we haven't flagged all of them as benefiting digestion or diabetes. Where fibre levels are higher, it is listed with the primary nutrients.

PROTEIN

Protein plays an essential role in the growth and development of every cell in the body. This includes brain development, healthy hair and nails, bone growth and hormone production, including insulin, which helps to regulate blood sugar and mood-enhancing endorphins. We only require 15 per cent of the calories we consume to come from protein, and the daily requirement for women is set at 45g per day (55g for men).

Proteins are made up of smaller molecules called amino acids. The human body needs 20 different amino acids in order to build the required proteins. Eleven of the amino acids can be made within the body, but the remaining nine must be obtained from the food we eat. These are referred to as 'essential' amino acids.

Although plant foods contain protein, they're known as 'incomplete' because they don't contain all of the essential amino acids as are found in meat. For this reason, non-meat-eaters must 'combine' plant sources of protein to get what they need, such as mixing rice and peas in a meal (see section on Vegetarians & Vegans, page 376).

Protein is useful when you are trying to lose weight because protein foods are very satiating. However, the trend to cut carbohydrate out of the diet completely in favour of large quantities of protein – as recommended by certain diet regimes – may lead to poor nutrient balance (especially of B vitamins) and variety, and is unlikely to be sustainable long term.

FAT

Fat has a key role to play in the normal functioning of the body. It is primarily used to store energy, but also provides insulation and protection to vital organs, produces essential hormones that promote growth and development, and is required for the absorption of fat-soluble vitamins such as A, D, E and K (you need a minimum of 25g fat per day to absorb these nutrients).

Of the three macronutrients, fat provides the greatest number of calories – twice the number per gram compared with carbohydrate and protein. However, it's a misconception that eating foods containing fat will make you fat. Including excessive fat in your diet may mean you're getting too many calories, but too much of any food beyond your energy requirements can have the same effect and lead to weight gain.

The particular problem with fat is that lots of high-fat foods are processed and come in partnership with refined sugar and salt. Also, certain fats are associated with an increased risk of disease. So it is most important to make the right choice of fat to get a healthy balance.

Fats are made up of fatty acids, of which there are two main types: saturated and unsaturated. It's recommended that total fat intake should account for about 35 per cent of the calories in our diet, which it does in the UK.

SATURATED FAT Saturated fatty acids are found in foods such as butter, full-fat dairy products and animal fats, all of which are often solid at room temperature, and in processed foods. Surveys show we eat too much saturated fat, mostly from dairy foods (in particular cheese) and meat. Excessive intake of saturated fat is associated with high cholesterol, and reducing the amount we eat has been at the forefront of healthy heart advice for many years.

Cholesterol, a waxy substance similar to fat, plays a number of important roles in the body, including the production of hormones and vitamin D. High cholesterol is a condition that can lead to atherosclerosis (blocked arteries), which is one risk factor for heart disease. However, not everyone with heart disease has high cholesterol, and some cultures with the highest levels of

TRANS FATS

Trans fats, which are artificially produced by a process that turns liquid vegetable oils into more solid fat, have been used by the food industry for their ability to prolong shelf-life and maintain the texture of food without affecting taste. They really are the 'bad guys' of the fat world and I would recommend trying to exclude them from your diet completely.

Trans fats upset the balance of cholesterol in the body by increasing the type often labelled 'bad' (LDL cholesterol) and decreasing that often labelled 'good' (HDL cholesterol). An imbalance of fats (called dyslipidaemia) that involves high LDL and low HDL, along with a high level of triglycerides (how fat is stored in the body), can have a negative effect on health, particularly that of the heart (see section on Heart, page 302). Trans fats also increase inflammation in the body (see section on Immunity, page 326), which has been implicated in a number of chronic health conditions contributing to insulin resistance (a precursor to diabetes) and possibly heart disease.

It is ironic that margarines were high in trans fats at a time when they were being marketed as a low-fat alternative to butter that would help to keep your heart healthy. Most manufacturers have now removed the trans fats from their margarines. Although trans fats can still be found in some snack foods and baked goods, and in fast foods, in recent years the food industry has voluntarily reduced the levels in their products and, on average, we eat within the recommended guidelines in the UK. To avoid trans fats look out for 'hydrogenated' or 'partially hydrogenated' vegetable fats on the food label. Avoiding processed foods is the best strategy.

cholesterol have the lowest levels of heart disease, which has led researchers to question the association between saturated fat, cholesterol and heart disease (we go into more detail about cholesterol on page 304).

Although our intake of saturated fats has caused concern, it appears that excessive trans fats (see page 293) in the diet, replacing saturated fats with refined carbohydrates (including sugar), or high intake of certain polyunsaturated fats (omega 6 fatty acids) could be just as – if not more – damaging to health.

Whilst it may be that foods naturally high in saturated fat, such as butter, cream and fatty meats, are not as bad as previously thought, I would still advise caution with high-fat foods, particularly processed ones, as they also usually contain considerable refined sugar and salt, and will lead to weight gain if you eat too much (this in itself is a risk factor for other health issues). Better to focus on the diet as a whole, balancing it with wholegrains, fruit, vegetables, lean proteins and healthy fats (such as olive oil and oily fish).

UNSATURATED FATS This type of fatty acids, often referred to as 'healthy fats', can be found in liquid oils as well as foods such as nuts, seeds, oily fish and avocados. There are two kinds: polyunsaturated and monounsaturated. The body is able to make monounsaturated fatty acids (these are found naturally in extra virgin olive oil) in the same way it makes saturated fatty acids, but polyunsaturated fats must be obtained from the diet. Both kinds should make up the majority of fat in the diet and can benefit your health in a number of ways, such as helping to balance levels of cholesterol.

Essential fatty acids Omega 3 and omega 6 are the polyunsaturated fats that must be obtained from the diet, as the body cannot produce them. The most significant nutritionally are the omega 3 fatty acids EPA and DHA, which can be found in oily fish (mackerel, trout, salmon, tuna, sardines), because they have a protective effect on the heart as they help to balance cholesterol levels, prevent clotting and reduce triglyceride levels in the blood (a risk factor for heart disease).

Another type of omega 3 fatty acid, called alpha-linolenic acid (ALA), can be obtained from plant foods such as flaxseeds and chia seeds and their oils (try crushing the seeds and sprinkle on breakfasts or add to smoothies), as well as walnuts and dark green leafy vegetables such as kale. The body is able to convert some of the fatty acid to EPA and DHA, which are essential in meat-free diets that avoid fish (such as those followed by strict vegetarians and vegans).

Omega 3 fatty acids help to reduce inflammation in the body, which can benefit a number of heath conditions and protect us against disease. However, omega 6 fatty acids can increase inflammation when eaten in excess. We tend to get too much omega 6 in the diet because its main source is certain oils, including sunflower, soya, vegetable and corn oil (all of which are much used in processed foods). Regularly eating plenty of foods rich in omega 3 will help to balance the ratio of omega 3 to 6, which will benefit health.

Omega 6 fatty acids still have a role to play – in proper brain function as well as normal growth and development. Not all of them cause inflammation. For example, gamma linolenic acid (GLA), which is found in evening primrose oil, may in fact help to reduce inflammation, which is why this oil is commonly used by women to help with symptoms of PMS.

Non-essential fatty acids Monounsaturated fats, which can be made within the body, are referred to as 'non-essential' fatty acids. One of these is omega 9, the main type of which is oleic acid. This fatty acid contains some unique antioxidants known as polyphenols, which are particularly heart-protective as they help reduce blood clotting and balance cholesterol levels. The highest source of oleic acid is extra virgin olive oil, often considered to be the healthiest of all the oils and a key component of the much publicised 'Mediterranean' diet.

MICRONUTRIENTS

Micronutrients, which are vitamins and minerals, are required in very small quantities but are essential for the proper functioning of your body's systems. Making your diet balanced and varied should ensure you get all the micronutrients you need. There will be times, though, when you don't manage to get everything you need from the food you eat (perhaps due to busy lives, illness, extreme dieting or greater physical demands put on the body, such as by intense training). Some people may experience the effects of deficiency, which can lead to poor health.

VITAMINS & MINERALS

These essential nutrients play a key role in your body's processes, such as the immune system, metabolism, and cell growth and repair (see the chart on pages 298–299).

Vitamins can be split into two groups: fat-soluble and water-soluble. The fat-soluble vitamins, which are found in the highest quantity in fatty foods, can be stored in the liver and fatty tissues, so do not need to be consumed every day. Water-soluble vitamins, which can be found mostly in fruit and vegetables, must be eaten on a daily basis because what we don't use will be flushed out of the body.

Minerals are found in all foods, with some foods higher in certain minerals than others, such as iron in red meat or calcium in dairy.

To avoid any possible deficiency, you might be tempted to take a vitamin and mineral supplement, but this isn't necessary as long as you eat a wide variety of foods (especially fruit and vegetables). The body can only use what it needs, so any beneficial effect from supplements doesn't increase exponentially with increased intake. Supplements do, however, have a role to play alongside food in the event of inadequate intake of vitamins and minerals, restrictive diets, medical conditions and deficiency.

ANTIOXIDANTS & PHYTONUTRIENTS An antioxidant is a molecule that prevents the oxidation of other molecules (a process that creates free radicals – see page 291). Certain vitamins and minerals hold antioxidant properties, as do other compounds that occur naturally in plants (these are known as phytonutrients; see below). The protective effect of antioxidant micronutrients, such as vitamins A, C and E and the mineral selenium, in helping to reduce free radicals in the body has been understood for some time.

Recent research has discovered the beneficial effects of other compounds known as phytonutrients (these are responsible for giving fruit and vegetables their colour). They are not considered essential to life, which is where they differ from micronutrients that we can't survive without. However, they can have a powerful effect on our health and reduce the risk of disease.

Phytonutrients (also referred to as phytochemicals) originally evolved to help plants protect themselves from diseases and insects, and research is beginning to show that in the same way they can also help to protect us from disease. There are thousands of phytonutrients found in fruit and vegetables, and as the research is fairly new, we're only just starting to unveil their identity and extremely complex action within the human body.

Lowering the risk of a number of diseases, including cardiovascular disease, cancer and dementia, has also been attributed to these antioxidants and phytonutrients.

MIXING COLOURS Although the science is complex, the message is very simple: to benefit from antioxidants and phytonutrients, eat a wide variety of plant foods of different colours. To maximise your uptake of phytonutrients in the body, it's a good idea to not only mix colours and types of plant foods but also preparation methods, combining raw with cooked (such as adding roasted sweet potato or tomatoes to a salad) because some phytonutrients may be more freely available to the body depending on the structure of the food.

- Red & pink foods Most red or pink fruit and vegetables contain the antioxidant **lycopene**, a member of the group of compounds known as carotenoids, which are converted into vitamin A within the body. This vitamin, along with vitamins C and E, helps to protect the body from free radical damage. Lycopene may reduce the risk of prostate cancer as well as helping to promote good colon health. Red berries contain **ellagic acid** (this helps to support the immune system) and **anthocyanins**, which help to reduce inflammation and may help preserve memory whilst slowing down

the degenerative processes of ageing. These antioxidants are also considered to be protective against certain cancers and cardiovascular disease, as well as offering antiviral and antibacterial properties.

- Yellow & orange foods The key antioxidant group found in orange and yellow fruit and vegetables is the **carotenoids** (also found in leafy green vegetables). These are converted to vitamin A in the body, which is essential for healthy skin and eyes. One of the carotenoids, **beta-carotene**, has been linked to a reduced risk of heart disease and certain cancers, as well as playing a role in the immune system, reducing cognitive decline and possibly dementia risk. You will also find a group of compounds with this hue known as **bioflavonoids**, which help to reduce inflammation in the body and may also work to slow down the development of cancer, heart disease and neurodegenerative diseases such as Alzheimer's and Parkinson's. Combining your orange foods with healthy fats found in avocados and olive oil will help with the absorption of carotenoids.

FOOD COLOURS

Choosing a variety of different foods to make up your diet ensures you will obtain a wide range of nutrients. As well as vitamins and minerals, brightly coloured fruit and vegetables contain health-giving plant compounds, which also dictate their hue. Whilst not essential to life, research shows these compounds can have a powerful effect on health and reduce the risk of disease. The graphic illustrates examples of the fruit and vegetables that fall into each colour band.

- Green foods Two antioxidants found in green vegetables – **lutein** (found also in yellow fruit and vegetables) and **zeaxanthin** – are major pigments in our eyes and therefore important for the maintenance of healthy vision. People who obtain higher amounts of these two compounds from their diet have been shown to have a lower risk of developing age-related macular degeneration (AMD), which is a major cause of blindness in older people. Zeaxanthin may also help to reduce the risk of breast and lung cancers, and play a role in the prevention of heart disease and stroke. Another antioxidant, **luteolin**, which is found in green peppers and celery, lowers inflammation in the brain and central nervous system. Green fruit and vegetables, such as green chilli peppers, also contain **quercetin**, which has an anti-inflammatory effect within the body.

- Purple & blue foods The antioxidant group known as **anthocyanins** is present in fruit and vegetables coloured purple and blue. These compounds are thought to reduce inflammation, which may in turn help with preservation of memory and reduced risk of certain cancers. Blueberries in particular have been the focus of research into the effects of anthocyanins and reduced mental decline (including Alzheimer's). Purple grapes are especially high in a type of polyphenol known as **resveratrol**, which appears to help protect against heart disease and promote a healthy circulatory system by reducing the levels of bad blood fats and blocking the formation of blood clots (which can cause heart attack and stroke). Blackberries contain **ellagic acid** and **catechins**, which may help to protect against cancer.

- White foods Onions, leeks and garlic contain **quercetin** and **allicin**, both of which are known to kill harmful bacteria and protect capillaries (the smallest of the body's blood vessels). You can find powerful **polyphenols** in mushrooms, which can help to reduce the risk of heart disease. **Glucosinolates** and **thiocyanates**, two antioxidants found in cauliflower, may also help to reduce the risk of heart disease and cancer, as well as helping with digestive disorders.

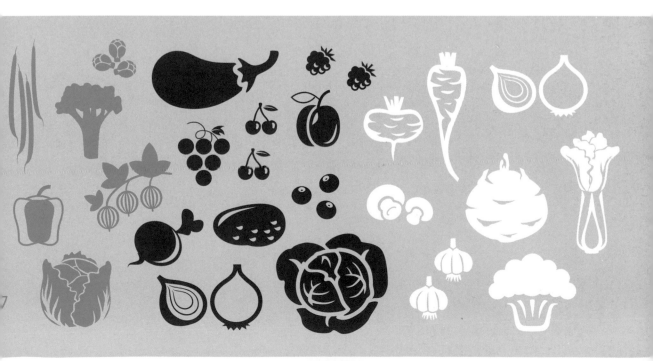

	VITAMIN	WHAT IT DOES	FOOD SOURCES
Fat-soluble vitamins	Vitamin A	Needed for healthy skin, hair and teeth. Antioxidant that protects against infection, heart disease and cancer	Retinol: liver, oily fish, eggs and dairy foods
			Beta-carotene: brightly coloured fruit and vegetables such as pumpkin, mangoes, tomatoes, peppers, carrots and dark green vegetables, including kale and broccoli
	Vitamin D	Required for the absorption of calcium, essential for maintaining strong bones. Also has a role in immune system and muscle function	Sourced mainly from sunlight but found in eggs, oily fish, fortified margarines and shiitake mushrooms
	Vitamin E	Antioxidant required for healthy skin, heart and immune system	Sunflower oil, avocados, papayas, broccoli, sunflower seeds, nuts (especially almonds), wholegrain foods, edamame beans and parsley
	Vitamin K	Essential for strong bones and proper blood clotting	Eggs, oily fish, avocados and dark green leafy vegetables such as Brussels sprouts, kale, spinach and broccoli
Water-soluble vitamins	Vitamin B1 (thiamin)	Needed for energy production, digestion of carbohydrates and heart function	Liver, wholegrain foods such as oats, rye and quinoa, pulses, kale, broccoli, avocados and spinach
	Vitamin B2 (riboflavin)	Helps to convert food into energy and essential for healthy hair and nails	Eggs, dairy foods, liver, asparagus, broccoli, chard, spinach and almonds
	Vitamin B3 (niacin)	Helps to convert food into energy and promote normal growth	Lean meat, poultry, eggs, mushrooms, asparagus, halibut, salmon, peanut butter and pulses such as red kidney beans and chickpeas
	Vitamin B5 (pantothenic acid)	Helps to convert food into energy and supports the adrenal glands (these control stress response in the body) and a healthy immune system	Wholegrain foods such as oats, brown rice and quinoa, nuts, chicken, eggs, liver, sunflower seeds, sweetcorn, broccoli and cauliflower
	Vitamin B6	Required for healthy immune and nervous systems	Poultry and lean red meat, eggs, oily fish, tofu, potatoes, cabbage, leeks, spinach, peppers, white fish and bananas
	Vitamin B12	Needed for energy production. Essential for growth, digestion and nerves, and to ensure healthy blood cells and prevention of pernicious anaemia	Meat, sardines, scallops, eggs, fortified soya milk, seaweed and spirulina
	Biotin	Required for energy production and healthy nails, hair and skin	Swiss chard, brewer's yeast, brown rice, nuts, edamame beans and egg yolks
	Folic acid (folate)	Prevents neural tube defects in unborn babies. Essential for a healthy immune system and preventing anaemia	Eggs, carrots, apricots, squash, melon, spinach, broccoli, okra, cauliflower and pulses such as lentils, chickpeas and black-eyed beans
	Vitamin C	Antioxidant essential for a strong immune system, good skin and wound-healing. Antioxidant properties linked to protection against cancer and heart disease	Fruit and vegetables, especially berries, kiwi fruit, oranges, pomegranates, peppers, potatoes, squash and broccoli

NUTRITION BASICS

	MINERAL	WHAT IT DOES	FOOD SOURCES
Minerals	Calcium	Essential for strong bones, teeth and heart. Also involved in muscle function and helps to maintain healthy blood pressure	Calcium-enriched soya products, dark green leafy vegetables (except spinach and Swiss chard), small boned fish such as sardines, tofu, almonds, sesame seeds (also tahini) and dried fruit
	Chromium	Enhances the activity of insulin in the body to help maintain normal blood glucose levels	Broccoli, liver, eggs, shellfish, nuts, seeds, prunes and wholegrain foods such as brown rice and quinoa
	Iron	Required for proper growth and development, and essential for the production of red blood cells (prevents iron-deficiency anaemia)	Lean red meat, liver, eggs, lentils, oats, dried fruit, kale, avocados, and dried herbs and spices
	Magnesium	Required to build healthy bones and helps the body to deal with stress. Associated with healthy muscle and nervous systems	Dark green vegetables, cashew nuts, sunflower and other seeds, halibut, meat, dried fruit, tomatoes, aubergines and onions
	Potassium	Required for proper muscle and nerve function. Lowers blood pressure and eases fatigue and irritability	Avocados, bananas, dried fruit and all vegetables (in particular chard and spinach)
	Selenium	Antioxidant that is essential for a healthy immune system. Also helps to regulate thyroid hormone activity	Brazil nuts, shellfish, bran, tomatoes and broccoli (found in most fruit and vegetables, depending on the soil they're grown in)
	Zinc	Essential for a strong immune system. Also involved in sexual development, brain function and nervous system; beneficial for men's health	Shellfish, lean red meat, turkey, wholegrain foods such as oats, brown rice, buckwheat and quinoa, eggs, cashew nuts, almonds, tahini, sesame seeds, lentils, miso, pumpkin seeds, pine nuts

THE DETOX PLANS

Although there's still a lot to know about how the body utilises food and the nutrients it contains, exciting findings from nutrition research so far have helped to improve both our health and the quality of the food we eat. What we know for certain is that diet is a key factor (along with an active, healthy lifestyle) in protecting against disease and ensuring optimal health and well-being.

This part of the book comprises a collection of common health issues and highlights where research has shown food may be beneficial in their management. Although nutrients don't work in isolation, eating certain foods – and thereby obtaining the compounds they contain – may help through the effect they can have on processes such as the immune system and hormone balance, and the availability of nutrients to cells in the body. The health issues are linked to our Detox Kitchen recipes, each of which indicates rich sources of specific nutrients and the conditions or problems for which they may be useful.

It's important to understand that no single food or pill is going to miraculously cure you of illness or suddenly undo years of damage caused by an unhealthy lifestyle. However, adopting a realistic approach to the way you eat (we like the 80/20 rule; see page 9) will make a huge difference to the way you feel, and will begin to reverse damage and promote long-term health. Following our Detox Kitchen principles will give you a renewed vision of healthy eating.

Within each of the sections that follow you'll find a detox plan that incorporates some of the dishes that have been highlighted as being useful for that particular health issue. These recipes are rich in some of the key nutrients that may be beneficial.

On the opposite page are two detox plans to try over three days. They are low in calories and not intended to be followed long term, but are a good way to kickstart one of our week-long detox plans that meets your needs.

For the detox plans below, and all of those on the following pages, drink fresh mint tea after meals, and herbal tea throughout the day to keep yourself hydrated and aid digestion.

KICKSTARTER DETOX

	DAY ONE	DAY TWO	DAY THREE
Breakfast	Cashew & goji berry flapjack (p80)	Baked eggs with spinach & tomato (p38)	Chia seed pudding with blackberry coulis (p35)
Juice	Carrot, beetroot, apple & celery juice (p57)	Cucumber, pear, mint & wheatgrass juice (p57)	Avocado, apple, kiwi & spinach smoothie (p55)
Lunch	Quinoa & cashew salad (p150)	Butter beans with cherry tomatoes & salsa verde (p160)	Baked aubergine with pomegranate (p121)
Mid-afternoon snack	Edamame & seed salad (p73)	Tenderstem & tahini (p66)	Pistachio oat bar (p79)
Dinner	Cabbage stuffed with chicken (p208)	Grilled salmon with ginger (p238) with Carrot & cucumber ribbons (p105)	Turkey burger with cabbage slaw (p214)
Sweet treat	Banana bread (p255)	Coconut macaroon (p263)	Raw cacao, ginger & avocado mousse (p276)

THE GREEN CLEANSE

	DAY ONE	DAY TWO	DAY THREE
Breakfast	Soft-boiled eggs with avocado salad (p38)	Apple, blueberry & cinnamon Bircher muesli (p28)	Avocado smash with toasted nuts & seeds (p36)
Juice	Cucumber, pear, mint & wheatgrass juice (p57)	Avocado, apple, kiwi & spinach smoothie (p55)	Carrot, beetroot, apple & celery juice (p57)
Mid-morning snack	Carrot & cucumber ribbons (p105)	Cabbage, apple & tarragon salad (p104)	Radish, cucumber & dill salad (p102)
Lunch	Green papaya salad (p101)	Courgette stuffed with beetroot & shallot (p118)	Fresh pea & raw courgette salad (p98)
Mid-afternoon snack with juice	Edamame & seed salad (p73) with Carrot, beetroot, apple & celery juice (p57)	Kale crisps with cashew nuts & paprika (p74) with Chia seed, coconut & pineapple smoothie (p52)	Broccoli stalk & cashew spread (p63) with Cucumber, pear, mint & wheatgrass juice (p57)
Dinner	Griddled courgette & asparagus with rocket pesto (p112)	Thai green curry (p137)	Pea & rocket soup (p95)

Cardiovascular disease (CVD) is the term used to describe a group of conditions that affect the arteries, including heart disease and stroke. As a group, it is the leading cause of premature death in the UK, even though it's largely preventable by making simple lifestyle changes such as adopting a healthy diet, maintaining a healthy body weight and taking regular exercise. Three of the most common risk factors for cardiovascular disease that can be attributed to the diet are high cholesterol, high blood pressure and type 2 diabetes. The risk of developing these conditions can be reduced by making the right food choices and adopting a diet that replaces unhealthy fats with healthy ones, limits refined carbohydrates (such as sugar) and contains plenty of fibre-rich plant foods and lean proteins.

The low-fat myth It has long been thought that a low-fat diet will help you to lose weight and control heart disease as well as other chronic conditions. Yet all the while this has been touted as the way we should be eating, nations have continued to gain weight and become less healthy. Food manufacturers have been producing low-fat and virtually-fat-free food products to help us to achieve

HEALTHY HEART DETOX

	DAY ONE	DAY TWO	DAY THREE
Breakfast with juice	Quinoa & oat porridge with blackberry compote (p33) with Carrot, beetroot, apple & celery juice (p57)	Beetroot & apple Bircher muesli (p25) with Raspberry, blueberry & coconut water smoothie (p49)	Quinoa & oat porridge with blackberry compote (p33) with Cucumber, pear, mint & wheatgrass juice (p57)
Mid-morning snack	Edamame & seed salad (p73)	almonds (30g)	Guacamole (p59) with crudités
Lunch	Pearl barley with cantaloupe melon (p151)	Nettle & kale broth (p92)	Butter beans with cherry tomatoes & salsa verde (p160)
Mid-afternoon snack	blueberries (80g)	Tenderstem & tahini (p66)	Cacao milk (p53)
Dinner	King prawn stir-fry (p230)	Tandoori chicken with pineapple salad (p201)	Turkey & cashew curry (p212)

this type of diet – but at the expense of adding larger quantities of salt, sugar and refined grains.

It seems that the total amount of fat in the diet is not linked to weight gain or disease but rather the *type* of fat (such as saturated and trans fats; see page 293) and total calories consumed. In a low-fat diet you may risk not eating enough of the healthy fats, which have been shown to have a protective effect on health, including that of the heart.

Another flaw with a low-fat diet is that when people stop eating so much fat, they can often compensate with quickly digested carbohydrates (such as refined sugar, white pasta and white bread), which cause rapid spikes in insulin that can encourage fat storage and, according to recent research, 'bad' cholesterol (see page 304). Over time, eating these types of carbohydrate foods in excess can increase your risk of heart disease and diabetes – just as much (if not more) as eating too much saturated fat.

It's because of this that we are now beginning to understand that a high level of saturated fat in the diet is not solely or as responsible for heart disease, and that trans fats and refined carbohydrates, including sugars, may be equally as damaging.

DAY FOUR	DAY FIVE	DAY SIX	DAY SEVEN
Apple, blueberry & cinnamon Bircher muesli (p26) with Carrot, beetroot, apple & celery juice (p57)	Strawberry soya yogurt (p29) with Avocado, apple, kiwi & spinach smoothie (p55)	Soft-boiled eggs with avocado salad (p38) with Raspberry, blueberry & coconut water smoothie (p49)	Chia seed pudding with blackberry & lime coulis (p35) with Carrot, beetroot, apple & celery juice (p57)
almonds (30g)	Pistachio oat bar (p79)	almonds (30g)	Cashew & goji berry flapjack (p80)
Butternut, coconut & chilli soup (p87)	Purple kale, broccoli, shallot & chilli salad (p108)	Grilled mackerel with ginger & saffron rice (p253)	Quinoa & cashew salad (p150)
Radishes & cauliflower with hummus (p66)	Beetroot hummus (p65) with crudités	Avocado & broad bean smash on brown rice cakes (p60)	Edamame & seed salad (p73)
Salmon, green beans, orange & hazelnut salad (p235)	Mexican bean stew (p139)	Thai green curry (p137)	Roasted pumpkin & tofu curry (p135)

① HIGH CHOLESTEROL

Cholesterol is a fatty substance that's made in the body, in the liver. Often portrayed as the villain, cholesterol has a very important role to play, being essential for the normal functioning of a number of processes, including the production of sex hormones (testosterone and oestrogens involved in reproduction), steroid hormones (such as cortisol, involved in regulating blood sugar levels) and vitamin D. We now know that cholesterol found naturally in the foods we eat does not increase cholesterol in the blood (if you eat more, the body produces less and vice versa, to maintain a balance).

The liver makes, packages and distributes cholesterol around the body as and when it's needed (for instance, to make hormones). The fact that the body *makes* cholesterol often surprises people. Even if you were to live on salads and other low-fat foods, you would still make cholesterol as it's essential for the body to work properly.

Cholesterol travels around the body as lipoproteins (made up of fat and protein). There are two types of lipoprotein, each defined by the ratio of fat to protein: those with more fat to protein are called low-density lipoproteins (LDL) and those with less fat to protein are called high-density lipoproteins (HDL).

Most of the cholesterol in the body is LDL cholesterol, which is ferried from the liver to other areas. Traditional thinking is that if you have too much LDL cholesterol in the bloodstream, it can deposit excess cholesterol into the arteries, which may lead to blockages (atherosclerosis) that put you at increased risk of heart attack and stroke.

HDL cholesterol travels the body 'hoovering up' as much excess LDL cholesterol as it can from the cells and tissues, then carries it back to the liver where the cholesterol is re-used or turned into bile salts (these are used in the digestion of fat in food). This process is considered to be heart-protective as it's helping to reduce the amount of LDL cholesterol in the blood.

For the sake of simplicity it's often easier to remember which cholesterol is which by their role. Because too much LDL can cause damage it is often referred to as 'bad', whilst HDL is called 'good'.

Fats to avoid Too much saturated fat in the diet does contribute to increases in LDL cholesterol and also raises the amount of blood fats in the body. These fats, called triglycerides, are stored around the body for energy (if you cut through a piece of raw steak, the white marbling of fat you see are triglycerides). A measurement of triglycerides in the blood is another marker used to identify someone's risk of heart disease. These fats are also associated with an increased risk of diabetes and fatty liver disease. Keeping an eye on the amount of fat (and refined carbohydrates) in your diet can help to reduce the amount of triglycerides in the blood. It's because of this association that dietary advice about cholesterol has focused on reducing saturated fat in the diet.

HEALING FOODS

Apples
Avocados
Butternut squash
Chia seed oil
Edamame beans
Extra virgin olive oil
Flaxseed oil
Foods fortified with plant sterols (see page 306)
Garlic
Ginger
Grapes
Miso
Nuts (brazils, walnuts)
Oatbran
Oats
Onions
Pears
Quinoa
Rapeseed oil
Raw cacao
Salmon
Sardines
Seeds (pumpkin, sunflower)
Sweet potatoes
Tamari
Tofu
Tuna

LIMIT

Processed foods
Refined carbohydrates (including sugar)

For an index of recipes that may help with high cholesterol, see page 398.

One of the worst types of fat you can eat are trans fats. These increase 'bad' LDL cholesterol and triglycerides whilst lowering 'good' HDL, and this ratio of fats is considered to be the most damaging to health. Trans fats are artificially produced when vegetable fats are 'hydrogenated' (turned from a liquid to a solid). They used to be found in margarines (see page 293), and are still used in some baked goods, crisps and frying fats. It's a good idea to check food labels so you can avoid eating trans fats.

Not all 'bad' cholesterol is the same   Too much saturated fat in the diet increases LDL cholesterol, but controversially it has been questioned whether this is as big a risk to heart disease as traditionally thought. Current research has identified that not all LDL cholesterol is the same. One variety exists in a large 'buoyant' form, which is thought to be benign, causing little damage to arteries. It is this type that is increased with saturated fat intake. Limiting saturated fat in the diet reduces this type of cholesterol, and the question is whether this is actually relevant. Reducing saturated fat will also lower HDL cholesterol, which it is also argued may not be a good thing.

The same theory highlights the effects of another variety of LDL cholesterol, formed from an excessive intake of refined carbohydrates (including sugar and refined wheat products), which may have a more negative effect on heart health. This smaller and denser LDL cholesterol is thought to be damaging because, given its size, it can pass from the bloodstream into blood vessels more easily, and it is much more susceptible to oxidation (caused by free radical damage; see page 291). Oxidation is further encouraged in the presence of excess omega 6 (from vegetable oils and food fried in these oils) and trans fats, as well as poor lifestyle (such as smoking and lack of exercise). Oxidised LDL then enters the arteries and causes inflammation and damage to the arterial wall, which results in fatty plaques (atherosclerosis) and increased risk of heart disease.

So eating foods naturally high in saturated fat, such as fatty meats, butter and other full-fat dairy foods, *may not* be detrimental to your health. However, it's worth remembering that processed foods high in saturated fat often co-exist with sugar and salt, which when eaten in excess are bad for your health.

Reducing high cholesterol The two theories explained above may seem a bit contradictory. It's worth remembering, though, that this is just one risk factor and other lifestyle factors, such as smoking, can have a greater impact on heart health. So let's make it simple. Here is my advice if you are concerned about your cholesterol levels:

- Continue to watch your saturated fat intake by cutting out processed foods from the diet.
- Choose wholegrain carbohydrates over refined 'white carbs' and avoid refined sugars where possible.
- Make the majority of your fat intake healthy fats, opting for extra virgin olive or rapeseed oil and other foods such as omega 3-rich oily fish (helps reduce inflammation, prevents blood clotting and balances cholesterol levels), nuts, avocados and seeds, whilst limiting vegetable oils and processed foods that are rich in omega 6.
- Get plenty of fruit and vegetables into your diet to ensure sufficient intake of the antioxidants that help to protect against ill health and disease.

In addition to choosing the right type of fats in the diet, specific foods may be useful if you're trying to reduce your cholesterol levels. Using 'functional foods', such as margarines, yogurts and drinks that contain **plant sterols**, has been shown to reduce blood cholesterol levels by up to ten per cent. You could also include foods naturally rich in plant sterols, such as avocado, almonds, fresh coriander, raw cacao, pumpkin seeds and olive oil, which all contain beta-sitosterol (shown to help lower cholesterol).

Eating foods high in **soluble fibre**, such as lentils, wholegrains and dried fruit (beta-glucan) as well as seeds, pulses and certain fruit high in pectin (apples, pears and grapes), can also help to lower cholesterol levels because they bind in the digestive tract and get carried away through the bowel. Aim for two to three servings of these foods per day – for example, oats for breakfast, a snack of grapes and a pulse-based dish for lunch. You should also eat plenty of fruit and vegetables, and make sure you're drinking enough water if you are going to increase your fibre intake.

Research into the cholesterol-lowering Portfolio Diet has highlighted the positive effects of soya foods, due to compounds known as **soy isoflavones**. To benefit from them, try including some soya foods, such as edamame beans, tofu, tamari and miso, in your diet. Note, though, that a very high daily intake of soy isoflavones (either from supplements or food) may not be suitable for men or premenopausal women who produce adequate levels of oestrogen.

The Portfolio Diet also recommends 30g of almonds daily, which appear to inhibit the manufacturing of LDL ('bad') cholesterol. Almonds also provide other heart-friendly fats (monounsaturated), as well as a large dose of the antioxidant vitamin E.

② HIGH BLOOD PRESSURE

Often referred to as the 'silent killer' because it doesn't cause any symptoms, high blood pressure puts you at increased risk of heart attack or stroke as blood vessels narrow. Having high blood pressure can be down to unlucky genes, but lifestyle factors such as smoking, drinking, being overweight and eating the wrong diet can all increase your risk.

One of the key things you can change in your diet is to reduce your salt intake to no more than 6g per day (check food labels). It's also important that you get enough **potassium** in your diet from fruit, vegetables and other foods such as lentils – another good reason to get your five-a-day (at least). **Calcium** and **magnesium** have a role to play in regulating blood pressure, so eating foods such as dark green leafy vegetables, seeds, soya products and dried fruit can ensure you get adequate amounts of these minerals.

Research has shown that soya protein (which contains **phytoestrogens** called soy isoflavones) may help lower blood pressure, so including some soya foods in your diet may be beneficial. Ongoing research is investigating the effect of beetroot on blood pressure, based on the theory that nitrates in the vegetable increase nitric oxide in the body, which helps to widen the blood vessels and reduce blood pressure.

HEALING FOODS

Almonds

Asparagus

Bananas

Beetroot

Broccoli

Brussels sprouts

Chilli

Cucumber

Dried fruit

Edamame beans

Fennel

Flaxseeds

Garlic

Grapes

Green beans

Kale

Lentils

Miso

Oranges

Spinach

Seeds (pumpkin, sunflower)

Swiss chard

Tamari

Tofu

Tomatoes

LIMIT

Alcohol

Caffeine

Salt

For an index of recipes that may help with high blood pressure, see page 397.

③ TYPE 2 DIABETES

Worldwide, type 2 diabetes is the most common long-term health condition. In the UK nearly three million people have been diagnosed with diabetes, 90 per cent of whom have type 2. It is most common after the age of 40, and the risk is greater in South Asians in whom it can occur from the age of 25. Usually attributed to being overweight, diabetes puts you at increased risk of heart disease, which is why it's included here in the section on heart health.

Diabetes affects the regulation of blood sugar levels. A hormone called insulin that transports glucose into cells in the body controls this process. In people with type 1 diabetes, the body doesn't produce insulin, so daily injections are required. In the case of type 2 diabetes, the body is either unable to produce enough insulin or has become resistant to it. In both cases, glucose builds up in the blood, which is used as an indicator of the condition.

Regulating blood sugar levels is essential because all tissues in the human body require a steady supply of glucose, meaning that diabetes can potentially affect every organ and result in health issues such as an increased risk of heart disease as well as kidney problems, reduced eyesight, nerve damage and immune system malfunctions. Some people with poorly controlled diabetes lose weight because not enough glucose is transported into cells for energy, so the body uses fat and protein (this causes muscle loss, which is a symptom of the condition).

Diagnosing diabetes It has been shown that a third of people in England have pre-diabetes (a term used to describe above-normal blood glucose levels that are not high enough to diagnose as indicating diabetes), which puts you at greater risk of developing type 2 diabetes. Many are unaware that they have pre-diabetes. It can be reversed by making lifestyle changes, such as losing weight and maintaining a healthy body weight, taking regular exercise and not smoking.

Not all overweight people get type 2 diabetes but it's thought that 85 per cent of those who do weigh more than they should. Abdominal fat (stored around the middle) is associated with insulin resistance (a reduced response to insulin), which is why your waist measurement is a good indicator of risk: it starts to increase if your waist is more than 94cm for men and over 80cm for women.

Symptoms of type 2 diabetes include:

- A frequent need to urinate
- Feeling thirsty and drinking a lot
- Tiredness and sleeping more than usual
- Losing weight without trying
- Blurred eyesight
- Slow-healing cuts

HEALING FOODS

Apples
Aubergines
Bananas
Broccoli
Brown rice
Chia seed oil
Chicken
Cinnamon
Eggs
Extra virgin olive oil
Flaxseed oil
Halibut
Hempseed oil
Kale
Lentils
Mushrooms
Nuts (cashews, walnuts)
Onions
Quinoa
Salmon
Spinach
Spring greens
Seeds (pumpkin, sunflower)
Sweetcorn
Sweet potatoes
Swiss chard
Tomatoes
Trout
Yeast extract

LIMIT

Foods high in saturated fat, trans fats and refined carbohydrates (including sugar)

For an index of recipes that may help with type 2 diabetes, see page 404.

How to reduce the risk Maintaining a healthy body weight and following a healthy balanced diet is the best way to reduce your risk of developing type 2 diabetes. Losing just five to ten per cent of your weight can reduce the risk by up to 60 per cent. If you already have pre-diabetes or type 2 diabetes, you can improve your condition by following the same basic principles of a healthy balanced diet.

- Opt for meals that have a low glycaemic load (GL; see page 290), which contain fibre-rich complex carbohydrates: food that is high in refined carbohydrates will cause sugar swings and put stress on the regulatory mechanism. Fibre-rich foods will also help you to control your weight.
- Because diabetics are at increased risk of heart disease, limit foods that are high in saturated fat and trans fats (to balance cholesterol levels), as well as foods high in salt (to reduce the risk of high blood pressure), and switch to more healthy fats (monounsaturated and omega 3), which can help to reduce inflammation and protect the heart.
- **Magnesium**, **zinc** and **vitamin B3** are all involved in blood sugar control, so include foods such as wholegrains, nuts, dark green vegetables, shellfish and pulses in your diet.
- The mineral **chromium**, which is found in small amounts in poultry, wholegrain foods and some fruit and vegetables (broccoli contains the greatest source), also plays a very important role in blood sugar control; deficiency has been associated with reduced glucose tolerance.
- There is some evidence that cinnamon may help to regulate blood sugar levels, so you could try adding it to your daily diet by sprinkling cinnamon over breakfasts, fresh fruit or hot drinks.

BONES

It is vitally important that you form as much bone as possible by eating enough calcium-rich foods during childhood and into young adulthood (mid 20s), which is when peak bone mass is achieved. Once this stage has been reached, you can't improve bone mass, but you can help to maintain your bone strength by getting plenty of vitamin D and eating foods rich in **calcium** (two to three portions per day). It's essential you have enough vitamin D as it's required to help the body absorb calcium.

Although our bones are in a constant state of renewal (known as bone turnover), beyond the age of 35 years we begin to gradually lose more bone than we gain because certain cells eat away calcium and deposit it into the bloodstream. Two of the key bone and joint health issues, especially as we age, are osteoporosis and arthritis.

The unique vitamin D There are two forms of vitamin D: that obtained from food (D2) and that from sunlight (D3). When your skin is exposed to sunlight, your body can make its own vitamin D (it cannot make other vitamins, which must come from the foods you eat). Your body turns vitamin D into a hormone, which is sometimes called 'activated vitamin D' or 'calcitriol'. This hormone regulates the body's level of calcium and phosphorus, and also plays a key role

HEALTHY BONES DETOX

	DAY ONE	DAY TWO	DAY THREE
Breakfast	Apple, blueberry & cinnamon Bircher muesli (p26)	Cashew & goji berry flapjack (p80)	Quinoa & oat porridge with blackberry compote (p33)
Juice	Carrot, beetroot, apple & celery juice (p57)	Strawberry & mango lassi (p55)	Avocado, apple, kiwi & spinach smoothie (p55)
Mid-morning snack	cashew nuts (30g)	Edamame & seed salad (p73)	raspberries (80g)
Lunch	Chicken & quinoa salad (p205)	Quinoa, kale & pistachio burger (p173)	Brown rice, pak choi & ginger broth (p83)
Mid-afternoon snack	Cucumber, mint & yogurt dip (p70) with Mixed seed crackers (p77)	Spicy nuts (p76)	Cucumber, mint & yogurt dip (p70) with crudités
Dinner	Tomato pesto with courgette spaghetti (p127)	Grilled mackerel with ginger & saffron rice (p253)	Mexican bean stew (p139)

in the mineralisation of bone (a process where new bone is formed as calcium is deposited in bone tissue).

The majority of the vitamin D we obtain is from sunlight – only about 20 per cent comes from food, and very few foods contain this vitamin. Those that do include oily fish (farmed fish contains much less vitamin D than fish caught in the wild), eggs and shiitake mushrooms (also mushrooms exposed to UV light after harvesting), as well as foods that are fortified with vitamin D.

In the UK we can only really absorb vitamin D from the sun between the months of April and September, and any that is stored in the body will be depleted within four to six weeks unless topped up. (Exposure to just 15 minutes per day during the summer months is adequate to absorb vitamin D for use and storage.)

Surveys have shown that 40 per cent of us have low levels of vitamin D during the winter months. Although not yet fully proven, deficiency has been linked to the development of multiple sclerosis (MS) and diabetes, and poor resistance to upper respiratory tract infections (as well as a resurgence of rickets in children). If you don't get a lot of sun or eat foods containing vitamin D, you might want to consider taking a 10mcg vitamin D supplement (also recommended for pregnant and breast-feeding women as well as the over-65s).

DAY FOUR	DAY FIVE	DAY SIX	DAY SEVEN
Beetroot & apple Bircher muesli (p25)	Chia seed pudding with blackberry & lime coulis (p35)	Poached eggs & sweet potato hash (p39)	Avocado smash with toasted nuts & seeds (p36)
Cucumber, pear, mint & wheatgrass juice (p57)	Carrot, beetroot, apple & celery juice (p57)	Cucumber, pear, mint & wheatgrass juice (p57)	Chia seed, coconut & pineapple smoothie (p52)
Spicy nuts (p76)	Edamame & seed salad (p73)	Cashew & goji berry flapjack (p80)	Edamame & seed salad (p73)
Raw vegetable & ginger salad (p107)	Butternut squash & butter bean stew (p138)	Purple kale, broccoli, shallot & chilli salad (p108)	Cajun chicken with avocado salad & mango salsa (p202)
Cashew & goji berry flapjack (p80)	Cacao milk (p53)	Cucumber, mint & yogurt dip (p70) with crudités	blueberries (80g)
Seared tuna & beetroot salad (p253)	Sweet potato & turkey Massaman curry (p213)	Salmon & dill fishcakes (p238)	Nettle & kale broth (p92)

① OSTEOPOROSIS

This condition occurs when bones become weak and very porous as a result of calcium breakdown, leaving them more susceptible to fracture. Post-menopausal women are particularly vulnerable because a key contributing factor to osteoporosis is a lack of the female hormone oestrogen.

Men are also at risk (although not as commonly) by way of many other factors shared with women, including family history, taking steroid medicines, not exercising, smoking or drinking too much alcohol, or by having low testosterone levels. The problem is made worse when coupled with a lack of vitamin D and calcium.

Osteoporosis is not an inevitable part of ageing, and although it is incurable, there are steps you can take to reduce your risk or slow down progression of the disease if it is already present.

Micronutrients for bones As we're talking about bone health then, naturally, **calcium** is essential, and you can maintain adequate levels by eating two to three portions of foods rich in this mineral daily. Dairy-free sources include fortified rice milk, dark green leafy vegetables, tahini, pulses, parsley and almonds. This calcium intake will need to be partnered with adequate vitamin D (see page 310).

Vitamin K has also been shown to help maintain bone density. This fat-soluble vitamin is partly made by bacteria in the intestine, which is a good reason to keep your gut healthy (see section on Digestion, page 316). Food sources of vitamin K include dark green leafy vegetables and eggs.

Soya foods contain **phytoestrogens** (a type of plant oestrogen similar to the one found in the body) called soy isoflavones. These bind to oestrogen receptors in the body and mimic the hormone's effect (although this effect is much weaker than the body's own oestrogen). Soy isoflavones may help to preserve bone mass in women during perimenopause and menopause (see section on Menopause, page 372). One downside is that a high daily intake of soya could affect absorption of calcium, magnesium, zinc and iron from food; however, a few servings of soya foods each day won't be a problem. Snacking on edamame beans or miso soup are easy ways to introduce soya into your diet.

If your bone mass is low and you have – or are at particular risk of – osteoporosis, then it's worth cutting down on foods that inhibit the absorption of calcium or increase its excretion from the body. This includes too much salt and caffeine. Large amounts of protein in the diet may also affect levels of calcium, as excess sulphate encourages loss of this mineral in urine (a criticism of very high protein diets). Foods rich in oxalates (such as spinach, rhubarb, Swiss chard and beetroot) and phytates (found in raw bran, certain nuts and beans) can also limit the absorption of calcium. Try to avoid combining these foods with those high in calcium so that you can maximise your uptake of this mineral.

HEALING FOODS

Asparagus
Avocados
Broccoli
Chicken
Dried figs
Dried herbs and spices
Edamame beans
Eggs
Halibut
Kale
Miso
Nuts (almonds, cashews)
Oranges
Parsley
Peas
Raisins
Raw cacao
Salmon
Spinach
Spring greens
Seeds (pumpkin, sunflower)
Tahini
Tamari
Tofu
Tomatoes
Trout
Tuna
Turkey

AVOID

Beetroot
Diet cola
Raw bran
Rhubarb
Spinach
Swiss chard

For an index of recipes that may help with osteoporosis, see page 408.

Magnesium and **phosphorus** are other key bone minerals. Magnesium can be found in foods such as dark green leafy vegetables, seeds, nuts (especially cashews), dried fruit, raw cacao and some white fish. Good sources of phosphorus include oily fish, poultry, nuts, seeds and soya products. Diet soda, especially cola, has been shown to promote bone loss as the phosphoric acid in the drink increases the ratio of phosphorus to calcium and stimulates a hormone that releases calcium from the bone (this is particularly relevant to teenage girls who tend not to drink milk and often further restrict their diet).

TOP BONE HEALTH TIPS

By your mid-20s peak bone mass is achieved as your skeleton reaches maturity (a process heavily influenced by diet). After this, bone turnover continues but you lose slightly more than you gain. Weak bones increase the risk of osteoporosis in later life. Some factors are unavoidable or difficult to control, such as your family history, age, disease and use of certain medications. However, the following tips can help to promote healthy bones:

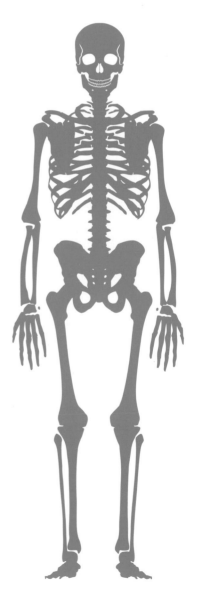

Include calcium-rich foods in your daily diet, such as fortified plant milks, tofu, sesame seeds, almonds, dried figs, pulses, tahini and dark green leafy vegetables.

Vitamin D is essential for strong bones. It is mostly gained from the sun but a little is found in oily fish, eggs and fortified foods.

Eat a wide variety of foods to glean other bone-friendly nutrients, including magnesium, phosphorus and vitamin K.

Extreme dieting limits nutrient intake, so always take a sensible approach if you are trying to lose weight.

Take up weight-bearing and muscle-building exercises such as jogging, dancing, using low-impact gym machines or light weight training.

Whilst food should always come first, in certain cases supplements might be helpful: vitamin D during the winter months, calcium for women during the menopause.

Stop smoking.

Limit alcohol to 3–4 units (men) and 2–3 units (women) daily. Examples of units: 25ml spirit measure = 1; 175ml glass of wine = 1.9; pint of beer = 2.

② ARTHRITIS

There are two types of arthritis: osteoarthritis and rheumatoid arthritis. Both are characterised by joint inflammation, stiffness, swelling and pain. Maintaining a healthy body weight through eating a balanced diet is the most effective way of providing some relief.

Osteoarthritis With this condition, the protective joint cartilage on the ends of bones (the smooth surface that lines the bones, allowing joints to move easily) breaks down over time. Osteoarthritis can affect any joint in the body but is most common in neck, knees, hips and hands. It is a degenerative condition with no cure; however, there are ways to slow down the progression, improve joint function and relieve pain, some of which are related to diet. As a start, maintaining a healthy body weight will ease the stress on joints.

Aside from the importance of getting plenty of calcium and vitamin D in your diet, as previously mentioned, other than losing weight, there is little evidence that specific foods can help relieve the symptoms associated with osteoarthritis. However, eating plenty of **vitamin C**-rich fruit and vegetables may help to slow the progression through the role this vitamin plays in the production of collagen (a protein that is the main component of joint cartilage). Foods high in vitamin C include citrus fruit, berries and dark green leafy vegetables; eating at least five servings of fruit and vegetables per day will provide you with all the vitamin C you need.

Rheumatoid arthritis Suffered by millions in the UK, this is a chronic inflammatory condition that affects the lining of joints, resulting in painful swelling (most commonly at the small joints in hands and feet). This can result in the erosion of bone and be crippling as the joint become deformed.

This type of arthritis is referred to as an autoimmune disease, which means your immune system attacks its own body tissues. The immune system sends antibodies, which bind to the lining of the joint. This in turn causes the cells of the immune system to seek out the antibodies and attack them, which produces inflammation (swelling and pain) and large amounts of free radicals (see page 291). Damage caused by free radicals underlies this condition due to the process of the inflammatory response.

Rheumatoid arthritis can also affect other organs in the body, such as the lungs as well as the skin and blood vessels. Including a wide variety of foods and plenty of brightly coloured fruit and vegetables in your daily diet will ensure that you get plenty of antioxidants (including beta-carotene, vitamin C, selenium and other phytonutrients) that can help to 'mop up' excess free radicals and reduce the inflammatory effect.

HEALING FOODS

Berries
Broccoli
Brussels sprouts
Chia seeds and oil
Citrus fruit
Curry powder
Flaxseeds and oil
Kale
Kiwi fruit
Lettuce
Nuts (brazils, walnuts)
Peppers
Pomegranate
Prawns
Pulses
Quinoa
Rapeseed oil
Salmon
Sardines
Spring greens
Tomatoes
Trout
Tuna
Turmeric

AVOID

No specific foods

For an index of recipes that may help with rheumatoid arthritis, see page 397.

Benefits from food People suffering from both types of arthritis are susceptible to anaemia as a side-effect of taking various pain-relieving drugs (these can cause bleeding and stomach ulcers). Those with rheumatoid arthritis are also susceptible to anaemia associated with chronic disease (this type of anaemia cannot be improved by taking iron supplements). It's important in both cases to eat plenty of **iron**-rich foods, such as meat (especially red), oily fish, pulses and dark green vegetables. You can help your body to absorb iron from non-meat sources by eating them with a source of vitamin C such as fresh orange juice.

A lack of **selenium** in the diet is fairly common in the UK diet and low levels have been associated with quickening the progression of rheumatoid arthritis. You can make sure you get plenty of selenium in your diet by eating foods such as nuts (brazils are the greatest source), shellfish and lots of vegetables, including tomatoes and broccoli. The antioxidant called **beta-cryptoxanthin**, found in red and orange peppers, has also been associated with slowing down the progression of rheumatoid arthritis.

There is compelling evidence that you can help to reduce the inflammation associated with rheumatoid arthritis by eating plenty of foods rich in **omega 3 fatty acids**, which are found in oily fish. Some studies have shown that the anti-inflammatory properties of these fatty acids have reduced swelling and pain of joints. Aim to eat up to four servings of oily fish per week (a maximum of two if you are pregnant). For vegetarians, vegans and those who don't like oily fish, try to include seed oils, seeds, walnuts and plenty of dark green leafy vegetables in your diet, or consider an omega 3 supplement.

It is also a good idea to try to achieve a balance of omega 3 to omega 6 as the latter can increase inflammation. Omega 6 is found mainly in vegetable oils such as sunflower and corn, and as such also appears in great amounts in manufactured food products. Cutting out processed foods and switching to extra virgin olive or rapeseed oil will help you to reduce the amount of omega 6 in your diet (but don't remove it completely because it is still an essential fatty acid with an important role to play in the body).

Certain spices such as turmeric may have an anti-inflammatory effect via compounds known as **curcuminoids**. Whilst not definitively proven, it's worth incorporating turmeric into your diet by adding it to curries, soups, stews, scrambled egg and even smoothies. You could try a level teaspoon daily to see if it helps.

DIGESTION

Digestion is the word used to describe the process by which food is broken down into forms that can be absorbed into the bloodstream and then transported to cells of the body. Maintaining a healthy digestive system is one of the most beneficial ways to promote good health and well-being.

It can take anywhere from two to six hours for a meal to be fully digested and nutrients absorbed. Once food is digested, it can take eight to 36 hours for waste to move through the colon. Although the intestine is able to heal itself and rid the body quickly of harmful substances, a diet rich in refined and processed foods of little nutritional value can lead to digestive problems.

The food we eat certainly influences our digestion. Some foods are known to help support the efficiency of the digestive system,

HEALTHY DIGESTION DETOX

	DAY ONE	DAY TWO	DAY THREE
Breakfast	Mango yogurt with dried apricots & banana (p29)	Apple, blueberry & cinnamon Bircher muesli (p28)	Pecan & coconut granola (p30)
Juice	Raspberry, blueberry & coconut water smoothie (p49)	Cucumber, pear, mint & wheatgrass juice (p57)	Carrot, beetroot, apple & celery juice (p57)
Mid-morning snack	blueberries (80g)	Broad bean & mint dip (p70) with crudités	Radishes & cauliflower with hummus (p66)
Lunch	Chicken & quinoa salad (p205)	Puy lentils & roasted aubergine with basil pesto (p161)	Red lentil soup (p89)
Mid-afternoon snack	Beetroot hummus (p65) with crudités	Pistachio oat bar (p79)	Cashew & goji berry flapjack (p80)
Dinner	Pasta with broad beans & mint pesto (p178)	Roasted pumpkin & tofu curry (p135)	Seared tuna & beetroot salad (p253)

such as those that are high in fibre or that contain live bacteria, as well as certain herbs and spices that have traditionally been used to help aid digestion (ginger and mint, for example). Diets that are made up mostly of processed foods (usually low in fibre and rich in saturated fat, salt and refined sugar) can often lead to digestive upset, ranging from indigestion and heartburn, which can adversely affect day-to-day life, to more serious conditions, such as irritable bowel syndrome (IBS) and diverticulitis.

It's not just the food you eat that influences your digestion but the way that you eat it. Dietary habits such as eating too quickly, eating very close to bedtime, slouching when eating or talking with your mouth full can all result in symptoms of poor digestion, such as bloating and reflux.

DAY FOUR	DAY FIVE	DAY SIX	DAY SEVEN
Beans on toast (p47)	Quinoa & oat porridge with blackberry compote (p33)	Chia seed pudding with blackberry & lime coulis (p35)	Mango cup with pomegranate (p33)
Chia seed, coconut & pineapple smoothie (p52)	Raspberry, blueberry & coconut water smoothie (p49)	Carrot, beetroot, apple & celery juice (p57)	Cucumber, pear, mint & wheatgrass juice (p57)
blueberries (80g)	Butter bean & spinach mash with crudités (p68)	Edamame & seed salad (p73)	Roasted curried chickpeas (p76)
Turkey burger with cabbage slaw (p214)	Prawn, cashew & black rice salad (p230)	Cauliflower risotto with pistachios (p130)	Chicken & vegetable pie (p219)
Avocado & broad bean smash on brown rice cakes (p60)	almonds (30g)	Beetroot hummus (p65) with crudités	Pineapple carpaccio & coconut shards (p273)
Brown rice & mushroom risotto (p182)	Sri Lankan butternut squash curry (p134)	Grilled salmon with ginger (p238) with Carrot & cucumber ribbons (p105)	Avocado salad (p97)

① CONSTIPATION

I doubt there'll be a single person reading this book who hasn't experienced constipation at some point in their life. Often people wrongly assume that they have constipation if bowel movements don't happen on a daily basis, but everyone's different – some may go daily and others less regularly. Constipation is usually defined by a change in pattern – going less regularly, with stools that may be hard, dry and lumpy.

A lack of fibre in the diet and dehydration are usually responsible for this condition, although a change in environment (such as travelling abroad), a sedentary lifestyle, stress or a medical condition such as irritable bowel syndrome can all play a role.

Diet is paramount to helping with constipation and your first step should be to increase the amount of fibre intake, both soluble and insoluble. **Insoluble fibre,** which is found in oat bran (try not to eat too much raw bran as it can inhibit the absorption of key nutrients, including zinc and iron), nuts and seeds, isn't digested in the gut, so it helps other foods to move through the digestive system more easily. As the name suggests, **soluble fibre** absorbs water, swells and softens stools. It is found in fruit and vegetables (eat these with peel and skin), oats, barley, flaxseeds and pulses.

Adults require about 24g of fibre per day – alongside your daily fruit and vegetable intake, a few servings of wholegrain foods or pulses will ensure you get all you need. In the UK it's not mandatory for food companies to include fibre on the nutrition label unless a claim is made, but many still do, so this is a useful way to keep an eye on your intake if you so wish.

Our cooking style at the Detox Kitchen involves using lots of vegetables, pulses and wholegrains, so most of our recipes offer a good source of fibre and as such will help to promote good digestion. Recipes that are particularly high in fibre are flagged in the 'rich in' list of nutrients.

If you are going to increase the amount of fibre in your diet, it's important that you do it slowly to avoid unwanted side effects, such as excess wind and bloating (although these will dissipate as your body adjusts to the increased fibre intake). You must also make sure you drink plenty of fluid, which enables soluble fibres to swell and do their job.

More ways to ease constipation

- Prunes are a traditional remedy for constipation, as is prune juice. For a gut-healthy breakfast, add some chopped prunes and seeds such as chia or crushed flaxseeds to live soya yogurt.
- Hot drinks can help to stimulate the bowel, so try drinking hot water with lemon, or herbal or rooibos teas first thing upon waking. You could try herbs such as senna (this can be

HEALING FOODS

All fruit, particularly blackberries, dried apricots, mangoes, and prunes and prune juice

All vegetables, particularly starchy vegetables such as butternut squash and sweet potatoes, Brussels sprouts, jerusalem artichokes and kale

Avocados

Barley

Flaxseeds

Nuts (almonds, cashews)

Oatbran

Oats

Pulses (beans, lentils)

Pumpkin seeds

Quinoa

Wholegrain rice (brown, black, red)

AVOID

Dairy foods

Refined and processed foods

For an index of recipes that may help with constipation, see page 401.

purchased as a tea), traditionally used for its laxative properties, which work by encouraging the muscles in your bowel to move stools through the body more easily.

- It's important you keep active – moving around will help to keep you regular.
- Avoid excess dairy and refined processed foods, which are notoriously low in fibre – eating too much of these can lead to constipation.
- Keep tea and coffee to a minimum because caffeine may cause mild dehydration, which will exacerbate the condition.

HOW MUCH FIBRE IS IN YOUR FOOD?

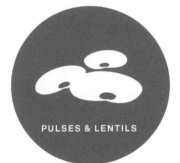

PULSES & LENTILS

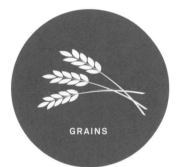

GRAINS

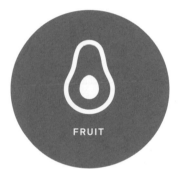

FRUIT

Puy lentils (40g)	8g
Black beans (40g)	6g
Aduki beans (40g)	6g
Chickpeas (40g)	6g
Red lentils (40g)	3g

Barley (60g)	7g
Porridge oats (50g)	5g
Quinoa (60g)	4g
Wholegrain rice (75g)	2g

Avocado (½)	4g
Dried prunes (5)	3g
Dried apricots (5)	3g
Mango (½)	3g
Blueberries (80g)	2g

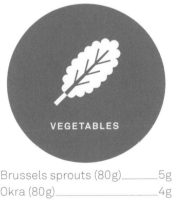

VEGETABLES

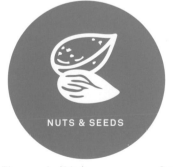

NUTS & SEEDS

Brussels sprouts (80g)	5g
Okra (80g)	4g
Jerusalem artichokes (80g)	3g
Kale (80g)	3g
Sweet potato (80g)	3g
Butternut squash (80g)	2g

Flaxseeds (30g)	8g
Almonds (30g)	3g
Sunflower seeds (30g)	2g
Pistachio nuts (30g)	2g

Your recommended daily intake of fibre is 24g. Often it can be tricky to know what that quantity looks like, so here are a few especially fibre-rich examples to give you a guide. The servings represent an average portion (the weight of dried pulses and lentils will yield an 80g cooked serving; the weight of uncooked grains will yield a 180g cooked serving; and for vegetables, prepared raw weights are given).

② BLOATING

Most of us have experienced abdominal bloating – a slight distension of the gut is perfectly normal after eating as gases are produced during digestion – but for some people it can be a much more regular occurrence. It can leave you feeling uncomfortable, puffy and, in some cases, visibly swollen in the abdomen. There are many reasons why you may experience bloating, including overeating, food intolerance, irritable bowel syndrome (IBS), excess bacteria in the bowel, constipation or simply taking in too much air whilst eating (due to talking or eating quickly).

Bloating is usually the result of too much gas in the gut, often overproduced by the bacteria that live there. A build-up of gas can also result from a reduced transit of waste in the colon, which is the case when you are constipated, or because of something you have eaten, such as a lot of fruit (bacteria will thrive on the sugars in broken-down fruit). It's important to keep your gut healthy. If you do experience frequent bloating, then foods such as live soya yogurt or live bacteria supplements can help by introducing more 'friendly' bacteria (look for strains of *Lactobacillus* and *Bifidobacteria*).

Ensuring your diet contains a source of food for friendly bacteria in the form of **prebiotics** (types of fibre that cannot be broken down or absorbed by the body, and that encourage good bacteria to flourish) will also help. These foods include asparagus, jerusalem artichokes, bananas, chicory, leeks and tomatoes.

Magnesium plays a role in maintaining a healthy gut, so try snacking on magnesium-rich foods such as nuts and seeds (sunflower, pumpkin). These are also a good source of fibre (see Constipation, page 318).

Foods to avoid   Refined sugars, alcohol and yeast all provide a feast for bad bacteria, too much of which can cause excess gas, which in turn can lead to bloating. Cutting out sugary foods and alcohol can help (this is something we at the Detox Kitchen advocate in general). Reducing the amount of yeast in your diet can be achieved by avoiding mushrooms, blue and aged cheeses, pickled or fermented foods and soy sauce (tamari is okay).

Some of the foods that are known to commonly cause bloating and wind include pulses (dried beans, peas and lentils), onions, broccoli, cabbage, cauliflower and, of course, Brussels sprouts. You could try to remove these foods from your diet to see if it helps, but be sure to still eat at least five-a-day from other fruit and vegetable sources. Limiting your dried fruit intake is another way to help with bloating and wind.

Food intolerances (wheat and dairy are the greatest offenders) often result in bloating. They can lead to the bowel not emptying properly, and excess gas as some or all of the broken-down food remains undigested and begins to be fermented by bacteria in the gut. If you avoid such foods (all of the recipes in this book are

HEALING FOODS

Asparagus

Aubergines

Bananas

Cashew nuts

Chicory

Cucumber

Fennel seeds

Fresh mint tea

Halibut

Jerusalem artichokes

Leeks

Live yogurt (dairy-free)

Papaya

Pineapple

Seeds (pumpkin, sunflower)

Tomatoes

AVOID

Alcohol

Certain vegetables, including broccoli, Brussels sprouts, cabbage, cauliflower and onions

Dairy foods

Pickled or fermented foods

Pulses (beans, lentils)

Refined sugar

Soy sauce

Wheat

For an index of recipes that may help with bloating, see page 397.

wheat- and dairy-free), it's important to understand which foods you must replace them with in order to glean the nutrients required to support good health (see Food Intolerance, page 325).

To get a good idea of the foods that might be causing you problems, it may be beneficial to keep a food and symptom diary, noting if there are any key culprits. Once you think you have identified them, you can remove them from your diet. But be sure not to remove too many foods at once, and try to maintain a balance of the key food groups (see page 287).

Ways to relieve bloating

- Fresh mint tea is traditionally associated with discouraging bloating as it relaxes the gut wall, offering relief as the 'valve' connecting your oesophagus to the gut is loosened (it also makes a delicious caffeine-free alternative to regular tea or coffee after meals). You could add a few teaspoons of fennel or caraway seeds for extra digestive relief.
- Pineapple and papaya contain specific enzymes that are thought to help digestion. Try serving these fruit with watermelon and finely chopped mint for a refreshing dessert.
- Try eating little and often, and take your time to eat. Sit at the table and make sure to chew your food properly so as not to put too much strain on the digestive system.

If your bloating lasts for more than a month, it might be a good idea to visit your GP to rule out any other underlying condition.

③ IRRITABLE BOWEL SYNDROME (IBS)

IBS is a common condition that affects up to 20 per cent of adults. It can have a big impact on daily life. The condition is characterised by abnormal muscle contractions in the intestine that result in bouts of either diarrhoea or constipation, or both. Other symptoms include bloating, abdominal cramps and pain, wind and nausea. Symptoms usually occur after eating, with the severity varying between people. There is no test for IBS, and diagnosis is normally done on the basis of symptoms and ruling out other conditions.

Food intolerances (see page 325) may play a role in causing IBS. Stress appears to exacerbate it, and sufferers are advised to take regular exercise and investigate different relaxation techniques to tackle stress levels.

There appear to be particular foods that can aggravate IBS, and the only way to identify if these are problem foods for you is by keeping a food and symptom diary. Common trigger foods include wheat and dairy, as well as foods that can cause bloating and wind, such as refined sugars, alcohol, soy sauce, pickled or fermented foods and certain vegetables (including pulses, onions, broccoli, cabbage, cauliflower and Brussels sprouts). Eliminating some of these foods from your diet can be a good starting point, but don't remove too much at once as you then may be at risk of inadequate nutrition. A dietitian or registered nutritionist can help here.

Other foods that you might want to avoid are those containing polyols (sugar alcohols such as sorbitol, which are used as artificial sweeteners), which can cause diarrhoea if eaten in large amounts, and processed foods.

A healthy gut Live bacteria, which help to promote a healthy gut, have been shown to be useful in relieving the symptoms of IBS, in particular bloating. You can find live bacteria in foods such as live yogurt (dairy-free) and supplements: look for strains such as *Lactobacillus* and *Bifidobacteria*.

A type of elimination diet known as FODMAPS (Fermentable Oligo, Di and Mono-saccharides and Polyols) has proven to be very successful in treating IBS. It must be carried out with the help of an experienced dietitian who will monitor your progress. The FODMAPS diet categorises foods by the amount of fermentable carbohydrates they contain: those with a high content cause an increase in the amount of liquid and gas in the gut and hence lead to the bloating, abdominal pain and diarrhoea associated with IBS. In general, foods that are high in the sugars from fruit (fructose) and dairy (lactose), as well as wheat in large quantities, are considered to be high in fermentable carbohydrates.

As with other digestive problems, it helps to eat smaller meals throughout the day and to take your time eating in order to avoid bloating from excess air taken in. Cutting down on fatty foods will also help as these take a long while to be digested.

HEALING FOODS

Chia seed oil

Flaxseed oil

Live yogurt (dairy-free)

Mackerel

Salmon

Sardines

Trout

Walnuts

AVOID

Alcohol

Certain vegetables, including broccoli, Brussels sprouts, cabbage, cauliflower and onions

Dairy foods

Fermentable carbohydrates (see below left)

Pickled or fermented foods

Pulses (beans, lentils)

Refined sugar

Sorbitol

Soy sauce

Wheat

For an index of recipes that may help with IBS, see page 406.

Monitoring your fibre intake is another way to help with IBS. Try to eat less fibre-rich food during bouts of diarrhoea, and try to take in more fibre (particularly the soluble type found in oats, pulses, fruit such as dates and apples, and vegetables) when experiencing constipation (soluble fibre swells to soften the stool and give it bulk to ease transit). If you are increasing your intake of soluble fibre, remember to drink plenty of water to help the fibre to swell.

You should avoid using raw bran, which is often taken to help with constipation, because it can irritate the gut and may prevent the absorption of key minerals, including iron and calcium. This is because compounds known as phytates (high levels of which are found in raw bran as well as in certain nuts, such as almonds and walnuts, and most dried beans such as pinto and red kidney) bind with minerals in the gut, causing them to be removed from the body.

Drink plenty of water to stay adequately hydrated, especially if you experience bouts of diarrhoea. You may also want to try digestive teas such as fennel seed, mint, chamomile and ginger, which can settle the stomach and help with bloating.

Possible inflammation It has always been thought that inflammation had no role to play in IBS, but a new theory suggests that in some cases IBS may be triggered by an infection within the intestines that causes diarrhoea and inflamed colon. (These symtoms may cause changes in the colon, affecting the way it functions and so leading to IBS.) Studies researching the theory have shown that some people with IBS may have ongoing inflammation, particularly those who predominantly suffer from diarrhoea. Making sure to include plenty of **omega 3**-rich foods in the diet, such as oily fish, nuts (walnuts), seeds (chia and flax) and seed oils, may prove to be helpful in reducing inflammation. In any case, these foods should always be a regular part of a healthy diet.

④ INDIGESTION & HEARTBURN

Occasional indigestion is a common complaint, but there are people who have to deal with the condition on a daily basis. It is normally caused by inflammation in the stomach – often the result of an excess of the acid that is produced to help digest food. Heartburn, which commonly occurs along with indigestion, happens when stomach acids flow backwards, or reflux, into the oesophagus.

The lining of the oesophagus has no protective layer (no mucus-producing tissues), so the acid from the stomach causes irritation. Heartburn is a particular problem for people who are obese or for women during pregnancy, when pressure from the abdomen forces fluids back up the oesophagus. Sufferers may also experience other symptoms of poor digestion, including bloating, wind, nausea and excessive burping.

Simple changes One of the easiest ways to help tackle indigestion and heartburn is to eat smaller meals throughout the day, and avoid large meals two to three hours before bedtime. It's also useful to eat quite slowly, chewing each mouthful thoroughly to stimulate the digestive enzymes.

Adopting a diet that is low in fat and has a good balance of starchy foods, protein (this stimulates the gall bladder to produce more bile, which will help to aid digestion), and fruit and vegetables will help to begin with. Getting a good supply of **omega 3 fatty acids** into the diet (from oily fish, seeds and seed oils, dark green leafy vegetables and nuts) can also help with any inflammation and may encourage better digestion.

Chocolate, peppermint, alcohol and fizzy drinks should be avoided when you have heartburn because they can relax the sphincter muscle, which acts like a valve between the oesophagus and stomach. Raw vegetables may also cause problems as they're difficult to digest, so try opting for cooked and then re-introduce raw veg slowly once indigestion becomes less regular.

Foods high in fat (particularly saturated, found in fatty cuts of meat and dairy foods) also take longer to be digested, which will slow the time it takes the stomach to empty and so increase the risk of reflux. Other dietary triggers for some people include certain fruit (such as citrus), coffee (both caffeinated and decaffeinated) and other caffeinated drinks including tea, cola and energy drinks, which can promote high acid production.

You may find that sipping chamomile or ginger tea between meals helps, as they soothe inflamed gastrointestinal tissue and may reduce oesophageal spasms.

HEALING FOODS

Brussels sprouts
Chamomile and ginger teas
Chia seed oil
Flaxseed oil
Kale
Salmon
Sardines
Spinach
Trout
Tuna
Walnuts

AVOID

Alcohol
Chocolate
Citrus fruit
Coffee
Fizzy drinks
Foods high in saturated fat, such as fatty cuts of meat, dairy foods and processed foods
Peppermint
Raw vegetables
Tea

For an index of recipes that may help with indigestion and heartburn, see page 405.

⑤ FOOD INTOLERANCE

Food intolerances are different from food allergies (see below). Intolerances are more common, and symptoms, which are usually related to digestion, such as bloating, cramping and diarrhoea, occur more slowly and can be longer lasting. It usually takes a significant portion of the trigger food to cause a reaction although there are some people who are particularly sensitive to even small quantities.

One of the most common food intolerances is lactose, a type of sugar found in dairy foods. The lack of an enzyme called lactase in the gut means not all of the lactose is digested, causing symptoms such as bloating. This condition is related to ethnicity: for example, those of Chinese descent have far higher lactose intolerance than those of Swedish descent.

Symptoms of food intolerances are often difficult to distinguish from those of other digestive disorders such as IBS, and as people can be intolerant to a number of foods, they can be difficult to diagnose. Apart from lactose intolerance, there are no reliable and validated tests to identify food intolerances. Because of this, the main tool used for diagnosis is an exclusion diet (also referred to as a diagnostic diet). This should be carried out by a dietitian who will remove the foods one by one and then re-introduce them over time. Most people with a food intolerance can eat a little of the culprit food, so an exclusion diet will help to establish tolerable levels.

Eating a mainly wheat- and dairy-free diet may be enough to prevent mild symptoms of food intolerance in some cases (where there are symptoms such as bloating), but if your symptoms persist you should visit a registered dietitian for professional advice.

Food allergy This is an abnormal immune response to one (or more) specific food and is brought about by a type of antibody known as immunoglobulin E (IgE). You can test if someone has an allergy and they will usually exhibit symptoms to trace amounts of the food within a few minutes. Symptoms can include facial swelling, hives, itching skin, nausea, diarrhoea and vomiting. In cases of extreme allergy, some individuals may go into anaphylactic shock, which can prove fatal.

Food allergies are relatively rare and in the UK have been estimated by the Food Standards Agency to affect one to two per cent of the adult population. The most common food allergens include peanuts, grains containing gluten, fish and shellfish, milk, mustard, celery, sesame seeds, soya products, eggs and sulphites.

IMMUNITY

The immune system helps to protect our bodies from attack by different organisms, viruses and bacteria. It has an army of cells that play a role in defending the body and, more remarkably, it has the ability to remember foreign substances and organisms, creating antibodies that offer protection against future attacks.

The right diet is critical to a strong and healthy immune system, and there are a number of nutrients that play a key role in supporting this. These include iron, zinc, selenium and vitamins A, C and E. Omega 3 fatty acids and the antioxidants found in brightly coloured fruit and vegetables also help by reducing inflammation and protecting immune cells from destructive free radicals.

Inflammation has been a buzzword in nutrition for a while now and the focus of much research. Put very simply, inflammation is the body's response to fight against something that may be harmful. The response may not always be helpful – in some conditions, such as psoriasis (which affects the skin), the immune system fights against its own cells by mistake. Inflammation may also be at the root of a number of chronic diseases, including that of the heart.

It's useful to first understand that inflammation is actually essential for survival in that it helps to protect the body from infection and injury. If you cut yourself, the immune system reacts by signalling for white blood cells to arrive at the scene and work to fight any potential infection as you experience swelling, redness and pain (key signs of inflammation).

HEALTHY IMMUNE SYSTEM DETOX

	DAY ONE	DAY TWO	DAY THREE
Breakfast	Mango yogurt with dried apricots & banana (p29)	Beetroot & apple Bircher muesli (p25)	Granola with pineapple & strawberries (p30)
Juice	Carrot, beetroot, apple & celery juice (p57)	Raspberry, blueberry & coconut smoothie (p49)	Cucumber, pear, mint & wheatgrass juice (p57)
Mid-morning snack	Cashew & goji berry flapjack (p80)	pomegranate seeds (80g)	Oven-baked asparagus & quail's eggs (p187)
Lunch	Shiitake mushroom & daikon stir-fry (p142)	Aduki bean stew (p170)	Chicken & quinoa salad (p205)
Mid-afternoon snack	Radishes & cauliflower with hummus (p66)	Avocado & broad bean smash on brown rice cakes (p60)	almonds (30g)
Dinner	Tandoori chicken with pineapple salad (p201)	Chickpea, pomegranate & pumpkin curry (p164)	Beetroot & carrot tagine with cauliflower cous cous (p132)

Inflammation can, however, have a negative effect on the body. Scientists are beginning to establish a strong association between something referred to as 'low-grade chronic inflammation' (caused by an overactive immune system) and accelerated ageing, along with its associated diseases. Excess fat and obesity are now thought to be linked to inflammation because fat cells are biologically very active, churning out hormones and immune system chemicals. These, in turn, can lead to insulin resistance (as cells become sensitive to insulin), a risk factor for diabetes and other conditions that increase your chances of heart disease.

Lifestyle factors (such as stress and smoking), a poor diet that includes an excess of foods containing trans fats, refined sugar and omega 6s, and food intolerances are thought to contribute to low-grade chronic inflammation as the immune system reacts to the consequences of 'modern living'.

The effects of this type of inflammation cause damage over a sustained period of time but can be reduced by adopting a healthy lifestyle, which includes diet. There are foods that may help to reduce inflammation in the body and these can be gleaned from a healthy balanced diet rich in wholegrain foods, fruit, vegetables, nuts and healthy fats (such as omega 3 and monounsaturated fatty acids). Certain anti-inflammatory foods may also be useful when dealing with conditions such as irritable bowel syndrome (IBS) or autoimmune diseases such as rheumatoid arthritis.

DAY FOUR	DAY FIVE	DAY SIX	DAY SEVEN
Soft-boiled eggs with avocado salad (p38)	Chia seed pudding with blackberry coulis (p35)	Mango cup with pomegranate (p33)	Mini frittatas (p41)
Chia seed, coconut & pineapple smoothie (p52)	Cucumber, pear, mint & wheatgrass juice (p57)	Avocado, apple, kiwi & spinach smoothie (p55)	Carrot, beetroot, apple & celery juice (p57)
raspberries (80g)	Broccoli stalk & cashew spread (p63) on rice cakes	almonds (30g)	Spicy nuts (p76)
Prawn, cashew & black rice salad (p230)	Butternut squash & sage risotto (p182)	Baked aubergine with pomegranate (p121)	Salmon, green beans, orange & hazelnut salad (p235)
Tenderstem & tahini (p66)	Pistachio oat bar (p79)	Kale crisps with cashew nuts & paprika (p74)	Butter bean & spinach mash with crudités (p68)
Stir-fried cauliflower rice with shiitake mushrooms and tofu (p143)	Pad Thai with brown rice noodles (p209)	Pollock & prawn fishcakes with courgette spaghetti (p247)	Broccoli & ginger soup (p84)

① COMMON COLD

Although not life-threatening, colds, coughs and sniffles can be a real pain in the winter months and, unfortunately, there's very little we can do once they've begun as there is no real cure. There are many different strains of colds and coughs, and most will get better of their own accord. But to help prevent you from contracting whatever is going round in the first place, you need to maintain a strong immune system. The correct diet will definitely go some way to ensuring this. If you do pick up a 'bug', there are certain foods that may help to relieve some of the symptoms.

Staying healthy **Vitamin C** is traditionally considered to help with colds, although this is yet to be definitively proven, particularly in the use of supplements. However, it does have a role to play in the maintenance of a strong immune system, and eating plenty of vitamin C-rich foods (fruit and vegetables) may help to increase disease-fighting antibodies.

Studies have shown that **zinc** may have a significant role to play in the prevention and alleviation of colds. As winter looms, try to eat more foods rich in zinc (shellfish, wholegrains such as oats and brown rice, dark green leafy vegetables, nuts and seeds).

Commonly referred to as the 'medicinal mushroom' in many Asian countries, shiitake have traditionally been used there for their perceived health benefits. Research has suggested that some compounds (**beta-glucan polysaccarides**) found in this variety of mushroom may help to stimulate the immune system and so protect against ill health (oats are also a good source of beta-glucans). In addition to this, shiitake mushrooms are among the few foods (with oily fish and eggs) to contain **vitamin D**, which has been linked to a reduced occurrence of upper respiratory tract infections (such as the common cold, flu and sinusitis). Many of us in the UK have low levels of vitamin D during the winter months (see page 310) so you might want to consider taking a supplement.

Most varieties of mushrooms offer a good source of **selenium**, one of the antioxidants required by the immune system, so it may well be beneficial to include mushrooms in your diet. Shiitake in particular work really well in hot spicy broths, which could also include garlic, ginger and chillies, all of which offer decongestant and anti-inflammatory properties.

What to do when you have a cold Vitamin-packed fruit smoothies and warming soups are useful when you have a poor appetite due to illness because they can deliver a powerhouse of nutrients in a small serving. This means they can help you to maintain a healthy diet even when you don't particularly feel like eating. You can also bulk up these dishes by adding super-nutritious ingredients such as pulses, rice and quinoa to soups, or tahini, chia seeds, spirulina and oats to smoothies.

HEALING FOODS

Asparagus
Broccoli
Brown rice
Buckwheat
Butternut squash
Cauliflower
Courgettes
Eggs
Kale
Kiwi fruit
Lean red meat
Lemons
Limes
Manuka honey
Miso
Mushrooms, especially shiitake
Nuts
Oats
Oranges
Parsley
Peas
Peppers
Pineapple
Pomegranates
Potatoes
Prawns
Quinoa
Raspberries
Seeds (pumpkin, sesame)
Spinach
Strawberries
Swiss chard
Tomatoes

AVOID

Alcohol
Milk

For an index of recipes that may help with the common cold, see page 400.

For some people, milk appears to aggravate cold and cough symptoms, making any phlegm associated with a cough thicker and more irritating. Switching to fortified soya or rice milk will help to ease this issue.

Drinking alcohol is probably the last thing on your mind when you have a cold, but if you're tempted, resist. It really is a bad idea as alcohol causes blood vessels to dilate, which can make your sinuses feel 'stuffed up'.

It's really important to stay adequately hydrated when you're ill. In addition to drinking plenty of water and other fluids, you could try some refreshing slices of a watery fruit such as melon or frozen berries. For hot drinks try adding fresh ginger, fresh mint, lemon, lemongrass or goji berries to hot water, or make weak caffeine-free tea such as rooibos. Stir in some honey to help soothe the throat and loosen mucus (you might want to try manuka honey, which is made by bees that take pollen from the tea tree plant, traditionally known for its antibacterial properties).

Another way to help to alleviate sore throats from a nasty cough is with a rosemary infusion (rosemary is considered antiseptic). Add 2 tablespoons of rosemary and 1 tablespoon mint to 600ml of boiling water and leave overnight; strain the mixture to remove the herbs and use as a mouthwash/gargle.

If you are prescribed antibiotics, you might want to consider a live bacteria supplement as these medications can destroy healthy bacteria in the gut.

Finally, some people swear by herbal remedies such as echinacea (to prevent a cold) or pelargonium (to relieve symptoms), although the evidence for their effectiveness is not conclusive.

② COELIAC DISEASE

Coeliac disease is an autoimmune disorder (not a food allergy to gluten, which is a common misconception), meaning that the body mistakenly attacks and destroys its own healthy body tissue. It's a common condition affecting one in a hundred people in the UK, with more reported cases occurring in women than men. The autoimmune response is triggered when someone with the condition eats a food containing the protein gliadin, which is one of the proteins that are collectively referred to as gluten (found in wheat, rye, barley, spelt and other cereal grains). Some people may be sensitive to gluten but do not have coeliac disease.

Gliadin combines with antibodies found in the digestive tract and damages the lining of the small intestine. This damage can inhibit the absorption of key nutrients, putting sufferers at risk of deficiencies, in particular anaemia from poor iron, folate and vitamin B12 absorption. There are many symptoms associated with coeliac disease, including diarrhoea, constipation, bloating, excessive wind, cramping, nausea and fatigue (see Constipation, page 318 and Bloating, page 320), and these can vary between individuals.

The only course of action for this condition is to remove gluten from the diet altogether – or almost completely for those people who are able to tolerate a little of certain grains (such as oats). A gluten-free diet is essential for people with coeliac disease but it's not a healthy option for everyone (there appears to be a growing trend to follow this type of diet and foods are marketed for this purpose). This is because cutting out large groups of foods can lead to insufficient intake of certain nutrients.

Getting enough nutrients Although there are lots of grains that a coeliac sufferer cannot eat, it's important to explore those that you can in order to obtain carbohydrate in your diet. Look to products made with corn, soya, buckwheat (try 100 per cent buckwheat soba noodles) and rice flours, as well as quinoa, millet and the many great varieties of rice. These foods will also make sure you are getting adequate **B vitamins** and fibre, which are traditionally found in wheat and other gluten-containing grains. You can also source B vitamins from foods such as lean meat, oily fish, wholegrains, eggs, dark green leafy vegetables, dried fruit, potatoes, nuts and pulses.

To avoid all forms of anaemia, make sure your diet contains plenty of foods rich in **iron**, **folate** and **vitamin B12**, such as lean red meat, poultry, oily fish, eggs, tofu, lentils, dried fruit, dark green leafy vegetables, dried herbs and spices, and spirulina. You can help the absorption of iron from non-meat sources by adding **vitamin C**-rich foods to meals – for example, a salad accompaniment, a glass of orange juice or fruit salad as a dessert. Both papaya and pineapple offer a good source of vitamin C, as well as containing enzymes (**bromelain**) that may help with digestion and thus alleviate certain symptoms of coeliac disease.

HEALING FOODS

Aduki beans
Asparagus
Bananas
Beetroot
Broccoli
Brown rice
Chia seed oil
Chicken
Chickpeas
Dried apricots
Dried figs
Dried marjoram and thyme
Eggs
Flaxseed oil
Ground cardamom
Kale
Kiwi fruit
Lean red meat
Lentils
Mackerel
Nuts (almonds, walnuts)
Oranges
Papaya
Pineapple
Potatoes
Raspberries
Red kidney beans
Salmon
Savoy cabbage
Soba noodles
Spinach
Spirulina
Strawberries
Tofu
Tuna
Turmeric

AVOID

Barley
Grain-based alcohols
Rye
Spelt
Wheat

Gluten-free recipes are marked by a (G) in the general index on pages 382–394.

Another nutrient that coeliac sufferers may not absorb properly is **calcium**, which is key to maintaining healthy bones. Undiagnosed coeliac disease therefore puts certain people at greater risk of developing osteoporosis (weakened bones; see page 312). The disease is also associated with lactose (milk protein) intolerance as it damages the part of the gut where lactase (the enzyme that digests lactose) is produced. To improve your calcium absorption, try looking to good non-dairy sources of calcium, which include dark green leafy vegetables (such as kale), almonds, fortified plant milks and tofu.

It's a good idea to include lots of foods rich in **omega 3 fatty acids** in your diet, including oily fish (adults can eat up to four portions per week, two if you are pregnant), as well as dark green leafy vegetables, chia seeds and flaxseeds and their oils, and walnuts. These healthy fats produce hormone-like substances called anti-inflammatory **prostaglandins**, which may help to control the inflammation associated with the disorder.

Hidden gluten Avoiding gluten can be tricky because it is 'hidden' in so many foods, especially stock cubes, packet and jarred sauces, certain alcoholic drinks and other processed foods. New legislation in the UK requires all food providers (including food manufacturers, restaurants and caterers) to flag up 14 key allergens, including gluten, for consumers, making it easier for coeliac sufferers to make the right food choices. Of course, cooking from scratch enables you to control what goes into your food and to make dishes that are as nutritious as possible to support your health. Most of the recipes in this book are gluten-free.

SKIN, HAIR & NAILS

What shows on the outside is definitely a reflection of your nutritional status and lifestyle. Healthy skin, in particular, is often the result of healthy lifestyle choices and a balanced diet (as well as good genes). Two of the worst things you can do for your skin are to smoke and to spend too much time in the sun – both will speed up the ageing process (as well as putting you at risk of something far more serious than a few wrinkles) as the body is exposed to free radical damage.

Free radicals are naturally produced as a byproduct of natural bodily processes; however, certain environmental factors (such as excess sunlight), poor lifestyle choices (such as smoking) and a bad diet can result in an overproduction of free radicals, which cause damage to cells in the body as it becomes overwhelmed.

HEALTHY SKIN DETOX

	DAY ONE	DAY TWO	DAY THREE
Breakfast	Quinoa & oat porridge with blackberry compote (p33)	Mango cup with pomegranate (p33)	Avocado smash with toasted nuts & seeds (p36)
Juice	Cucumber, pear, mint & wheatgrass juice (p57)	Carrot, beetroot, apple & celery juice (p57)	Avocado, apple, kiwi & spinach smoothie (p55)
Mid-morning snack	Cashew & goji berry flapjack (p80)	Avocado & broad bean smash on brown rice cakes (p60)	Red pepper & butter bean mash (p68) with red pepper crudités
Lunch	Dal with roasted fennel (p163)	Wild rice salad with jerusalem artichokes & heirloom tomatoes (p154)	Aduki bean stew (p170)
Mid-afternoon snack	Butter bean & spinach mash with crudités (p68)	cantaloupe melon slices (80g)	Candied walnuts (p81)
Dinner	Grilled salmon with ginger (p238) with Fresh pea & raw courgette salad (p98)	Sweet potato & turkey Massaman curry (p213)	Poached trout with fennel gratin (p241)

Antioxidants that are obtained from the food we eat can help to fight damage being caused by free radicals. Including plenty of antioxidant-rich fruit and vegetables (the more vibrant their colour the better) in the diet and drinking enough water (about two litres each day), as well as including skin-friendly foods such as avocados (rich in good fats and vitamin E), oily fish (rich in anti-inflammatory omega 3 fatty acids) and berries, kiwi fruit and pineapple (rich in vitamin C), will all help to lessen the damage to your skin and soften the ageing process.

Cutting out processed foods with poor nutritional quality will also help to keep your skin looking its best because foods high in refined sugar and less healthy fats (trans and saturated) will have a negative effect.

DAY FOUR	DAY FIVE	DAY SIX	DAY SEVEN
Quinoa & oat porridge with blackberry compote (p33)	Mango cup with pomegranate (p33)	Beans on toast (p47)	Avocado smash with toasted nuts & seeds (p36)
Cucumber, pear, mint & wheatgrass juice (p57)	Carrot, beetroot, apple & celery juice (p57)	Avocado, apple, kiwi & spinach smoothie (p55)	Raspberry, blueberry & coconut water smoothie (p49)
Butter bean & spinach mash with crudités (p68)	Cashew & goji berry flapjack (p80)	mango slices (80g)	Tenderstem & tahini (p66)
King prawn, noodle & lemongrass broth (p84)	Cajun chicken with avocado salad & mango salsa (p202)	King prawn & mango salad (p227)	Salmon, green beans, orange & hazelnut salad (p235)
toasted pumpkin & sunflower seeds (25g)	Beetroot hummus (p65) with Mixed seed crackers (p77)	Red pepper & butter bean mash (p68) with carrot crudités	Candied walnuts (p81)
Warm quinoa, squash & spinach risotto (p179)	Roasted pumpkin & tofu curry (p135)	Sweet potato cake with kale & green beans (p113)	Beetroot falafel (p115)

① ACNE

Acne is a common condition that can affect you psychologically, resulting in low self-esteem, social withdrawal and, in some cases, depression. It occurs as pores within the skin become blocked due to an overproduction of sebum, an oily substance that keeps your skin smooth. When this happens, bacteria that normally live happily on the surface of the skin begin to colonise the area, which causes the characteristic inflammation and pustules typical of the condition (your immune system responding to the infection).

This overproduction of sebum is due to hormonal changes, in particular an increase in the activity of sex hormones called androgens (testosterone is the main androgen produced by both men and women; in women it is converted to the female hormone oestrogen). Although acne commonly occurs in teenagers as they experience a surge of androgen hormones during puberty, it can continue into adulthood. Women are much more likely than men to develop adult acne, due to hormonal changes experienced during their period. Pregnancy and conditions such as polycystic ovary syndrome (see PCOS, page 374) can also cause changes to hormone levels that may result in acne.

It's worth stressing that there are no foods known to *cause* acne (although there may be foods that can worsen the condition or help to ease it, and more research is emerging to back this up). It's a misconception that eating foods such as chocolate, sweets and chips will result in acne or aggravate it – no evidence supports this. However, having said that, if your diet is made up predominately of refined and processed foods of poor nutritional quality, it's unlikely that you're eating a varied and balanced diet of nutrient-rich foods that will help to ensure the health of your skin and balance out hormone levels.

To promote healthy skin Try eating foods with a low glycaemic load (see GL, page 290), which are generally wholegrains and foods low in sugar, to help regulate blood sugar levels. Foods with a high GL lead to spikes in blood sugar that cause an increase in the hormone insulin. In some cases, if these foods are eaten to excess it could result in weight gain and reduced insulin sensitivity as cells becomes less responsive to the effect of insulin in lowering blood sugar levels. This, along with a cascade of other responses, may unbalance hormones, and stimulate the sebaceous glands found under the skin to produce more sebum, which will aggravate the condition.

Brightly coloured fruit and vegetables contain antioxidants, including **beta-carotene**, which is converted to **vitamin A** in the body and is essential for the maintenance and repair of skin (vitamin A is also found in oily fish and eggs). Every day try to eat plenty of dark green vegetables (kale, spinach, broccoli) as well as orange and yellow fruit and vegetables (butternut squash, mangoes, yellow peppers, sweet potatoes).

HEALING FOODS

Apricots
Asparagus
Avocado
Broccoli
Brown rice
Brussels sprouts
Butternut squash
Cabbage
Carrots
Chia seed oil
Courgettes
Eggs
Extra virgin olive oil
Flaxseed oil
Kale
Mackerel
Mango
Melon
Miso
Mushrooms
Nuts (cashews, walnuts)
Oats
Peppers
Prawns
Pulses (beans, lentils)
Quinoa
Salmon
Samphire
Seeds (pumpkin, sunflower)
Spinach
Sweet potatoes
Trout

LIMIT

Dairy foods
Omega 6-rich foods

For an index of recipes that may help with acne, see page 395.

Oily fish is rich in **omega 3 fatty acids**, which may be useful to help with acne through their role as an anti-inflammatory. You can also find vegetarian sources of omega 3 in seeds (chia and flax) and their oils, nuts (walnuts) and dark green leafy vegetables. Eat plenty of these foods throughout the week – up to four servings of oily fish; nuts and seeds as daily snacks; or a little chia oil in smoothies. Also, use extra virgin olive or rapeseed oil for cooking rather than vegetable or sunflower oil, which are high in omega 6 fatty acids (these can promote inflammation if eaten in excess).

There is research to suggest that many acne sufferers may be deficient in **zinc**, a mineral that can help to regulate sebaceous gland activity, and thus reduce the production of sebum. You can ensure adequate zinc intake in the diet by including foods such as shellfish, nuts, seeds, eggs and wholegrains.

Dairy foods contain hormones from milk-bearing animals such as cows and sheep, which research suggests could have an impact on your own hormone balance, and thus affect the condition of your skin. If you cut back on dairy, it's important you eat plenty of other calcium-rich foods to ensure the health of your bones (see Food Intolerance, page 325).

② PSORIASIS

A fairly common autoimmune condition (when the body's immune system attacks its own healthy cells), psoriasis affects about one in 50 people. It causes inflammation that presents itself as scaly, pink patches, usually on elbows, shins and scalp, that are the result of an increased rate of skin cell growth. Skin cells are formed at the bottom layer of the skin and then move upwards to replace dead cells on the surface in a process that usually takes around a month. In the case of psoriasis, the process of skin cell growth happens in the space of a few days.

The condition usually runs in the family and treatment consists of ointments and following a healthy diet to help to control the symptoms. Outbreaks of psoriasis can be triggered by factors such as stress, smoking and eating certain foods. To identify dietary triggers you would need to carry out an exclusion diet, which is best done with the help of a dietitian or nutritionist. Be warned that seeking advice on the internet will provide you with a whole raft of 'trigger foods' that may not be relevant to you, and cutting out lots of foods from your diet at once will put you at risk of vitamin and mineral deficiencies.

There are a few, commonly shared dietary factors that it may be sensible to avoid. These include alcohol, which can cause problems because it widens blood vessels, encouraging flow to the skin; this can make itching and flaking worse as the skin warms and reddens. Another factor is an omega 6 fatty acid known as arachidonic acid (ARA), which promotes inflammation. As the symptoms of psoriasis are inflammatory, causing its characteristic skin manifestations, cutting down on foods that contain ARA might help, as this fatty acid may worsen the condition. Foods that contain ARA include fatty cuts of meat (especially liver), eggs and dairy foods. You will also find this fatty acid in vegetable oils (try switching to extra virgin olive oil or coconut oil for cooking), margarines and processed foods.

Omega 3 fatty acids are essential when it comes to relieving inflammatory conditions. In the case of psoriasis they can be very useful to help reduce the symptoms – it has been shown to help patches look less aggravated through the effect of a hormone-like groups of substances known as **prostaglandins**. There are two types of prostaglandins: one that encourages inflammation (made from omega 6 fatty acids) and one that eases inflammation (from omega 3 fatty acids). It's beneficial to try to offset the amount of omega 6 in your diet by eating more omega 3-rich foods, as well as making changes to your diet, such as switching to extra virgin olive oil or coconut oil for cooking and avoiding processed foods (these often use vegetable oil, which is high in omega 6, as their main source of fat). Make sure you include plenty of oily fish in your diet (up to four portions per week, two if you're pregnant) or a vegetarian source of omega 3, such as dark green leafy vegetables, chia and flax seeds and their oils, and walnuts.

HEALING FOODS

Broccoli
Brussels sprouts
Butternut squash
Cantaloupe melon
Carrots
Chia seed oil
Flaxseed oil
Kale
Mackerel
Mangoes
Peppers
Quinoa
Salmon
Spinach
Sweet potatoes
Trout
Tuna
Walnuts

AVOID

Dairy foods
Eggs
Fatty cuts of meat
Liver
Margarine
Vegetable oils

For an index of recipes that may help with psoriasis, see page 412.

As always, plenty of fresh fruit and vegetables in the diet will provide an abundance of antioxidants. Particularly useful are those antioxidants that can be absorbed by the fat found beneath the surface of the skin, like the carotenoids such as **beta-carotene** found in orange, yellow and green fruit and vegetables. These may help with redness and swelling through their mild anti-inflammatory effect.

BALANCING OMEGA 3 AND OMEGA 6

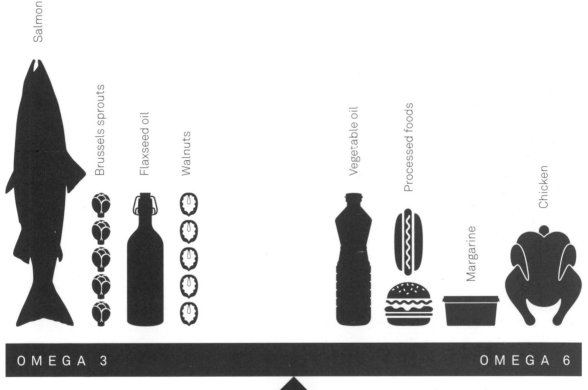

Most people get much more omega 6 (from margarine, meat, vegetable oils used for cooking and processed foods) in their diet than omega 3 (found in oily fish, dark green vegetables, walnuts and certain oils such as flaxseed), and this could influence the effect of inflammation on the body. Both of these fatty acids have an important role to play, but it can benefit your health to try to get a better balance of the two. The foods richest in these fats are shown on either side of the scales above. To achieve a good balance of the omegas, try to eat more oily fish and dark green leafy vegetables, to increase omega 3 intake. To decrease omega 6, cut out processed foods (including margarine) and switch to oils such as olive or rapeseed.

③ ECZEMA

This condition is characterised by an itchy, scaly and inflamed rash. It is common in children, and many people grow out of the condition during their teens. However, eczema still affects around one in 12 adults in the UK. There are two varieties: contact eczema, which is a type of allergy that causes a nasty red rash when your skin has been irritated by something touching it (this could be a type of metal or the material of your clothing), and atopic eczema.

It is not clear exactly what causes atopic eczema. It can run in families but also appears to be linked to the immune system (which is affected by stress), to allergies and changes in hormone levels. Environmental factors can play a part in the increased risk of a 'flare-up' – these could include a skin lotion (particularly if it contains lanolin), cleaning products, materials (especially wool, which naturally contains lanolin) or extremes in temperature.

Certain foods have been known to aggravate atopic eczema, but these may be different for each individual case. Common culprits include eggs, dairy products, nuts (especially peanuts), wheat and certain food additives. The only way you can identify what may be 'trigger foods' for you is by keeping a food diary and noting if any ingredient has worsened your eczema. You can then eliminate one food at a time for a month to see if this helps, and then reintroduce it to be sure that particular food was responsible. Cutting out whole food groups can be tricky, and could lead to nutritional deficiencies if not done properly, so you might find it easier to work with a registered nutritionist or dietitian.

Eating well to improve atopic eczema As with skin conditions such as psoriasis, foods rich in the omega 6 fatty acid arachidonic acid (ARA) should be avoided because they will encourage inflammation within the body and worsen the condition. Such foods include fatty cuts of meat (especially liver), eggs and dairy products, as well as vegetable oils (switch to cooking with extra virgin olive oil), margarines and processed foods.

You should also eat plenty of foods rich in **omega 3 fatty acids** to try to balance out the ratio of fatty acids in the body, as well as reducing inflammation through the action of anti-inflammatory **prostaglandins**. Adults can eat up to four servings of oily fish per week (two if you're pregnant) without any risk of toxic heavy metal build-up. If you don't eat fish, you can source your omega 3 from dark green vegetables, seeds (chia and flax) and their oils (add these to smoothies and dressings), and nuts (walnuts).

Fat-soluble antioxidants such as **beta-carotene** may have a mild anti-inflammatory effect, especially as they can target the layer of fat found below the surface of the skin. In general, we should all be eating plenty of brightly coloured fruit and vegetables to harness their potential to reduce free radical damage, which in the case of eczema may be the result of dryness in the skin.

HEALING FOODS

Asparagus

Bananas

Broccoli

Brussels sprouts

Butternut squash

Cantaloupe melon

Carrots

Chia seed oil

Chicory

Flaxseed oil

Garlic

Globe artichokes

Kale

Live yogurt (dairy-free)

Mackerel

Mangoes

Onions

Peppers

Quinoa

Salmon

Spinach

Sweet potatoes

Trout

Tuna

Walnuts

AVOID

Dairy foods

Eggs

Fatty cuts of meat

Liver

Margarine

Vegetable oils

For an index of recipes that may help with eczema, see page 404.

There is research to suggest that live bacteria cultures, such as *Lactobaccillus* or *Bifidobacterium*, which you can find in some yogurts (check the ingredients list) and as a supplement, may help to reduce the effects of eczema, although the findings are at present limited to infants. Regardless of whether the effects can be seen in adults, maintaining a balance of good bacteria in the gut with live bacteria foods such as yogurt (you can find dairy-free versions) and promoting their growth with **prebiotic** foods (bananas, onions, garlic, chicory, asparagus, globe artichokes) is beneficial for overall health.

④ HAIR & SCALP

Healthy, glossy hair is always a good indicator of someone's health and nutritional status –those with particularly poor diets tend to have hair that appears dull and brittle and, in some cases, that may be thinning or falling out. Whilst diet alone is not the only reason for someone to have a poorly conditioned scalp and hair, it can have a big influence.

For the best-looking hair, it's important to get a good supply of **omega 3 fatty acids** in the diet because these will help to reduce inflammation and improve the condition of the scalp. B vitamins are also important as they help to maintain healthy skin and circulation, which can keep your scalp healthy.

BALDNESS Male-pattern baldness is related to the hormone testosterone, which causes the hair follicles to shrink. As a result, they produce thinner hair over time until it becomes so fine that it fails to make it above the surface of the skin. Such baldness is very common in men and, unfortunately, there is nothing that can be done with diet to improve the condition. Your chances of losing your hair are very closely related to genetics and the degree of hair loss experienced by other men in your family.

Women can also experience male-pattern baldness, sometimes as the result of excessive testosterone (as in the case of polycystic ovary syndrome; see page 374). Other causes include an underactive thyroid or crash dieting – the possibility of thinning hair is another reason for losing weight slowly and steadily over time – as well as stress (make sure you are eating plenty of **vitamin B**-rich foods as these are essential for supporting healthy adrenal glands and nervous system).

In terms of diet, poor **zinc** levels have been associated with hair loss. You can boost your intake of zinc by eating foods such as shellfish, nuts, seeds, eggs and wholegrains. Anaemia may also result in hair loss, as well as making you feel run-down and lacking in energy. This condition can be the result of low **iron** (found in lean red meat, oily fish, eggs, lentils, dark green leafy vegetables, dried herbs and spices), **folate** (in most fruit and vegetables) or **vitamin B12** (oily fish, eggs, spirulina), so it's important that you maintain healthy levels of each of these.

Vitamin A also plays a small part through its role in healthy sebum production (sebum is the waxy substance that lubricates and moisturises the skin and hence the scalp). You can glean plenty of this vitamin from foods rich in **beta-carotene** (dark green, yellow and red fruit and vegetables).

HEALING FOODS

Aduki beans
Asparagus
Avocados
Beetroot
Brown rice
Butternut squash
Cantaloupe melon
Carrots
Cauliflower
Chickpeas
Dried fruit, especially apricots
Edamame beans
Eggs
Kale
Lean red meat
Lentils
Mackerel
Mangoes
Oats
Oranges
Parsley
Peas
Peppers
Salmon
Sardines
Seeds (pumpkin, sunflower)
Spinach
Spirulina
Sweet potatoes
Tuna
Turkey

AVOID

Processed foods (lacking in vitamin and mineral quality)

For an index of recipes that may help with hair and scalp problems, see page 405.

⑤ WEAK, BRITTLE NAILS

Healthy nails are those where the bed appears pink and the tips white. Many of us can't help damaging our nails by biting, picking or overusing corrosive nail varnish removers, and these are the most likely culprits for poor nail health. However, a weak, brittle or ridged appearance may indicate a nutritional deficiency or even underlying medical condition.

Mineral deficiencies It's commonly thought that a lack of **calcium** and **zinc** is responsible for poor nail health, and you will see many supplements on the shelves of healthfood shops that promote these minerals as being effective at 'strengthening' and 'repairing' poor nails (be aware that excessive calcium intake from supplements could also prevent the absorption of other key minerals). Zinc in particular has been associated with the white spots commonly found on nails (in fact, these are most likely the effect of damage from day-to-day activities).

    Whilst it is true that zinc and calcium will play a role in the health of your nails, it is small because nails contain very little of these minerals. As long as you are getting two to three servings of dairy alternatives (fortified rice milk, dark green leafy vegetables, almonds, sesame seeds) and foods containing zinc, such as shellfish, nuts and seeds, it's unlikely they will be responsible.

Other causes As nails are made from a protein known as keratin, inadequate amounts of protein in the diet can result in weak nails. It's very unlikely that meat-eaters would be lacking in the amino acids that make up the proteins in the body, but for those such as strict vegans, who are on restrictive diets that don't include animal products, this may be an issue. For vegans it's important to combine plant proteins such as pulses, grains and soya products to make sure you get all the essential amino acids needed (see section on Vegetarians & Vegans, page 376).

    One of the more likely causes of weak, brittle nails is anaemia, which can develop from a lack of iron, folate or vitamin B12, and can lead to the blood delivering inadequate nutrition to the nails. Iron deficiency is the most common, particularly in women (see page 354), and can be diagnosed by a blood test on the recommendation of your GP. Eating foods rich in iron (such as lean red meat, dark green leafy vegetables, pulses, dried fruit, herbs and spices) will help get your iron stores back up to healthy levels. Try combining these foods with those that contain **vitamin C**, such as fruit and vegetables, as they can help to increase absorption of iron. To ensure you have adequate levels of **folate** and **vitamin B12**, include foods such as seafood, eggs, dark green leafy vegetables, pulses and orange juice.

HEALING FOODS

Aduki beans

Asparagus

Avocados

Beetroot

Broccoli

Cauliflower

Chickpeas

Dried fruit, especially apricots

Dried herbs and spices

Edamame beans

Eggs

Kale

Kiwi fruit

Lean red meat

Leeks

Lemons

Lentils

Limes

Parsley

Peas

Peppers

Pineapple

Poultry

Prawns

Sardines

Spinach

Spirulina

Sunflower seeds

Tofu

AVOID

No specific foods

WEIGHT

Put very simply, weight gain is usually a result of eating more calories than you are burning off. (There are conditions that make people more prone to weight gain, such as polycystic ovary syndrome or underactive thyroid, but these are relatively uncommon.) Most of us don't like to admit what we've eaten, or we underestimate the portion size – research has shown that people trying to lose weight under-report their calorie intakes by as much as 500 calories a day, which is potentially the amount required to lose 450g (one pound) a week. In addition, we may simply forget the extra little nibbles, sips and bites of food and drink – at our desks, off a child's plate or when preparing meals – that can all add up at the end of the day.

There is a great deal of information out there about how to lose weight, some of it particularly bad, involving prolonged fasting or complicated elimination regimes, offering quick-fix solutions and encouraging negative attitudes to food. Although we don't intend the Detox Kitchen to be a diet regime, many people do lose weight when they eat our food as they begin to adopt healthier eating practices.

For anyone who is trying to shift the pounds, this section offers helpful advice and includes a weight-loss plan based on an intake of 1500 calories per day (it's very difficult to support an active lifestyle and get all the nutrients for good health on less than this). You will

1500-CALORIE DETOX

	DAY ONE	DAY TWO	DAY THREE
Breakfast	Blueberry & apple muffin (p43)	Apple, blueberry & cinnamon Bircher muesli (p28)	Pecan & coconut granola (p30)
Juice	Carrot, beetroot, apple & celery juice (p57)	Cucumber, pear, mint & wheatgrass juice (p57)	Carrot, beetroot, apple & celery juice (p57)
Mid-morning snack	Radishes & cauliflower with hummus (p66)	Edamame & seed salad (p73)	Butter bean & spinach mash with crudités (p68)
Lunch	Pinto bean chilli (p168)	Avocado salad (p97)	Pearl barley with cantaloupe melon (p151)
Mid-afternoon snack	mixed berries (80g)	Beetroot hummus (p65)	Sesame seed cookie (p81)
Dinner	Grilled mackerel with ginger & saffron rice (p253)	Cabbage stuffed with chicken (p208)	Baked sea bream with braised leeks (p244)

also find two three-day plans on page 301. Intended to 'kickstart' all of our detox plans, these short plans are low in calories and not intended to be followed long term, but may be a good way to begin your weight-loss regime. In addition, you'll find calorie information for each recipe, which will help you to monitor your energy intake.

Those who take regular exercise will tend to burn more calories. People who are heavily muscular typically have a higher resting metabolic rate, meaning they burn more calories whilst carrying out their daily activities. Exercising regularly is a good way to lose fat and increase body muscle, and thus increase your metabolism.

Being overweight usually means you're eating too many foods with a high calorie content, which are inevitably rich in fat, salt and sugar – all associated with a diet closely linked to a number of health conditions, including heart disease and diabetes. It's worth remembering, though, that you can gain weight on 'healthy' foods if you eat too much of them because some are high in calories (for example, there are around 600 calories in 100g of nuts and seeds; however, they're very nutritious, meaning you can glean a high amount of key nutrients from just a small quantity). This is why people often say that they don't understand why they're putting on weight when they eat really healthily.

DAY FOUR	DAY FIVE	DAY SIX	DAY SEVEN
Apple, blueberry & cinnamon Bircher muesli (p28)	Strawberry soya yogurt (p29)	Poached eggs & sweet potato hash (p39)	Mango cup with pomegranate (p33)
Chia seed, coconut & pineapple smoothie (p52)	Avocado, apple, kiwi & spinach smoothie (p55)	Cucumber, pear, mint & wheatgrass juice (p57)	Carrot, beetroot, apple & celery juice (p57)
Kale crisps with cashew nuts & paprika (p74)	Spicy nuts (p76)	Pistachio oat bar (p79)	Edamame & seed salad (p73)
Butternut squash & butter bean stew (p138)	Mung bean curry with onion, cucumber & cashew nut salad (p167)	Nettle & kale broth (p92) with Quinoa bread (p44)	Wild rice salad with jerusalem artichoke & heirloom tomatoes (p154)
Pistachio oat bar (p79)	Coconut macaroon (p263)	Avocado & broad bean smash on brown rice cakes (p60)	Tenderstem & tahini (p66)
Chicken & quinoa salad (p205)	Seared tuna & beetroot salad (p253)	King prawn stir-fry (p230)	Turkey burger with cabbage slaw (p214)

Maintaining a healthy body weight is not only one of the best ways to protect your future health against disease, but it also helps you retain a good level of self-esteem. This is something that can easily be lost when you're unhappy about the way you look – a feeling that can filter into all aspects of your life.

A food diary Keeping a food diary – and being honest in writing down what you've eaten (or, better still, taking pictures of your meals on your phone) – is the only way to find out what's going on. Often it can be a revelation as patterns of food intake begin to emerge. A registered nutritionist can help you assess your food diary and work out your calorie intake each day. Or you could use one of the many online apps to enter the information (remember, though, that estimating portion sizes and establishing what was in a recipe can be rather tricky).

Once you see it all on paper, it's usually pretty obvious where the excess calories are coming from. Then you can begin to establish a few diet goals and make simple changes that will help you to cut down on your energy intake, such as reducing portion size, eating more fruit and vegetables, or switching to wholegrain foods.

Comfort eating We all like to eat for comfort occasionally and the foods we choose are often those that can raise serotonin levels in the brain, making us feel relaxed and less anxious. Such foods are generally high in sugar and refined carbohydrates, which can cause spikes in blood sugar levels and then quickly leave us feeling worse as the effect wears off.

Eating these foods regularly can become a habit and lead to weight gain, so trying to understand what triggers you to reach for them, and at what moment, will help you to establish a healthier way of eating. If you are going to keep a food diary, it's useful to write down how you felt each time you ate. This will help you to get to grips with the problem and look for healthier food options or other ways to boost mood (exercise releases 'feel-good' hormones in the brain).

Checking if you are overweight A quick way to establish whether you're overweight is to check your body mass index (BMI) using the chart on page 347. This guide uses a simple equation based on your height and weight. A normal BMI range is shown in blue – anything below or above this range means you're carrying too little or too much weight. There are some instances, though, such as if you're pregnant or very muscular, where the BMI is not a reliable measure because the equation is based simply on weight and doesn't differentiate between fat and muscle mass. Saying that, you wouldn't be looking to start losing weight whilst you are pregnant, and if you did have a high muscle to fat ratio it's very likely you are already leading an active healthy lifestyle. Maintaining a healthy body weight is essential for everyone.

If your BMI indicates that you need to lose weight, start by setting a realistic weight-loss goal. Losing 450g to 1kg (one or two pounds) each week is a sensible target. Although it may take longer to slim down to your ideal weight, there is less chance of you giving up and putting the weight back on. Try not to obsess over the scales – weigh yourself weekly, not daily, because there are factors such as water retention that might cause fluctuations over the course of a day.

Rather than worrying too much about the grams or stones, it's often better to set a practical goal, such as fitting back into an old pair of jeans you love or other favourite item of clothing. It's achievements like these that can give you a real boost.

Some useful tips

- Be mindful about food. It's been shown that people who eat mindfully eat fewer calories. Simple steps include sitting down to eat, chewing your food slowly and putting your cutlery down between mouthfuls. All of these give your brain time to register that you're eating and when you're full.
- Eat a balance of foods with plenty of variety so you can glean as many nutrients from your diet as possible. Try to eat mostly plant foods (fruit, vegetables and wholegrains) accompanied by lean proteins and healthy fats (oils, avocados, nuts and oily fish). Make sure you are also eating a few servings of dairy alternatives (fortified rice milk, tahini, almonds, dark green vegetables) each day to make up for the lack of dairy foods.
- Opt for foods with a low glycaemic load (GL; see page 290) as these will help you to maintain balanced blood sugar levels, which will moderate your mood and cravings.
- Feel fuller for longer by including protein (animal and plant) and high-fibre foods (wholegrains and vegetables) in each meal. Foods with a high water content can also be a useful way to help you feel full on fewer calories. Try eating soup or tomato/stock-based dishes, such as stews, casseroles and curries.
- Eat regularly to maintain steady blood sugar levels and prevent hunger pangs. Don't forget about breakfast – research has shown that people who don't eat breakfast are more likely to be overweight.
- Keep foods that are high in saturated fat and sugar to a minimum: fat is high in calories, so when eaten in excess will encourage weight gain, and excess sugar will be stored in the body as triglycerides (the main storage fat in the body). Don't cut fat out completely, though, as a little can help to satiate you as well as adding to the flavour and texture of food. Opt for extra virgin olive oil or small servings of avocado, nuts and seeds.
- Don't get dehydrated because this can often be misread as hunger and encourage you to eat. Be sure to drink plenty of water throughout the day.

- Avoid alcohol as it contains nearly as many calories as fat (with little nutritional benefit), and can unbalance blood sugar levels. Alcohol can also disrupt sleep (a lack of sleep has been linked to weight gain or difficulty in losing weight).
- Keep active because this will help to increase your metabolism and promote weight loss. It doesn't mean you need to train for a triathlon – simply incorporating some activity into your daily regime will help, and in the long term is more sustainable than training full on for short periods of time.

Trying to gain weight For some people, trying to gain weight can be just as difficult and frustrating as losing it. A bout of illness, surgery, digestive conditions, stress or a very active lifestyle can make it difficult to maintain a healthy body weight. Although it's tempting to fill up on calorie-laden foods high in fat, salt and sugar, this is not the best strategy to adopt and will likely leave you feeling sluggish and unhealthy.

Being a member of the 'skinny genes' club, I feel qualified to share a few tips for gaining weight in a healthy way:

- Don't skip meals, and opt for three meals plus plenty of nourishing snacks. People trying to gain weight often have small appetites, so instead of large portions it may be more useful to think about your daily food intake as six mini-meals.
- Choose higher calorie, nutrient-rich healthy foods such as nuts, seeds, avocados, oils, oily fish, nut butters, tahini (found in hummus), bananas, granola, dried fruit and home-made dressings and marinades. Quinoa and edamame beans are a little higher in calories than other grains and pulses.
- Eat nourishing snacks such as nut butter and sliced banana on wheat-free bread; small grain-based salads; omelettes; guacamole or a tomato and avocado salad drizzled with extra virgin olive oil; porridge with chopped nuts and dried fruit; coconut yogurt with granola. Nuts and dried fruit are another good snack, as are edamame beans with chilli and sesame oil. Smoothies are also a great way to boost calories – try adding avocado, nut butters or tahini.
- Boost dishes by getting into the habit of always adding one more ingredient. This could be chopped nuts or pulses; cooked foods like quinoa or sweet potato to salads; flavoured oils and grains to soups; dried fruit to grain-based salads; dried coconut flakes to fruit salads; or coconut milk to curry.

BODY MASS INDEX (BMI) CHART

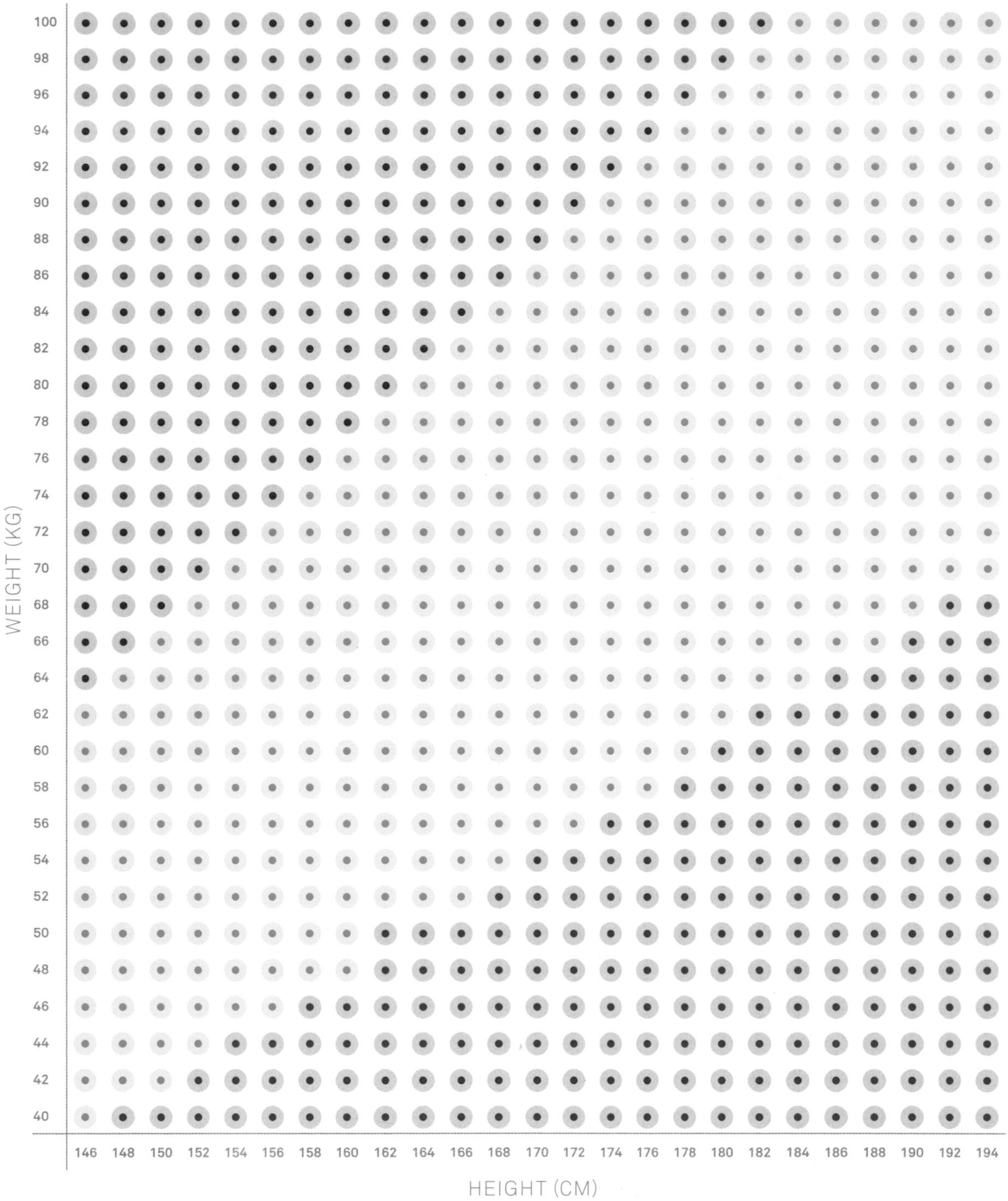

WEIGHT (KG)

HEIGHT (CM)

The BMI chart is a measure of body fat based on your height and weight. To use the chart, run your finger along a line from your weight and another finger up from your height until they converge. The point at which they meet shows which zone (see explanation right) you fall into.

- Underweight
- Normal weight
- Overweight
- Obese

1 stone = 6.35kg
1 pound = 450g

1 foot = 30cm
1 inch = 2.5cm

We all lead busy lives that can get really stressful at times. Working out how best to cope with that stress, so it doesn't affect our ability to do the important things in life, is vital to our well-being. Factors that influence stress levels include relationship and financial problems, as well as an inability to establish a healthy work-life balance.

Stress can occur in three stages. The initial phase produces adrenaline and is often characterised by the 'fight or flight' response. The second stage is resistance to stress as the body develops coping mechanisms, and stage three is exhaustion when the body becomes depleted of resources. It's when we are unable to cope that the risk of long-term damage increases and certain conditions, such as anxiety and depression, which can badly affect quality of life, begin to appear.

HEALTHY MIND DETOX

	DAY ONE	DAY TWO	DAY THREE
Breakfast	Apple, blueberry & cinnamon Bircher muesli (p28)	Soft-boiled eggs with avocado salad (p38)	Granola with pineapple & strawberries (p30)
Juice	Cucumber, pear, mint & wheatgrass juice (p57)	Carrot, beetroot, apple & celery juice (p57)	Cucumber, pear, mint & wheatgrass juice (p57)
Mid-morning snack	Avocado & broad bean smash on brown rice cakes (p60)	Cashew & goji berry flapjack (p80)	Butter bean & spinach mash with crudités (p68)
Lunch	Wild rice salad with jerusalem artichoke & heirloom tomatoes (p154)	Quinoa & cashew salad (p150)	Salmon, green beans, orange & hazelnut salad (p235)
Mid-afternoon snack	Edamame & seed salad (p73)	Radishes & cauliflower with hummus (p66)	dried figs (50g)
Dinner	Salmon & brown rice noodles (p237)	Minced chicken in lettuce wraps (p211)	Roasted pumpkin & tofu curry (p135)

Stress, anxiety and depression can affect appetite. If it diminishes, you may not be able to get everything you need to help keep yourself properly nourished. These psychological conditions can also cause you to overeat the wrong types of food, which can send blood sugar levels awry, and to drink too much coffee (coffee increases adrenaline). Stress can also deplete the body of key nutrients, including B vitamins and magnesium.

In some cases, eating the right foods can help to manage the adverse conditions that may arise. Omega 3 fatty acids have been shown to have a beneficial effect by helping to balance out the levels of stress hormones. A good diet and regular exercise are simple ways to help promote good mental health as well as a healthy body.

DAY FOUR	DAY FIVE	DAY SIX	DAY SEVEN
Banana muffin (p43)	Quinoa & oat porridge with blackberry compote (p33)	Mango yogurt with dried apricots & banana (p29)	Baked eggs with spinach & tomato (p38)
Avocado, apple, kiwi & spinach smoothie (p55)	Raspberry, blueberry & coconut water smoothie (p49)	Carrot, beetroot, apple & celery juice (p57)	Chia seed, coconut & pineapple smoothie (p52)
Radishes & cauliflower with hummus (p66)	Cashew & goji berry flapjack (p80)	cashew nuts (30g)	Edamame & seed salad (p73)
Kale, edamame & fennel frittata (p199)	Butternut squash & butter bean stew (p138)	Quinoa, asparagus & almond salad (p150)	Lemon chicken (p220)
blueberries (80g)	Tenderstem & tahini (p66)	Avocado & broad bean smash on brown rice cakes (p60)	Cacao milk (p53)
Pinto bean chilli (p168)	Halibut with chickpea stew & pesto (p242)	Thai green curry (p137)	Mexican bean soup (p88)

① DEPRESSION

Depression is very common: at least one in ten of us will experience severe depression that will last for several weeks or even months. There are many triggers for depression, including a life event such as bereavement or the breakdown of a relationship. Other lifestyle triggers include smoking and alcohol or drug use. Symptoms of depression vary and can involve both physical and psychological factors, such as a lack of appetite, poor sleep, constipation, weight gain or loss, and a lack of energy and enthusiasm.

Whilst food won't cure your depression, a healthy diet containing the right foods can help to ease symptoms and promote well-being. It's important that you make every effort to keep your appetite up and eat regularly so you can glean all the nutrients you need. Aside from food, exercise can provide a useful way to deal with mild to moderate depression as it releases serotonin, the brain's 'feel-good' hormone.

Combating symptoms of depression There is strong evidence that **omega 3 fatty acids** may help to relieve symptoms. Research has shown rates of depression to be lower in countries with high omega 3 intake, and that levels of this fatty acid tend to be markedly lower in sufferers. To increase your omega 3 intake you could try eating up to four portions of oily fish per week (two if you're pregnant) plus dark green leafy vegetables, walnuts, seeds (flax and chia) and their oils.

As with all conditions that involve mood, it's important to maintain steady blood sugar levels, which can affect concentration, ability to focus and energy levels. Combining complex carbohydrates such as wholegrain foods (brown rice, buckwheat, barley and oats) with protein will facilitate a slow, maintained release of energy.

Certain foods contain significant levels of the amino acid **tryptophan** (poultry, oily fish, eggs, pulses), which is converted in the brain to the hormone **serotonin**. The relaxing effect of this hormone is useful to relieve anxiety and encourage sleep. As tryptophan uptake requires carbohydrate, you could try a carbohydrate snack before bed, such as a small bowl of porridge, or oatcakes with honey.

Deficiencies in **magnesium** and **B vitamins** (in particular vitamin B12) have also been linked to depression: B vitamins are involved in the production of neurotransmitters in the brain. These nutrients can be found in dark green leafy vegetables, lentils, oily fish, nuts, seeds and spirulina (a type of algae).

PMS-related depression has been associated with a lack of **vitamin B6** (found in poultry, eggs, oily fish, quinoa and green leafy vegetables), which may have to do with the function this vitamin plays in converting the amino acid tryptophan to serotonin in the brain. Be careful if considering a supplement because high doses (over 50mg) can result in unwanted symptoms such as numbness.

There are two compounds found in raw cacao, one considered to act as a mild mood enhancer (**phenylethylamine**) and the other a mild stimulant (**theobromine**); however, their effect is small.

HEALING FOODS

Aubergines
Avocados
Beetroot
Broccoli
Brown rice
Brussels sprouts
Cabbage
Cantaloupe melon
Chia seed oil
Chicken
Dried figs
Edamame beans
Eggs
Flaxseed oil
Halibut
Kale
Leeks
Lentils
Mackerel
Mung beans
Nuts (cashews, walnuts)
Oats
Onions
Oranges
Quinoa
Raisins
Raw cacao
Salmon
Seeds (pumpkin, sunflower)
Soba noodles
Spirulina
Sweetcorn
Tomatoes
Tuna
Turkey

AVOID

Alcohol
Caffeine
Refined sugar

For an index of recipes that may help with depression, see page 402.

② ANXIETY

Most people have experienced anxiety at some point in their life, triggered by a situation (public speaking), phobia (fear of heights) or post-traumatic stress (after a terrifying experience), or as a generalised disorder (continual feeling of anxiety without any triggers present). Anxiety often accompanies depression but can exist on its own, and symptoms include sweating, shortness of breath, dizziness and heart palpitations. In some cases, it can result in panic attacks.

As with depression, food cannot treat anxiety, but making the right food choices and maintaining a healthy diet will help to ensure the best possible mental health and well-being. It's important that you try to maintain steady blood sugar levels when you suffer from anxiety because foods that are metabolised quickly in the body (such as refined carbohydrates, including sugar) can cause blood sugar imbalances. 'Sugar highs' can have a detrimental effect, leaving you a little on edge, which will affect concentration and your capacity to focus. To promote a slow, maintained release of energy and balance out blood sugar levels, opt for a low GL diet by choosing complex carbohydrates such as wholegrains (brown rice, soba noodles, barley, quinoa, oats), root vegetables and pulses.

Studies have shown that the mineral **magnesium** (involved in muscle relaxation) is useful when dealing with anxiety, although whether this is directly related to the nervous system is not fully understood. However, it will do you no harm to include plenty of magnesium-rich foods in your diet such as nuts, seeds, dark green vegetables and some white fish.

Low levels of the amino acids **L-lysine** (found in edamame beans, poultry, pulses, seeds and eggs) and **L-arginine** (oily fish, shellfish, oats, nuts, pulses) have also been linked with anxiety, so consuming more may benefit the condition. You can get a steady supply of these nutrients by eating foods rich in good-quality proteins. **Omega 3** has been shown to be beneficial for anxiety but exactly how is not yet fully understood. It may be related to the release of serotonin (the 'feel-good' hormone) in the brain, which can improve mood, or the fact that omega 3 may help to prevent surges in stress hormones (adrenaline and cortisol).

As you would expect, caffeine will aggravate anxiety, leaving you edgy (caffeine releases the hormone adrenaline), so should be avoided. Instead opt for herbal teas, including chamomile, bergamot and lemon balm, all of which can have a calming effect. If you have difficulty dropping off to sleep, you could try valerian or blue vervain tea in the evenings to encourage relaxation.

HEALING FOODS

Aduki beans
Aubergines
Bergamot, chamomile, valerian and vervain teas
Brown rice
Butternut squash
Cabbage
Chicken
Chickpeas
Citrus fruit
Dried figs
Edamame beans
Eggs
Garlic
Green beans
Kale
Nuts (cashews, peanuts, pine nuts)
Oats
Onions
Prawns
Quinoa
Raisins
Seeds (pumpkin, sunflower)
Soba noodles
Sweetcorn
Sweet potatoes
Swiss chard
Tomatoes

AVOID

Alcohol
Caffeine
Refined sugar

For an index of recipes that may help with anxiety, see page 306.

FATIGUE

Feeling 'run down' or completely depleted of energy is a common complaint that can occur for many different reasons – sometimes as a result of lifestyle and sometimes because of diet, in particular low levels of B vitamins, needed for converting food into energy (these may be used up in response to stress, which can also leave you fatigued). Or it can be as simple as not eating enough food to supply the energy required to complete your daily tasks.

The mid-afternoon energy slump is classic for someone who eats a lunch with a high glycaemic load (GL) – food that is quickly

FIGHTING FATIGUE DETOX

	DAY ONE	DAY TWO	DAY THREE
Breakfast	Beetroot & apple Bircher muesli (p25)	Granola with pineapple & strawberries (p30)	Quinoa & oat porridge with blackberry compote (p33)
Juice	Avocado, apple, kiwi & spinach smoothie (p55)	Carrot, beetroot, apple & celery juice (p57)	Chia seed, coconut & pineapple smoothie (p52)
Mid-morning snack	Cashew & goji berry flapjack (p80)	mixed berries (80g)	Quail's eggs, celery salt & cherry tomatoes (p73)
Lunch	Sweet potato cake with kale & green beans (p113)	Quinoa & cashew salad (p150)	Butternut squash & sage risotto (p182)
Mid-afternoon snack	Tenderstem & tahini (p66)	Edamame & seed salad (p73)	Candied walnuts (p81)
Dinner	Salmon & brown rice noodles (p237)	Roasted pumpkin & tofu curry (p135)	Cajun chicken with avocado salad & mango salsa (p202)

broken down by the body, causing a rapid increase in blood sugar, usually followed by slump and hunger (baked potatoes have this effect as a result of their high GL) – plus sweet snacks. Avoiding 'sugar highs' and maintaining steady blood sugar is the way to keep your energy levels up.

For some people there can be a more deep-rooted reason for fatigue, including poor mental health (depression and anxiety), a medical condition such as chronic fatigue syndrome, food intolerance, or vitamin and mineral deficiency.

DAY FOUR	DAY FIVE	DAY SIX	DAY SEVEN
Mango yogurt with dried apricots & banana (p29)	Avocado smash with toasted nuts & seeds (p36)	Chia seed pudding with blackberry & lime coulis (p35)	Baked egg with spinach & tomato (p38)
Cucumber, pear, mint & wheatgrass juice (p57)	Raspberry, blueberry & coconut water smoothie (p49)	Carrot, beetroot, apple & celery juice (p57)	Avocado, apple, kiwi & spinach smoothie (p55)
Spicy nuts (p76)	Cashew & goji berry flapjack (p80)	Guacamole (p59)	Edamame & seed salad (p73)
Sweet potato frittata (p196)	Stir-fried cauliflower rice with shiitake mushrooms & tofu (p143)	Brown rice, pak choi & ginger broth (p83)	Quinoa pizza (p148)
mixed berries (80g)	Beetroot falafel (p115)	brazil nuts (30g)	Roasted curried chickpeas (p76)
Halibut with chickpea stew & pesto (p242)	Turkey burger with cabbage slaw (p214)	Pollock & prawn fishcake with courgette spaghetti (p247)	Grilled mackerel with ginger & saffron rice (p253)

① IRON DEFICIENCY (ANAEMIA)

Iron plays a key role in the production of red blood cells, whose job it is to transport oxygen around the body. Anaemia is an umbrella term used to describe a group of disorders that are characterised by the inability of red blood cells to carry out this function. The most common type of anaemia is related to iron deficiency, but others do exist that involve low levels of folate and vitamin B12. All three of these nutrients are involved in the production of red blood cells.

The symptoms of anaemia are related to the lack of oxygen in the bloodstream. In mild cases this can leave you feeling weak and fatigued and looking pale. In more severe cases, you could experience shortness of breath or fainting. Iron deficiency is common in women as a result of their monthly blood loss, and pregnant women can be at particular risk due to the demands the growing baby places on them (during the third trimester and after birth). Other groups at greater risk are those with high physical demands on their body, such as sports people, and those on meat-free diets such as vegans.

Including plenty of iron-rich foods in your diet is an obvious place to start. You should also make sure you're getting enough **vitamin B12** (from oily fish, eggs, spirulina) and **folate** (found in most fruit and vegetables). In more severe cases, you might want to visit your GP, who will carry out blood tests and then may prescribe iron supplements.

It's simple to fortify your cooking with **iron**, such as by including pulses or dark green vegetables in cooked dishes and salads, adding dried fruit to cooked dishes or as a breakfast topping (try making a dried fruit compote) and opting for pulse-based dips as snacks. Foods with the highest iron content include lean red meat, poultry, oily fish and eggs. You can also find useful amounts of iron in non-meat foods, such as pulses, dried fruit, soya products, dark green leafy vegetables, oats, avocados, and dried herbs and spices (even in small quantities – just a couple of teaspoons of dried thyme or marjoram, cumin seeds or turmeric can add up to 2g of iron).

Eating non-meat iron sources with a food rich in **vitamin C** (citrus fruit, berries, red peppers) will help you to absorb more of the iron – include a glass of orange juice with your breakfast; spoon fruit compote on to your porridge; or serve green vegetables with your meal. **Copper** also aids in the absorption of iron and you will find this mineral in foods such as kale, cashew nuts, mushrooms and pulses (chickpeas, soya beans, aduki beans).

It's good to be aware of those foods that can prevent the absorption of iron (and iron supplements). These include tea (contains tannins), caffeine drinks and compounds called phytates, found in raw bran, certain nuts and beans. It's best to avoid these foods with iron-rich meals.

HEALING FOODS

Asparagus
Avocados
Beetroot
Broccoli
Butternut squash
Carrots
Cauliflower
Chicken
Dried apricots
Dried figs
Dried marjoram and thyme
Eggs
Ground cardamom
Kale
Kiwi fruit
Lean red meat
Lemons
Limes
Oats
Oranges
Parsley
Pineapple
Pomegranates
Pulses (beans, lentils)
Pumpkin
Raspberries
Red peppers
Salmon
Spinach
Spirulina
Strawberries
Swiss chard
Tofu
Trout
Tuna
Watercress

AVOID

Caffeine
Raw bran
Tea

For an index of recipes that may help with anaemia, see page 395.

② CHRONIC FATIGUE SYNDROME (CFS)

It is not yet fully understood how or why chronic fatigue syndrome (CFS), also known as myalgic encephalopathy (ME), develops. One theory is that it occurs in some people after a bout of viral illness such as glandular fever or flu (as the immune system never fully recovers). Other possible contributing factors are prolonged stress from a traumatic experience, such as bereavement or depression, or even hormone imbalances or immune system disorders.

The symptoms are primarily debilitating fatigue, as well as headaches, muscle aches, joint pain, poor concentration, prolonged exercise recovery time and sleep that doesn't refresh. Many of these symptoms could be linked to any number of other problems, such as anaemia, thyroid issues, diabetes or obesity, so a doctor will go through a series of tests to rule these out before diagnosing CFS.

There is no cure for CFS, but symptoms may improve over time, and a well-balanced diet can play a big role in improving mood and energy levels. Ensuring you maintain blood sugar levels by eating regularly throughout the day and including plenty of complex carbohydrate foods (brown rice, quinoa, pulses, soba noodles) will ensure you have an adequate energy supply. **Omega 3 fatty acids** are also useful because symptoms such as joint inflammation and swollen glands may be temporarily eased by eating foods rich in this nutrient (oily fish, chia seeds and flaxseeds and their oils, dark green leafy vegetables and walnuts).

Maintaining a strong immune system is also important, to make sure you're able to resist infection. Try to get plenty of **zinc** (from seafood, poultry, eggs, oats and nuts) and **vitamin C** (most fruit and vegetables, including kiwi fruit, berries and peppers) as these will help to promote good immunity.

It's worth avoiding foods that contain the artificial sweetener aspartame (found in low-fat and other diet foods) and the flavour-enhancer monosodium glutamate (MSG) because both have been shown to make the symptoms of CFS worse.

HEALING FOODS

Berries
Broccoli
Brown rice
Cauliflower
Chia seed oil
Chicken
Chickpeas
Courgettes
Crab
Eggs
Flaxseed oil
Kale
Lemons
Limes
Miso
Mushrooms
Nuts (brazils, walnuts)
Oats
Oranges
Peas
Peppers
Pineapple
Pomegranates
Prawns
Quinoa
Rapeseed oil
Salmon
Sardines
Seeds (pumpkin, sesame)
Soba noodles
Spring greens
Tomatoes
Trout
Tuna
Turkey

AVOID

Foods containing aspartame and MSG

For an index of recipes that may help with CFS, see page 400.

③ INSOMNIA

Poor sleep (insomnia), which affects around one in five people, can mean difficulty nodding off, staying asleep or waking up too early. The result is that you don't feel refreshed when you get up in the morning, and the lack of sleep will leave you tired during the day, unable to concentrate and, most likely, irritable with mood swings. The amount of sleep you need varies between people, with some managing perfectly well on three to four hours per night, but in general six to eight hours is the average.

There are many reasons why you may not be able to sleep, and it could occur for no particular reason at all. It may be a temporary issue, such as a work- or family-related problem, or a particular condition such as indigestion, cramp or the common cold. It could also be related to something more long term, such as anxiety and depression.

Basic steps such as simple relaxation techniques or reading before bed can help, as can making sure your bedroom is in complete darkness (the brain secretes more of the 'sleep hormone' melatonin in the dark). Cutting out stimulants, such as alcohol and caffeine, and avoiding exercise close to bedtime are other ways to ensure you are fully relaxed. You could also try herbal teas such as chamomile, valerian and passion flower, which are known to help aid relaxation.

With respect to diet, eating plenty of foods that are rich in the amino acid **tryptophan** (poultry, nuts, edamame beans, avocados, chickpeas) will ensure you have adequate levels in the body to be converted to **serotonin** in the brain (which in turn is used to make **melatonin**, which regulates sleep and wake cycles). In order for tryptophan to pass across the blood/brain barrier, it requires the action of carbohydrates, which raise insulin levels to help pave the way. So to aid relaxation and induce sleep at bedtime, you could opt for an evening meal rich in complex carbohydrates; or try a small carbohydrate-rich snack a short time before bed (something like a couple of oatcakes with a little honey, or a small bowl of porridge).

Magnesium deficiency has been linked to insomnia, so try to include plenty of foods rich in this mineral, such as white fish, dark green leafy vegetables, dried fruit, and nuts and seeds (which make great snacks or additions to breakfasts and salads). **Calcium** is another mineral that combats insomnia in that it helps the brain to use tryptophan to manufacture melatonin. Try a small bowl of porridge with fortified rice milk before bed – the calcium in the milk will help the body to take up tryptophan from the oats (they are a good source).

HEALING FOODS

Aubergines
Avocados
Broccoli
Brown rice
Brussels sprouts
Cabbage
Cashew nuts
Chamomile and valerian teas
Chicken
Chickpeas
Courgettes
Cucumber
Dried figs
Edamame beans
Fortified rice milk
Garlic
Halibut
Kale
Mung beans
Oats
Quinoa
Seeds (pumpkin, sesame, sunflower)
Soba noodles
Sweetcorn
Swiss chard
Tahini
Tofu
Tomatoes

AVOID

Alcohol
Caffeine

For an index of recipes that may help with insomnia, see page 405.

④ HEADACHES

Headaches are one of the most frequent health complaints. The most common type is the tension headache when you feel as though there's a build-up of pressure around the front or sides of the head. You may also develop a headache as the result of a cold or swollen sinuses, which can be felt behind the eyes.

Tension headaches are usually the result of stress, but other factors can include dehydration, lack of sleep, insufficient exercise and alcohol. Women often experience hormonal headaches around the time of their period, which in some cases can lead to migraine (see page 358). You can also experience headaches after a sudden release of tension, which might occur after a particularly traumatic time. The sudden drop in stress hormones causes neurotransmitters to be released, making blood vessels dilate and contract, which manifests as headache.

Most people become dehydrated through the day. This not only causes headaches, but a drop in concentration and ability to focus, which can occur with even the mildest of cases. To avoid dehydration make sure you drink at least two litres of fluid a day, opting primarily for water, which you could have hot or cold, plain, or flavoured with fresh mint, lemon, cucumber, fresh basil or fresh ginger. Soups and some fruit (such as melon) also have a high water content and can help to keep you hydrated. Caffeine-free teas, such as rooibos or herbal varieties, are good too because caffeine has been linked to the onset of headaches, as has the sweetener aspartame found in many diet drinks such as cola. As a rule of thumb, if you feel thirsty, you are already experiencing the effects of dehydration.

Other ingredients that may trigger headaches are monosodium glutamate (MSG) and the amino acid tyramine, which can be found in foods such as red wine, chocolate and pickled foods such as sauerkraut. Nitrates, commonly found in processed meats, have also been linked to headaches.

If you think your headaches are a result of certain foods and drinks then it's worth keeping a food diary for a week, noting which seemed to trigger an event. If your headaches appear to be constant (considered chronic if they occur more than half the days of the month), whether or not you eat certain food and drinks, and especially if the headaches are accompanied by other symptoms, it may be worth visiting your GP.

HEALING FOODS

No specific foods but keep well hydrated

AVOID

Alcohol

Caffeine

MSG

Nitrates (in processed meat)

Tyramine (in chocolate, pickled foods and red wine)

⑤ MIGRAINE

Although the primary symptom of a migraine is a painful headache, the condition is much more complex and involves other symptoms, including disturbed vision, feeling sick, vomiting, sensitivity to light and tingling in the arms. Often during an attack, the sufferer may have to lie still in a darkened room for several hours.

It's thought that people are genetically predisposed to migraine and unfortunately there's no cure. The symptoms can differ greatly between people, so looking for preventative measures relative to your situation is the key. Identifying what are known as 'triggers' can help manage the occurrence of your migraines; the most common ones include stress, lack of sleep, environment (flickering lights, loud noise or cigarette smoke), hormonal changes in women (possibly related to the hormone oestrogen), certain foods and alcohol. In addition, dehydration can lead to migraine.

Trigger foods Food can play a role in the onset of migraines for some people, with the most common triggers being chocolate and caffeine, as well as red wine (all of these contain high amounts of the amino acid tyramine). So you could start by removing these foods and drinks from your diet to see if it helps.

Many people experience a craving for sweet foods just before the onset of a migraine and assume that this is a trigger for them, when in fact the sweet cravings may just be a symptom of the condition. It's worth bearing this in mind if you are trying to identify your own trigger foods.

Certain foods contain chemicals and additives that are often mentioned by migraine sufferers as causing problems, the most common being monosodium glutamate (MSG, used as a flavour-enhancer), nitrates (found in processed meats) and aspartame (used to sweeten low-calorie food and drinks).

Keep a diary In order to identify any possible triggers, it's worth keeping a detailed symptom and trigger diary, noting down all of the factors that may be involved, which could include environmental issues (weather conditions, flickering lights or loud noise) or food. You will need to keep the diary for a sufficient amount of time (such as a month) to see if any patterns emerge, at which point you can begin to remove the trigger (where possible) and then to see if there is any improvement in the frequency and intensity of your migraine attacks. Don't be disheartened if you can't identify a trigger – many people don't find any.

One of the most common dietary migraine triggers is insufficient food, so it is very important that you don't skip meals. Try eating little and often to maintain steady blood sugar levels, and opt for foods with a low glycaemic load (GL; see page 290) such as complex carbohydrates, which are found in wholegrain foods (brown rice, oats, barley, quinoa, starchy vegetables such as sweet potatoes).

HEALING FOODS

Asparagus
Aubergines
Avocados
Broccoli
Cabbage
Carrots
Courgettes
Dried figs
Eggs
Flaxseeds
Garlic
Green beans
Halibut
Kale
Mackerel
Nuts (almonds, cashews)
Onions
Raisins
Salmon
Seeds (pumpkin, sesame, sunflower)
Spinach
Squid
Sweetcorn
Swiss chard
Tomatoes

AVOID

Caffeine (in coffee, tea, cola and energy drinks)
Food containing aspartame and MSG
Tyramine (in chocolate, pickled foods and red wine)

For an index of recipes that may help with migraine, see page 408.

Foods that are rich in **vitamin B2** (also known as riboflavin) have been shown to help some people who suffer from migraines; such foods include fish, eggs and dark green leafy vegetables. **Magnesium** deficiency has also been linked to the onset of migraines, so you could try including plenty of magnesium-rich food in your diet, such as white fish, nuts, seeds, dried fruit and dark green leafy vegetables.

KNOW YOUR TRIGGERS, PLAN YOUR STRATEGIES

Have regular meals

Hormonal changes (for women)

Foods with the amino acid tyramine: red wine, chocolate, pickled foods

Eat foods rich in vitamin B2: mackerel, salmon, squid, eggs, mushrooms, spinach, almonds

Eat foods rich in magnesium: nuts (especially cashews), seeds (pumpkin, sunflower), oily fish (mackerel, salmon), avocados, dried figs

Sleep well and reduce stress

Drink plenty of water

Weather changes (humidity), flickering lights, loud noise

Additives and chemicals: MSG, nitrates (in processed meats), aspartame sweetener

Whilst there is no such thing as a 'cure' for migraine, identifying your triggers (purple circles) will allow you to develop strategies (white circles) that may help to prevent the onset of an attack.

MEN

There's growing concern over the state of men's health because men tend to die at a significantly younger age than women, and health statistics show they have a greater risk of developing cancer, as well as higher rates of obesity and diabetes. Apart from heart problems, which affect both sexes, the main areas of men's health that cause concern are prostate problems, male-specific cancers (prostate and testicular) and mental health issues, in particular depression (see page 350). Many of the risk factors connected to these can often be reduced by eating the right diet, reducing alcohol intake and keeping physically active.

The reasons for men's poor health are numerous and complex – often the issues come with stigma and embarrassment – but may include those listed opposite.

HEALTHY MAN DETOX

	DAY ONE	DAY TWO	DAY THREE
Breakfast	Apple, blueberry & cinnamon Bircher muesli (p28)	Mango cup with pomegranate (p33)	Soft-boiled egg with avocado salad (p38)
Juice	Cucumber, pear, mint & wheatgrass juice (p57)	Avocado, apple, kiwi & spinach smoothie (p55)	Carrot, beetroot, apple & celery juice (p57)
Mid-morning snack	Spicy nuts (p76)	Edamame & seed salad (p73)	Tomato & cashew cream (p62) with Mixed seed crackers (p77)
Lunch	Baked aubergine with pomegranate (p121) and a green salad with seeds	Prawn, cashew & black rice salad (p230)	Brown rice & mushroom risotto (p182)
Mid-afternoon snack	Guacamole (p59) with Mixed seed crackers (p77)	kiwi fruit (80g)	Tenderstem & tahini (p66)
Dinner	Turkey burger with cabbage slaw (p214)	Roasted pumpkin & tofu curry (p135)	Halibut with chickpea stew & pesto (p242)

- men lack awareness and understanding of their health issues
- men are less likely to discuss their health and feelings
- men are reluctant to take action when they're feeling unwell or depressed
- men are more likely to engage in risky behaviours
- men are affected by the stigmas surrounding their health issues (including prostate health and impotence)

A discussion of these factors is beyond the scope of this book; however, there are some key ways that men can improve their health by changing the way they eat, in particular to deal with prostate problems, reduce the risk of cancer, enhance male fertility and help with impotence.

DAY FOUR	DAY FIVE	DAY SIX	DAY SEVEN
Banana muffin (p43)	Baked egg with spinach & tomato (p38)	Avocado smash with toasted nuts & seeds (p36)	Chia seed pudding with blackberry & lime coulis (p35)
Chia seed, coconut & pineapple smoothie (p52)	Cucumber, pear, mint & wheatgrass juice (p57)	Carrot, beetroot, apple & celery juice (p57)	Strawberry & mango lassi (p55)
Red pepper & butter bean mash (p68) with Mixed seed crackers (p77)	Cashew & goji berry flapjack (p80)	brazil nuts (30g)	Avocado smash with toasted nuts & seeds (p36)
Puy lentils & roasted aubergine with basil pesto (p161)	Avocado & quinoa salad (p147)	Quinoa pizza (p148)	Pad Thai with brown rice noodles (p209)
Cacao milk (p53)	Edamame & seed salad (p73)	Red pepper & butter bean mash (p68) with crudités	Quail's eggs, celery salt & cherry tomatoes (p73)
Turkey & cashew curry (p212)	Grilled mackerel with ginger & saffron rice (p253)	King prawn stir-fry (p230)	Pinto bean chilli (p168)

① PROSTATE

The prostate, which is a small gland located beneath the bladder, can cause urinary problems, including benign enlargement, cancer and inflammation. After a man reaches the age of about 50, the prostate begins to enlarge in a process called benign prostatic hyperplasia (BPH). In most cases this is perfectly harmless, but it can cause inconvenient urinary issues as the gland pushes against the bladder. Urinary tract infections, poor diet and lifestyle habits (smoking and drinking) can predispose men to problems.

Although there appears to be little that food can do to slow down the growth of an enlarged prostate, research suggests that the **beta-sitosterol** found in foods such as flaxseeds, pumpkin seeds, olive oil, avocados, almonds, raw cacao and fresh coriander may help to relieve the urinary symptoms of BPH. It's also good for men to make sure they are getting plenty of **zinc** in their diet (found in foods such as shellfish, wholegrains, eggs, nuts and seeds) as this mineral is beneficial for men's health as a whole – including reproductive health – and the overall functioning of the prostate.

Prostate cancer is one of the most common forms of cancer in men. It tends to occur in later life and early diagnosis is key to successful treatment. Maintaining a healthy diet may help to reduce the risk of developing the disease as well as promoting overall good health. Although no single food will definitively prevent you from developing prostate cancer, there is a lot of research highlighting several foods and nutrients that may play a role in the reduction of risk. In their own right, these foods are also healthy additions to any balanced diet and you'll find plenty of recipes in this book that incorporate these ingredients.

A lot of the research investigating the links between prostate cancer and diet has looked at tomatoes, which contain the powerful antioxidant **lycopene**. The World Cancer Research Fund has concluded that foods rich in this antioxidant are likely to help to reduce the risk of developing prostate cancer. It appears that the greatest effect comes from cooked and processed varieties, such as tinned tomatoes, tomato purée and tomato soup, suggesting that the lycopene from these foods is more readily absorbed in the body. You will also find this antioxidant in other red foods, such as watermelon, pomegranate, pink grapefruit and red peppers.

Soya contains **phytoestrogens** (plant hormones) that may play a key role in prostate health. Soya products such as tofu, tamari, edamame beans and miso contain a particular type of phytoestrogen called **soy isoflavones**. Studies have shown that these may help with BPH and protect against, or slow down, cancerous tumours through their ability to lower a male hormone that stimulates the overgrowth of prostate tissue. Although more research is required to definitively show the effect of soya on prostate health, incorporating moderate amounts into your diet will provide you with a healthy protein alternative to meat.

HEALING FOODS

Avocados
Blueberries
Broccoli
Brown rice
Brussels sprouts
Cauliflower
Chia seeds and oil
Chickpeas
Crab
Dried thyme
Edamame beans
Eggs
Extra virgin olive oil
Flaxseeds
Fresh coriander
Kale
Lentils
Mackerel
Miso
Nuts (almonds, brazils, cashews, pine nuts, walnuts)
Oats
Papayas
Parsley
Prawns
Quinoa
Raw cacao
Red peppers
Salmon
Seeds (sesame, sunflower)
Tahini
Tamari
Tofu
Tomatoes, particularly cooked, tinned, purée or paste, and sun-dried
Tuna
Turkey
Watermelon

AVOID

No specific foods

For an index of recipes that may help with prostate health, see page 411.

Other foods that may have a protective effect against prostate cancer include those rich in **selenium**, such as nuts (particularly brazils), seafood, bran and poultry. Research is also investigating **vitamin E** – foods rich in this nutrient (including nuts, sunflower seeds and wholegrains) may offer benefits such as a reduction in inflammation and protection against cancer.

It has long been known that cruciferous vegetables, such as broccoli, cabbage, Brussels sprouts, kale and cauliflower, have a protective effect on the prevention of cancer, and there is strong evidence to back this up. It's thought that this is down to a group of compounds known as phytonutrients (plant chemicals) that possess antioxidant properties, in particular **isothiocyanates** found in cruciferous vegetables – another reason to include plenty of fresh vegetables (and fruit) in the diet.

TOP FOODS FOR PROSTATE HEALTH

There has been a lot of research into the effect of diet on prostate health, especially cancer risk. Some nutrients are helpful for men's health generally, such as zinc, and others appear to be of particular benefit to prostate health, such as lycopene and selenium. Here are our top food heroes for these nutrients.

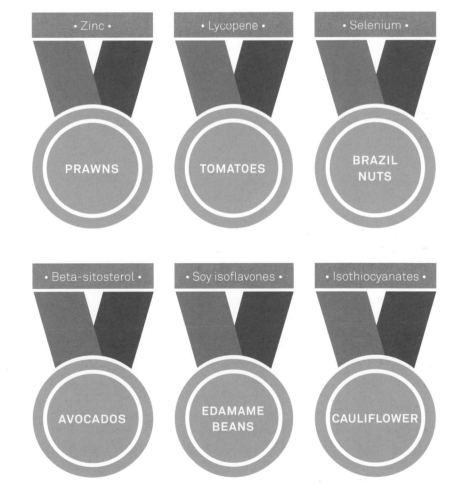

• Zinc •
PRAWNS

• Lycopene •
TOMATOES

• Selenium •
BRAZIL NUTS

• Beta-sitosterol •
AVOCADOS

• Soy isoflavones •
EDAMAME BEANS

• Isothiocyanates •
CAULIFLOWER

② FERTILITY

In the last decade sperm counts in men have dropped considerably and more sperm abnormalities are being seen, both of which can make conception more difficult. It's often not how many sperm are being produced but the quality of the sperm (whether they are strong enough to fertilise the egg). When there are problems in conceiving, it can be just as much the responsibility of men as it is of women. The one common denominator associated with infertility in men is lifestyle factors: the quality of the diet, smoking, drinking and stress.

Smoking in particular makes conceiving difficult as it not only affects all aspects of sperm health (probably due to the heavy toxic metal in tobacco called cadmium), but it can lead to impotence, which for obvious reasons will make natural conception very difficult. Alcohol can also affect the shape of sperm, and a heavy drinking session can wipe them out for several months as it reduces the hormones required to make sperm. The hormones produced as a result of stress are also thought to interfere with sperm-producing hormones, so it is a good idea to factor some relaxation techniques into your fertility regime.

It takes at least three months for sperm cells to mature, so if you and your partner are trying for a baby, you need to allow enough time to get your diet and lifestyle on track in preparation. Overweight and obese men are less fertile – a third less than their slimmer counterparts – which may be a result of lower testosterone levels. Obese men also have sperm of low quality. So if you need to lose some weight, this is a great time to do so. Often simply giving up the booze and snacks results in a fairly significant weight loss when partnered with some exercise.

Zinc is top of the list of minerals beneficial to male fertility. It is used for the production of male sex hormones, and sperm is thought to contain high levels of zinc. Choosing plenty of zinc-rich foods (seafood, poultry, beans, eggs, nuts, wholegrains) will help to increase your sperm levels, as will reducing negative lifestyle habits, such as heavy drinking, that can deplete the body of zinc.

Getting plenty of **vitamin C** in your diet is also important, as it has been shown to reduce the tendency of sperm to clump together (common with infertility). You will get all the vitamin C you need by eating at least five portions of fruit and vegetables each day, especially citrus fruit, berries and red peppers. Eating a variety of fruit and vegetables will also ensure you are getting a good selection of **antioxidants** (including **selenium**, which is involved in making certain proteins found in sperm). These will help to reduce the damage done by free radicals, which some experts believe may be a contributory factor leading to infertility in men.

A lack of **omega 3 fatty acids** in the diet may also be involved in fertility problems. Make sure you are getting enough by eating a few servings of oily fish each week. You will also find these fats in dark green leafy vegetables, walnuts, and seeds and oils (chia and flax).

HEALING FOODS

Asparagus
Avocados
Beetroot
Blueberries
Broccoli
Brown rice
Cauliflower
Chia seeds and oil
Chickpeas
Crab
Dried thyme
Eggs
Flaxseeds
Kale
Kiwi fruit
Lemons
Lentils
Limes
Mackerel
Miso
Mushrooms
Nuts (almonds, cashews, pine nuts, walnuts)
Oats
Oranges
Parsley
Peas
Peppers
Prawns
Quinoa
Raspberries
Salmon
Samphire
Seeds (pumpkin, sesame, sunflower)
Spinach
Spring greens
Strawberries
Tahini
Tuna
Turkey

AVOID

Alcohol

For an index of recipes that may help with male fertility, see page 406.

③ IMPOTENCE

There are psychological reasons why men experience impotence, but it has also been shown that it often can occur as a result of physical factors. Adopting good healthy lifestyle habits and improving the diet will go some way to tackling the problem of impotence.

Diabetes, high blood pressure and atherosclerosis (blocking of the arteries caused as a result of factors such as high cholesterol) are key contributory factors that can reduce blood flow and cause impotence. Maintaining a healthy weight will help to reduce the risk of diabetes, and cutting down on saturated and trans fats (as well as refined carbohydrates including sugar) will help to prevent atherosclerosis. As with all male health issues, eating plenty of **zinc**-rich foods (seafood, poultry, beans, eggs, nuts, wholegrains) is important for reproductive health, even if not directly linked to impotence.

Lifestyle choices, such as drinking and taking illegal substances and certain medications, as well as smoking, can also affect male sexual function. Nicotine is a particular problem, as it impedes blood flow by constricting small arteries (such as those found in the penis).

HEALING FOODS

Broccoli
Chickpeas
Crab
Dried thyme
Eggs
Lentils
Miso
Mushrooms
Nuts (almonds, cashews, pine nuts)
Oats
Peas
Prawns
Quinoa
Samphire
Seeds (pumpkin, sesame, sunflower)
Spinach
Swiss chard
Tahini
Turkey

LIMIT
Foods high in saturated fat, trans fats and refined sugar

Women's health covers many conditions particular to females. Often these can be the result of a disruption in the delicate balance of hormones, which alters naturally at different stages of a woman's life (including puberty, pregnancy, lactation and menopause). Hormonal disturbances are frequently beyond control; however, eating a poor diet, an unhealthy lifestyle (smoking and drinking), being overweight, disrupted sleep and stress can have an effect and, if left untreated, can lead to long-term health consequences.

Hormonal imbalances are often complicated. Whilst diet alone doesn't offer a cure, adopting a healthy lifestyle will have an effect on the complex balance. Research also indicates that certain foods may be useful for the effect they have on hormones, whilst others may help reduce the inflammation that underpins or aggravates certain conditions.

The menstrual cycle To understand the role of female hormones, it's useful to start with the menstrual cycle, which involves the two main female sex hormones, oestrogen and progesterone. At the beginning of the cycle, the levels of oestrogen and progesterone are low. This signals the pituitary gland (the 'master gland' that plays a major role in regulating vital body functions including hormone control) to produce another hormone called follicle stimulating hormone (FSH).

HEALTHY WOMAN DETOX

	DAY ONE	DAY TWO	DAY THREE
Breakfast	Quinoa & oat porridge with blackberry compote (p33)	Mango cup with pomegranate (p33)	Soft-boiled eggs with avocado salad (p38)
Juice	Cucumber, pear, mint & wheatgrass juice (p57)	Carrot, beetroot, apple & celery juice (p57)	Carrot, beetroot, apple & celery juice (p57)
Mid-morning snack	Edamame & seed salad (p73)	Beetroot hummus (p65) with crudités	Pistachio oat bar (p79)
Lunch	Baked aubergine with pomegranate (p121)	Pesto chicken with quinoa & peach salad (p206)	Salmon, green beans, orange & hazelnut salad (p235)
Mid-afternoon snack	Cucumber, mint & yogurt dip (p70) with crudités	Candied walnuts (p81)	Edamame & seed salad (p73)
Dinner	Seared tuna & beetroot salad (p253)	Roasted pumpkin & tofu curry (p135)	Baked aubergine with pomegranate (p121)

FSH begins the process of maturing a follicle (a sac filled with fluid in the ovary, which contains an egg). This follicle produces more oestrogen, which gets the uterus ready for pregnancy.

Usually at around day 12 to 14, ovulation occurs. This causes an increase in oestrogen levels that triggers a sharp rise in luteinising hormone (LH) from the pituitary gland, causing release of the egg from the follicle. The ruptured follicle then secretes progesterone and oestrogen, preparing the uterus for pregnancy. If the egg is not fertilised, oestrogen and progesterone levels drop and on day 28, menses begins.

In some conditions, such as polycystic ovary syndrome (see page 374), the balance of these hormones is upset, which causes a number of symptoms such as a disrupted menstrual cycle. Excess of certain hormones (such as oestrogen) may aggravate symptoms of other conditions such as heavy painful periods or endometriosis. Being overweight or obese can cause excessive hormone production (oestrogen is produced in body fat), which can increase a woman's risk of developing female cancers. As a woman enters menopause, changes in hormones (reduced oestrogen) can leave her more susceptible to conditions such as heart disease and osteoporosis.

Understanding the effect of hormones on women's health and the importance of a good, well-balanced diet can help with the management of female-specific conditions.

DAY FOUR	DAY FIVE	DAY SIX	DAY SEVEN
Strawberry soya yogurt (p29)	Avocado smash with toasted nuts & seeds (p36)	Mango cup with pomegranate (p33)	Chia seed pudding with blackberry & lime coulis (p35)
Avocado, apple, kiwi & spinach smoothie (p55)	Cucumber, pear, mint & wheatgrass juice (p57)	Carrot, beetroot, apple & celery juice (p57)	Avocado, apple, kiwi & spinach smoothie (p55)
Tenderstem & tahini (p66)	raspberries (80g)	Radishes & cauliflower with hummus (p66)	almonds (30g)
Avocado & quinoa salad (p147)	Mexican bean stew (p139)	Cabbage stuffed with chicken (p208)	Turkey burger with cabbage slaw (p214)
Beetroot, apple, carrot & ginger cake (p262)	Cacoa milk (p53)	Guacamole (p59) with red pepper crudités	Cashew & goji berry flapjack (p80)
Grilled mackerel with ginger & saffron rice (p253)	Kale, edamame & fennel frittata (p199) with Lentil sprout & celery salad (p161)	Mung bean curry with onion, cucumber & cashew nut salad (p167)	Red lentil soup (p89)

① PREMENSTRUAL SYNDROME (PMS)

Many women of child-bearing age have experienced some form of PMS that begins in the run-up to their period. There are many symptoms associated with the condition, and most women fall into either the category that revolves around anxiety (mood swings, irritability and tension) or cravings (increased appetite, sugar cravings, fatigue and headaches). Women often talk about having these kinds of feelings, but it's not until they get their period that they attribute them to their monthly cycle. Other symptoms include breast tenderness, back pain and bloating.

For one in five women, the symptoms are severe enough to disrupt daily life. There are plenty of theories about the origin of PMS but none of these has been proven. The condition is likely due to fluctuations in hormone levels during each monthly cycle. However, as symptoms differ between women, it would suggest other factors are involved.

Some women are prescribed medication, such as the contraceptive pill, to balance out hormones, and in some cases antidepressants are used to help increase levels of the 'feel-good' hormone serotonin in the brain.

The Detox Kitchen can't offer women an antidote to PMS as there are no foods that can prevent it, but maintaining a balanced diet will definitely help with overall health and well-being. And there are foods that may help by relieving the associated symptoms.

Steady blood sugar levels As with any condition that can affect your mood, ensuring blood sugar levels remain constant is important to avoid rapid spikes and dips (these will exacerbate feelings such as irritability and anxiety). Maintaining a diet that contains mostly foods with a low glycaemic load (GL; see page 290) – those rich in complex carbohydrates, such as wholegrains, pulses and starchy vegetables including butternut squash and sweet potatoes – will ensure a slow release of sugar into the blood. This is because the fibre in these kinds of foods causes them to be digested slowly and thus limits the amount of insulin the body produces (slowing the transport of glucose into cells).

Carbohydrate cravings (especially sugar) are thought to be the result of low levels of serotonin (which requires carbohydrate for uptake into the brain), as well as low progesterone and high oestrogen causing a drop in blood sugar. Including plenty of low GL foods (of plant origin) can be beneficial because the fibre present in them balances blood sugar and helps to lower oestrogen levels (this is particularly relevant if you get heavy, painful periods that can be exacerbated by surges in oestrogen).

Cutting back on sugar, salt and saturated fat is not only good for your overall health but will help with bloating and fluid retention (and inflammation). This is something to bear in mind when you're in the midst of a sugar craving. Trans fats (see page 293) are the worst type

HEALING FOODS

Afalfa sprouts

Bananas

Broccoli

Brown rice

Cabbage

Chia seeds and oil

Dried fruit

Edamame beans

Eggs

Flaxseeds

Fortified rice milk products

Halibut

Kale

Lentil sprouts

Lettuce

Nuts (almonds, cashews)

Oats

Oily fish

Peppers

Pulses (beans, lentils)

Seeds (pumpkin, sesame, sunflower)

Spinach

Tamari

Tinned salmon

Tofu

Tomatoes

Turkey

LIMIT

Foods high in salt, refined sugar, trans fats and saturated fat

For an index of recipes that may help with PMS, see page 410.

of fat because they decrease the levels of compounds that help to prevent inflammation and subsequently fight pain, so it makes sense to avoid these fats altogether.

Phytoestrogens from plant foods The effects of increased oestrogen on the body (such as breast tenderness) are thought to be reduced in the presence of phytoestrogens (also known as plant oestrogens; these are similar to the oestrogen hormones produced by the body, but have a much weaker effect). These phytoestrogens bind to oestrogen receptors in place of the body's own oestrogen.

Phytoestrogens can be found in soya foods (edamame beans, tofu and fermented soya products such as miso), pulses (particularly chickpeas and lentils), fruit (dried apricots, red and purple berries), seeds (flax, sesame, sunflower) and nuts (pistachios, walnuts). Premenopausal women should moderate intake of soya, but a few servings each day is fine. If you suffer from heavy, painful periods then it's advisable to avoid soya altogether (including soy isoflavone supplements) because it may raise oestrogen levels to a point that makes matters worse.

Vitamin & mineral intake is important Some women experience low iron stores, which can partly be attributed to their monthly blood loss (as well as low dietary intake of iron). During your period it's important to ensure your diet contains plenty of iron-rich foods, especially if you experience heavy bleeding each month. A lack of iron may put you at risk of anaemia, which if not addressed can leave you feeling tired, lethargic and depressed. You can get plenty of **iron** from foods such as lean meats, pulses, dried fruit and dark green leafy vegetables. Try teaming your non-meat iron-rich foods with a source of vitamin C, which is found in all fruit and vegetables, especially citrus fruit, berries and red peppers. Also, avoid drinking tea with meals as the tannins can affect iron absorption.

There is research suggesting women who have higher levels of **calcium** tend to get fewer of the symptoms associated with PMS (such as mood disturbances, cramping and bloating). If you are going to forgo dairy products in your diet then it's important that you get a healthy supply of this mineral from dairy alternative foods such as fortified rice milk, dark green leafy vegetables, almonds, dried fruit and tahini (two to three servings per day).

Magnesium is another mineral associated with symptoms of PMS, particularly in women with inadequate amounts. Snacking on seeds and nuts is a useful way to increase your intake of magnesium, as is including foods such as pulses (lentils and beans), dried fruit, nuts and dark green leafy vegetables.

Lots of women opt for **vitamin B6** supplements, which have been shown to be helpful in relieving the emotional symptoms associated with PMS, such as mood swings. Be aware, though, that if vitamin B6 is taken in large amounts, it may lead to nerve damage

– this has been observed with intake that exceeds 50mg, which is the recommended dose to get a therapeutic effect. Vitamin B6 can be found in a lot of foods, but is particularly rich in wholegrains, poultry, eggs, oily fish and dark green leafy vegetables.

Prostaglandins Another theory related to PMS is that inflammation may be involved, in particular hormone-like compounds called prostaglandins produced in areas where symptoms originate, such as breast, brain and gastrointestinal tract (the long tube in the body that passes food), suggesting a role in problems such as cramping, breast tenderness, bloating, diarrhoea and constipation. Derived from omega 3 and omega 6 fatty acids, prostaglandins have a number of different functions in the body, including a role in the inflammatory response.

There are two types of prostaglandins: those that promote inflammation (made from omega 6) and those that reduce it (made from omega 3). The key is for your body to produce more of the anti-inflammatory and less of the inflammatory prostaglandins in order to help relieve PMS pain. Foods rich in **omega 3 fatty acids** include oily fish, seeds, seed oils, walnuts and dark green leafy vegetables; those rich in omega 6 are oils such as vegetable and sunflower. As always, getting plenty of brightly coloured fruit and vegetables in your diet will ensure you're getting adequate **antioxidants**, which will also help with inflammation.

Many women swear by the effect evening primrose oil has on the symptoms of PMS. If you haven't already tried it, you could take a supplement for a few months to see if it helps.

☾ URINARY TRACT INFECTIONS (CYSTITIS)

A urinary tract infection (UTI) can occur in any part of the urinary tract, and the symptoms are the result of an inflamed bladder (in some cases it can affect the kidneys). In women the condition is more commonly referred to as cystitis; men can get a similar condition known as urethritis.

Cystitis occurs as bacteria (*E.coli*) make their way up along the urethra and into the bladder, usually as a result of wiping from back to front after a bowel movement. Irritation caused by heavily scented soaps, body washes and perfumes can also play a part in developing cystitis, and in some cases it can be the result of a sexually transmitted infection such as chlamydia. The main symptom experienced during an attack of cystitis is an urgent need to pee – regardless of whether the bladder is full or not – which is accompanied by a stinging pain.

Cystitis is more common in women than men as they have a shorter urethra; older women are more vulnerable as changing oestrogen levels affect the body's tissues, making them thinner and thus more prone to damage and infection. The hormonal changes experienced during pregnancy also make women more vulnerable to cystitis at this time (under the influence of the hormone progesterone, the bladder becomes larger and more relaxed, so it does not empty as efficiently, leaving it vulnerable to bacterial infection).

The most effective first step you can take is to drink plenty of water (two litres daily) because this will help you to pee and 'flush out' some of the invading bacteria from the urinary tract. Second, you might like to invest in some **cranberry juice**: substances found in cranberries play a role in preventing the bacteria from sticking to the bladder wall (this will not help to *treat* the current infection but will help to prevent a recurrence). You need to choose a cranberry juice with minimal or no sugar and a high concentration of fruit, not the watered-down, very sweet juice drink available in most shops. If you don't like the taste of cranberries, try a cranberry extract capsule, which you can find in most healthfood shops.

As you are trying to avoid dehydration, it's worth avoiding drinks that contain caffeine, such as colas, tea, coffee, energy drinks and alcohol. Some people also find that spicy foods can trigger an attack of cystitis. If you're getting recurrent attacks, you might want to keep a food and symptom diary to help you identify possible trigger foods.

More often than not, doctors will prescribe antibiotics to cure bacterial UTIs. These drugs can upset the balance of bacteria in the gut, so it's a good idea to try 'live' yogurt products (you can get dairy-free varieties) and live bacteria supplements. These may also help to inhibit the growth of micro-organisms that cause UTIs.

HEALING FOODS
Cranberry juice
Live yogurt (dairy-free)

AVOID
Caffeinated drinks (coffee, tea, cola and energy drinks)
Spicy foods

③ MENOPAUSE

The menopause can be defined as when a woman no longer has her monthly periods. The process usually begins around the age of 45–50 (the perimenopause) and is the result of a decline in the hormone oestrogen, which helps to release eggs from the ovaries and regulates periods. This hormone also has a role in other functions, including bone density, skin temperature and keeping the vagina moist.

Irregular and fluctuating hormone patterns, such as dips and surges in oestrogen levels, are responsible for symptoms such as hot flushes, night sweats, loss of sex drive (libido), mood swings and irritability, and thinning bone (which can increase the risk of osteoporosis and fractures). The degree and severity of menopausal symptoms can differ between women, with some experiencing few if any symptoms and others being severely affected. The process normally concludes around the age of 55 and the stage after this is known as postmenopause.

HRT Hormone replacement therapy (HRT), a combination of oestrogen and progesterone, is used to treat symptoms of the menopause. HRT has had its fair share of controversy over time, with suggested links to breast cancer and cardiovascular disease. However, current advice is that if the severity of symptoms is adversely affecting a woman's quality of life, then the benefits of taking HRT alongside a healthy lifestyle outweigh the risk. It's also recommended that HRT should be used in the lowest possible dose for the shortest period of time. The decision is ultimately left to the individual, but those with a history of oestrogen receptor positive breast cancer will be advised against HRT.

A healthy, helpful diet Eating the right type of foods may help to alleviate the milder symptoms of menopause and protect women against the risk of any potential health conditions. Although it may take a bit of effort at first, once you understand which foods to include, you can begin to make changes in your diet. Adopting a way of eating that includes plenty of wholegrains, fruit and vegetables (these contain **B vitamins** that help with hormone balance), and a minimum of saturated fat and refined carbohydrates will ensure you get all the essential micronutrients you need, as well as phytoestrogens and bioflavonoids.

Before the menopause, oestrogen helps to protect women against the risk of developing heart disease, so it's important to eat a heart-healthy diet (see section on Heart, page 302). **Omega 3 fatty acids** play a key role in protecting the heart, so be sure to include foods such as oily fish, seeds (chia and flax) and their oils, dark green leafy vegetables and walnuts for their anti-inflammatory properties. These fatty acids have also been shown to help reduce the effect of hot flushes.

HEALING FOODS

Alfalfa sprouts
Aubergines
Avocados
Barley
Blueberries
Broccoli
Chia seeds and oil
Chickpeas
Dried figs
Edamame beans
Eggs
Flaxseeds and oil
Fortified rice milk products
Halibut
Kale
Lentils
Lentil sprouts
Mackerel
Miso
Mung beans
Nuts (almonds, cashews, walnuts)
Papayas
Red kidney beans
Salmon
Sardines
Seeds (pumpkin, sesame, sunflower)
Shiitake mushrooms
Spring greens
Strawberries
Tahini
Tamari
Tofu
Tomatoes
Trout

LIMIT

Alcohol
Caffeine
Foods high in refined sugar, trans fats and saturated fat

For an index of recipes that may help with menopausal problems, see page 407.

Obtaining the necessary nutrients Menopause accelerates the loss of bone mass as a result of falling oestrogen levels. This, along with less efficient calcium absorption, can put you at greater risk of osteoporosis in later life. It is therefore imperative to maintain good bone health. Key bone nutrients include the minerals **calcium** (found in fortified rice milk, nuts, dark green leafy vegetables and tahini) and **magnesium** (from lentils and beans, dried fruit, nuts and dark green leafy vegetables), as well as **vitamin D** (in eggs, oily fish and shiitake mushrooms). You can read more about this in the section on Bones (page 310).

Soya foods, such as edamame beans, tofu, tamari and miso, contain soy isoflavones, a type of **phytoestrogen** (plant oestrogen). These behave in the same way as the oestrogen found in the body but with much less effect, so may help to reduce the severity of hot flushes. If you have, or are at particular risk of, oestrogen receptor positive breast cancer, it may not be suitable to eat a diet rich in soy isoflavones; speak with your GP about any potential risks to your health before including lots of these foods in your diet.

Phytoestrogens are also found in pulses (chickpeas, lentils), sprouts (lentil, alfalfa), fruit (dried apricots, red and purple berries), seeds (flax, sesame, sunflower) and nuts (pistachios, walnuts). Including these foods in the diet may help to balance out hormone levels, as well as offering many other health benefits.

Vitamin E has been considered as a useful way to alleviate hot flushes, so you could try incorporating foods rich in this nutrient into your diet. You can find vitamin E in foods such as avocados, seeds, nuts, eggs and wholegrains.

Caffeine and alcohol, as well as spicy foods, will exacerbate symptoms of the menopause (such as hot flushes, night sweats and mood swings) because these dilate the blood vessels, bringing heat to the surface of the skin. Excess alcohol can also put pressure on the liver, which may make it less effective at removing oestrogen from the body.

Maintaining balanced blood sugar levels will help with mood swings and irritability, so try to eat regularly, avoid sugary foods and opt for low GL foods (complex carbohydrates; see page 290). Ensuring your diet is also low in refined carbohydrates (including sugar), saturated fat and trans fats will help to maintain a healthy heart and contribute to a healthy body weight.

④ POLYCYSTIC OVARY SYNDROME (PCOS)

PCOS is a condition characterised by harmless cysts that form on the ovaries. These cysts are follicles containing eggs that haven't formed properly. Symptoms of PCOS typically include irregular periods, weight gain, acne (see page 334), excessive facial hair and difficulty conceiving, although not all women with the condition get these symptoms.

It isn't fully clear what causes PCOS, but hormone imbalances and insulin resistance are key factors and thought to result in the inflammation that underpins the condition (excess insulin is thought to cause an inflammatory response that doesn't switch off, causing damage to the body, known as low-grade inflammation). These are two areas where the right diet may have a beneficial effect.

How the hormones work Insulin resistance occurs when the hormone (insulin), which is released to help control blood sugar levels, has less of an effect on the tissues in your body, resulting in overproduction of insulin to compensate. Higher than normal levels of luteinising hormone (which stimulates the ovaries to ovulate) work alongside insulin, causing the ovaries to produce excess testosterone, which negatively affects ovulation and egg development. You can reduce your risk of developing insulin resistance by maintaining a healthy body weight and following a diet with a low glycaemic load (GL; see page 290). This, in turn, will reduce the levels of testosterone in the body.

Helping hormone balance To balance out hormones and lessen the effect of oestrogen you could try including some soya foods (edamame beans, tofu, miso) in your diet. These contain soy isoflavones, which are the most potent of plant oestrogens – otherwise known as **phytoestrogens**. They are similar to the body's own hormone but with a much weaker effect (about a thousand times). They bind with oestrogen receptors in the body and thus reduce the effect of naturally occurring oestrogen.

You can also find phytoestrogens in pulses (chickpeas, lentils), fruit (dried apricots, red and purple berries), seeds (flax, sesame, sunflower) and nuts (pistachios, walnuts). By following a diet rich in plant foods, you will also be getting plenty of fibre, which can help to rid the body of excess oestrogen.

Maintaining a diet with a low glycaemic load (GL), rich in complex carbohydrates (such as brown rice, oats, pulses and starchy vegetables, including butternut squash), helps to balance out blood sugar levels and prevent dips and spikes in insulin, which is especially important when you have PCOS. Following this type of diet can also be a useful weight-loss strategy: when you have PCOS, it is critical to maintain a healthy weight in order to reduce the risk of conditions such as insulin resistance (although weight loss can be difficult because PCOS is often accompanied by a slower metabolism and increased

HEALING FOODS

Alfalfa sprouts
Apples
Barley
Black-eyed beans
Blueberries
Broccoli
Brown rice
Buckwheat
Chia seed oil
Chicken
Chickpeas
Cinnamon
Dried apricots
Edamame beans
Eggs
Extra virgin olive oil
Flaxseed oil
Lentil sprouts
Lentils
Miso
Mung beans
Mushrooms, particularly shiitake
Nuts (pistachios, walnuts)
Oats
Quinoa
Raspberries
Red kidney beans
Salmon
Seeds (pumpkin, sesame, sunflower)
Strawberries
Sweet potatoes
Sweetcorn
Tamari
Tofu
Trout
Tuna

LIMIT

Alcohol
Foods high in refined sugar, trans fats and saturated fat

For an index of recipes that may help with PCOS, see page 409.

production of the hunger hormone). You can further balance out blood sugar by including proteins and healthy fats (such as extra virgin olive oil, avocados and oily fish) in your meals, as these will also help to put the brakes on carbohydrate absorption and thus keep insulin levels low.

Don't be tempted by 'low carb' diets because these usually involve eating foods that are high in saturated fat, an excess of which increases the risk of heart disease (PCOS itself puts you at greater risk of heart disease), as well as very high levels of protein that can further encourage insulin production. It's also beneficial to avoid high GL foods (refined sugars, white bread and pasta) as these will increase insulin production and, along with foods high in saturated and trans fats, will encourage inflammation.

More beneficial foods Getting plenty of **omega 3 fatty acids** from foods such as oily fish, dark green leafy vegetables, nuts (walnuts), and seeds (chia and flax) and their oils can be helpful as omega 3s reduce inflammation and also balance out the inflammatory effects of too much omega 6 in the diet (most people tend to take in a lot more omega 6 from vegetable oil).

Chromium is a mineral that plays a role in the formation of a glucose tolerance factor, which helps to make the hormone insulin more effective. You can find small amounts of chromium in poultry, wholegrain foods, mushrooms, sweetcorn, apples, sweet potatoes and eggs, with the highest content in broccoli.

Vitamin D is also now recognised to help control blood sugar and improve insulin sensitivity. Most of this vitamin is obtained from sunlight (see page 310) but you will find it in a few foods such as eggs, shiitake mushrooms, oily fish and fortified margarines. Many of us have low levels of vitamin D during the winter months, which can influence all aspects of health, so you might want to take a supplement once the clocks go back and we get less sunlight.

B vitamins have an important role to play as they not only help to control weight by converting macronutrients into energy but are essential for the liver to convert old hormones into harmless substances that can then be expelled by the body.

Cinnamon is a useful spice, shown to help control blood sugar. It can easily be added to your diet by sprinkling on fruit or adding to hot drinks. Due to the effect on blood sugar, you should take care if you're diabetic, and avoid being tempted by cinnamon supplements.

As part of your healthy eating regime, do watch the amount of alcohol you drink. Excess alcohol can lead to weight gain and raise blood sugar levels; it can also put a strain on the liver, which will render it less effective at clearing away excess hormones.

VEGETARIANS & VEGANS

Traditionally, neither vegetarians nor vegans eat fish or meat, although there are many definitions of a vegetarian diet, some of which do include fish. Vegans also exclude all other foods of animal origin, including eggs, dairy products, gelatine and, in some cases, honey. Many people choose non-meat diets for health reasons, and it has been shown by studies, including those of the Seventh Day Adventists (strict vegetarians), that for people on such regimes there is a decreased incidence of cardiovascular disease and cancer (particularly colorectal and prostate cancers).

It's not unusual for people who adopt a vegan diet to lose weight because plant-based diets are often high in fibre and low in calories. If you are thinking of going vegan, make sure you get the energy balance right to match your daily needs. Include energy-dense foods in your diet, such as nuts, nut butters, seeds, avocados, oils and dried fruit, all of which also offer vitamins, minerals and healthy fats that will help you to feel well and maintain a healthy weight.

Combining non-meat proteins Although plant foods contain protein, they're called 'incomplete' as they don't contain all of the essential amino acids found in meat. It's important that you combine your non-meat proteins together so the amino acid profiles complement

HEALTHY VEGAN DETOX
(REPLACE HONEY IN RECIPES WITH MAPLE OR AGAVE SYRUP)

	DAY ONE	DAY TWO	DAY THREE
Breakfast	Pecan & coconut granola (p30)	Mango cup with pomegranate (p33)	Avocado smash with toasted nuts & seeds (p36)
Juice	Cucumber, pear, mint & wheatgrass juice (p57)	Avocado, apple, kiwi & spinach smoothie (p55)	Carrot, beetroot, apple & celery juice (p57)
Mid-morning snack	Edamame & seed salad (p73)	Tenderstem & tahini (p66)	Mango cup with pomegranate (p33)
Lunch	Acocado & quinoa salad (p147)	Puy lentils & roasted aubergine with basil pesto (p161)	Quinoa, asparagus & almond salad (p150)
Mid-afternoon snack	Broad bean & mint dip (p70) with cucumber crudités	Cacao milk (p53)	blueberries (80g)
Dinner	Pearl barley with cantaloupe melon (p151)	Vegetable lasagne (p124)	Sri Lankan butternut squash curry (p134)

each other (a lack of essential amino acids could impact on your body's ability to build certain proteins and affect many aspects of health as they are vital for the growth and repair of cells and tissues).

Known as 'food combining', this is simple to do by making meals that contain two or more of the non-meat protein sources: pulses (chickpeas, black-eyed beans, lentils, split peas), soya products (tofu, miso, edamame beans), nuts and seeds.

Ensuring adequate micronutrients There are a few key vitamins and minerals that may be lacking in a non-meat diet, especially a vegan diet (most vegetarians are able to eat highly nutritious foods such as eggs to increase their intake of key nutrients). Vitamin B12, iron, zinc and calcium are four essential nutrients that are commonly found in foods of animal origin and as such can often be lacking in a plant-based vegan diet.

Iron and vitamin B12 are particularly important as they are involved in red blood cell production, and a lack can result in anaemia. Strict vegetarians and vegans, especially new converts, might want to consider taking a multivitamin and mineral supplement to ensure they get all the micronutrients required to support good health and well-being.

DAY FOUR	DAY FIVE	DAY SIX	DAY SEVEN
Quinoa & oat porridge with blackberry compote (p33)	Strawberry soya yogurt (p29) with 30g almonds	Beans on toast (p47)	Cashew & goji berry flapjack (p80)
Chia seed, coconut & pineapple smoothie (p52)	Cucumber, pear, mint & wheatgrass juice (p57)	Carrot, beetroot, apple & celery juice (p57)	Strawberry & mango lassi (p55)
Banana bread (p255)	blueberries (80g)	Radishes & cauliflower with hummus (p66)	Edamame & seed salad (p73)
Pearl barley, peas, spinach, broad beans & hazelnuts (p176)	Quinoa, Brussels sprouts & cashews (p175)	Wild rice salad with jerusalem artichoke & heirloom tomatoes (p154)	Cauliflower risotto with pistachios (p130)
Edamame & seed salad (p73)	Red pepper & butter bean mash (p68) with Mixed seed crackers (p77)	Mixed seed crackers (p77)	Beetroot hummus (p65) with red pepper crudités
Roasted pumpkin & tofu curry (p135)	Mexican bean stew (p139)	Stir-fried cauliflower rice with shiitake mushrooms & tofu (p143)	Dal with roasted fennel (p163)

Non-meat sources of **iron** include foods such as tofu, pulses, dried fruit, dark green leafy vegetables (except spinach, which can inhibit mineral absorption), wholegrains (such as oats and brown rice), nuts and spices (even a small quantity such as 2 teaspoons can add up to 2g of iron). You can increase your body's absorption of iron from non-meat sources by eating them with a source of **vitamin C** (see Iron Deficiency, page 354). Some of these foods also provide a useful non-meat source of **zinc**.

Dairy products, which are the main provider of **calcium** in a normal diet, are excluded from a vegan diet, but there are plenty of non-dairy sources of this mineral, such as fortified rice milk, tofu, almonds, sunflower seeds, sesame seeds and tahini, and dark green leafy vegetables (again with the exception of spinach, which can inhibit mineral absorption). Include plenty of these foods in your diet to ensure you get adequate calcium to support healthy bones.

Vitamin B12 is predominantly found in foods of animal origin but can be obtained from a few plant-based sources, including yeast extract, seaweed, spirulina (which can be added to smoothies and shakes) and fortified foods such as rice milk (this is often fortified with B12). These should be eaten on a daily basis because a lack of B12 can put you at risk of pernicious anaemia, causing tiredness, lethargy and fatigue.

Vegetarians and vegans may also find it difficult to get enough **omega 3 fatty acids** from their diet (this beneficial fat is found predominantly in oily fish). Foods such as seeds (chia and flax) and their oils, dark green leafy vegetables and certain nuts (walnuts) contain a fatty acid known as ALA (alpha-linolenic acid), which can be converted in the body to the heart-protective omega 3 fatty acid EPA (eicosapentaenoic acid) and DHA (docosahexaenoic acid), both found in oily fish. In addition to protecting the heart, EPA and DHA reduce triglyceride levels in the blood (a risk factor for heart disease) and reduce inflammation. If you're worried about not getting enough omega 3 from your diet, you could consider a supplement suitable for vegetarians/vegans as a back-up.

HEALING FOODS

Avocados
Broccoli
Brown rice
Brussels sprouts
Buckwheat
Cabbage
Chia seeds and oil
Dried fruit
Extra virgin olive oil
Flaxseeds and oil
Green beans
Herbs and spices, especially dried marjoram, ground cardamom and turmeric
Kale
Nuts (almonds, walnuts)
Nut butters
Pulses (beans, lentils))
Quinoa
Rapeseed oil
Rice milk
Seaweed
Seeds (sesame, sunflower)
Spirulina
Tahini
Tamari
Tofu
Yeast extract

LIMIT

Foods rich in oxalates (rhubarb, spinach and Swiss chard)

Vegan recipes are marked by a (V) in the general index on pages 382–394.

GLOSSARY OF HEALTH TERMS

AMINO ACIDS The building blocks of proteins found in food and the end product of protein digestion in the body, which allows them to be absorbed into the bloodstream. Essential for growth and repair of the body, there are 20 amino acids in total. Eleven of them can be made in the body (these are called 'non-essential' amino acids), but the remaining nine must be obtained from the diet ('essential' amino acids).

ANTIOXIDANTS Nutrients that help to reduce the amount of free radicals in the body. Vitamins such as A, C and E, as well as certain minerals, including selenium, are all considered to be powerful antioxidants and can be obtained from the food we eat.

BETA-GLUCAN A type of soluble fibre found in oats that can help protect against heart disease by positively balancing out cholesterol levels.

BLOOD SUGAR LEVEL The amount of sugar (glucose) in the blood. Resistance to insulin (the hormone that controls blood sugar levels) can lead to higher than normal levels and is an indicator of diabetes.

CARBOHYDRATE One of the three nutrients that provide energy (calories) in the diet, which are known as macronutrients. Carbohydrates provide four calories per gram and are recommended to make up half of the energy obtained from the diet. They can be split into starches, sugars and fibre. Unlike sugars and starches, only a small amount of fibre can be digested and yields less energy (two calories per gram).

CHOLESTEROL Vital for the production of hormones in the body and the manufacturing of vitamin D. Cholesterol occurs in two forms: as LDL (low-density lipoproteins), which is ferried from the liver to other parts of the body, and HDL (high-density lipoproteins), which mops up LDL and transports it back to the liver for processing. LDL is often referred to as 'bad' cholesterol for the negative effect it has on heart disease, and HDL is referred to as 'good' for its role in removing LDL from the bloodstream.

CHRONIC INFLAMMATION Occurs in the body when it is unable to overcome the effects of an attack. This causes the immune system to become overactive, often referred to as low-grade chronic inflammation. This has been linked to excess body fat (obesity) and is thought to be a contributory factor to a number of diseases.

COMPLEX CARBOHYDRATES These are fibre-rich carbohydrates that are broken down slowly in the body, thus helping to regulate blood sugar levels. You will find them in naturally starchy foods such as butternut squash, sweet potatoes, wholegrain varieties of rice, barley and pulses.

ENZYMES Proteins that speed up the rate of chemical reactions in the body. Digestive enzymes are required for the reactions involved in the breakdown of food.

FATTY ACIDS These are the building blocks of fats found in food and the end product of fat digestion in the body, which allows them to be absorbed into the bloodstream. They are the main storage of energy in the body and are essential for a number of its functions.

FIBRE Obtained from plant foods, fibre provides bulk to the diet and encourages proper bowel function.

FLAVONOIDS A group of phytonutrients (compounds that benefit health) that give plants their colour (pigment), such as anthocyanins found in purple and blue fruits. Flavonoids are considered to have a protective effect on health by way of their ability to reduce inflammation, which is thought to be at the root of many chronic conditions, including heart disease and cancer.

FODMAPS Treatment for IBS that eliminates fermentable carbohydrates from the diet.

FOOD ALLERGY An immune response to a food that causes symptoms such as hives, facial swelling, cramping, diarrhoea and, in some severe cases, anaphylaxis, which can cause the throat to swell and may result in death if not treated quickly enough.

FOOD INTOLERANCE Different from a food allergy, intolerance to food can result in the onset of symptoms such as cramping and bloating, which occur more slowly and often many hours after eating the offending food.

FREE RADICALS Unstable molecules produced naturally as a byproduct of bodily processes. An increased level of free radicals is thought to damage body cells and increase the risk of chronic diseases. Lifestyle and environmental factors, such as smoking and pollution, can also impact on free radical damage.

GLYCAEMIC INDEX (GI) A classification of carbohydrate foods according to the effect they have on blood sugar levels. All carbohydrates are broken down in the body to glucose, which cells use as a primary energy source. The speed at which these foods are broken down relates to their rating on the glycaemic index. Complex carbohydrate foods would be rated low on the index as their fibre content prevents them from being broken down too quickly.

INFLAMMATION A protective response of the immune system to an attack on the body that may occur as a result of injury or illness. It presents itself as heat, redness, swelling and pain.

INSULIN Hormone that regulates blood sugar levels after we eat carbohydrate foods, by transporting glucose (the end product of carbohydrate digestion) into cells for energy, as well as to the liver and muscles for storage.

LIVE BACTERIA 'Friendly' bacteria (found in live yogurt) that help to promote gut health. Effective strains of this bacteria include *Lactobacillus* and *Bifidobacterium*.

LYCOPENE Powerful antioxidant found in tomatoes that may have a protective effect against the development of prostate cancer.

MACRONUTRIENTS The three main food groups (carbohydrate, fat and protein) that contribute to the amount of calories in the diet.

MICRONUTRIENTS Vitamins and minerals, which are essential to life. They are needed in small amounts and must be obtained from the diet as they cannot be made in the body.

NEUROTRANSMITTERS Chemicals that send messages between cells by way of nerve endings.

OMEGA 3 FATTY ACIDS Essential fatty acids that must be obtained from the diet. The most crucial fatty acids, eicosapentaenoic acid (EPA) and docosahexaenioc acid (DHA), are found in oily fish. Alpha-linolenic acid (APA), found in plant foods such as flaxseed and rapeseed oil, walnuts and kale, can be partially converted to EPA and DHA in the body and is the primary source of omega 3 for those on meat-free diets.

OMEGA 6 FATTY ACIDS Like omega 3s, these fatty acids must be obtained from the food we eat as the body cannot produce them. They have an important role to play, in proper brain function as well as normal growth and development. However, they are thought to increase inflammation when eaten in excess of omega 3. Main food sources are those made with refined vegetable oils, such as margarines and processed foods.

PECTIN A type of soluble fibre found in apples, pears and grapes that may help to protect against heart disease by positively balancing out blood cholesterol levels.

PHYTOESTROGENS Naturally occurring plant oestrogens such as soy isoflavones found in foods such as edamame beans and miso. They have been associated with reducing levels of LDL (bad) cholesterol and have the potential to help balance female hormones.

PHYTONUTRIENTS Chemical compounds (also called phytochemicals) that occur naturally in plants. Phytonutrients are not essential for life but may play a key role in protecting us against disease. Fruit and vegetables are rich sources of phytonutrients, including the flavonoid group and the phytoestrogen group, which includes the soy isoflavones.

PREBIOTICS Non-digestible fibres found in certain foods that stimulate the growth of 'friendly' bacteria in the gut. These fibres can be found in foods such as bananas, chicory, garlic, onions, globe artichokes and asparagus.

PROSTAGLANDINS Hormone-like chemicals that are made in the body from fatty acids. There are two types of prostaglandin: one (made from omega 6 fatty acids) encourages inflammation and the other (made from omega 3 fatty acids) eases inflammation. Maintaining a balance of omega 3 and omega 6 fatty acids is considered to be beneficial to health.

RECOMMENDED DAILY ALLOWANCE (RDA) The amount of nutrients in the diet necessary to maintain good health, as decided by health professionals.

REFINED STARCHES Starchy foods where the hull, bran and fibre have been removed from the grain during processing. These foods are often referred to as 'simple' carbohydrates because they are broken down quickly by the body to be used for energy (they rapidly raise insulin levels and cause spikes in blood sugar).

REFINED SUGAR Sugar found in confectionery, soft drinks and sweet snacks (this includes all types of white and brown sugar, as well as agave and maple syrups). Like refined starches, these sugars are referred to as simple carbohydrates.

SATURATED FATS These fats tend to be solid at room temperature, such as butter or the hard white fat found on meat; processed foods are often high in saturated fat. Excess of saturated fats in the diet is considered to be a risk factor for heart disease as a result of the negative effect they have on blood cholesterol.

SEROTONIN Hormone produced in the brain that is thought to have a positive influence on mood, emotion and sleep.

SIMPLE CARBOHYDRATES These require little digestion (providing a quick source of energy), have the greatest impact on blood sugar levels and contain no other nutrients or fibre. All sugars are simple carbohydrates, and this includes glucose and fructose.

SOY ISOFLAVONES Antioxidants from the flavonoid family found in soya foods (tofu, tamari, edamame beans, miso). They behave the same way in the body as oestrogen but with less effect, which may help with hormonal balance in females. Soy isoflavones are also associated with positively balancing cholesterol levels, which will help to protect against heart disease.

TRANS FATS A type of fat (found mostly in processed foods) that can have a negative effect on health by increasing LDL (bad) cholesterol and reducing HDL (good) cholesterol, and by promoting inflammation within the body, which can impact on heart health. A small amount of trans fats occurs naturally in foods such as red meat and dairy products, but the majority are produced by a process (called 'hydrogenation') used by food manufacturers that converts liquid oils into solids.

UNSATURATED FATS These fats have a different chemical structure to saturated fat and are considered to be a healthier type of fat. They are either monounsaturated or polyunsaturated. Commonly associated with good heart health, they are found in foods such as oils, nuts, seeds, avocados and oily fish.

VITAMINS AND MINERALS A group of compounds vital for the body to function properly. They are required in small amounts and must be obtained from the diet as they can't be made by the body.

GENERAL INDEX

menstrual cycle 366–7
Mexican bean soup (V)(G) 88
Mexican bean stew (V)(G) 139
micronutrients 295, 380
migraine 358–9
    For an index of recipes that may help with,
      see p408
milk 10, 289; *see* almond milk; coconut milk; oat milk;
    rice milk
Mince pies, Mini (G) 258
Minced chicken in lettuce wraps (G) 211
minerals 295; *see* calcium; chromium; iron; magnesium;
    potassium; zinc
Mini carrot & orange muffins (G) 256
Mini frittatas (G) 41
Mini mince pies (G) 258
mint 12, 317
    Lemon & mint yogurt (V)(G) 128
    Mint pesto (V)(G) 178
    Mint tea (V)(G) 12, 321
miso 142, 306, 373
monosodium glutamate (MSG) 233, 355, 357, 358
monounsaturated fats *see* fats
morning sickness 52
mousse
    Raw cacao, ginger & avocado mousse (V)(G) 276
MSG *see* monosodium glutamate
muesli
    Apple, blueberry & cinnamon Bircher muesli (V) 26
    Beetroot & apple Bircher muesli (V) 25
muffins 18
    Banana muffins 43
    Blueberry & apple muffins 43
    Mini carrot & orange muffins (G) 256
    Spiced muffins (V)(G) 261
multiple sclerosis (MS) 311
mung beans 15
    Mung bean curry with onion, cucumber & cashew nut
      salad (V)(G) 167
mushrooms 297, 311, 328
    Braised lettuce, mushrooms & prawns 233
    Brown rice & mushroom risotto (V)(G) 182
    Mushroom salad (V)(G) 228
    Pointed cabbage & mushroom stir-fry (V)(G) 142
    Shiitake mushroom & daikon stir-fry (V)(G) 142
    Stir-fried cauliflower rice with shiitake mushrooms
      & tofu (G) 143
myalgic encephalopathy (ME) *see* chronic fatigue
    syndrome

N

nail problems 292, 341
nausea 52, 324
Nettle & kale broth (V)(G) 92
neurotransmitters 380
niacin *see* vitamin B3
nitrates 57, 307, 357

nut butter 17
nut oils 11
nuts 16, 24, 288, 290, 292, 294; *see also specific nuts*

O

oat milk 17
oats 10, 19, 287, 289, 290, 292, 319
    Cashew & goji berry flapjacks (V) 80
    Oat scones (V) 259
    Pistachio oat bars (V) 79
    Quinoa & oat porridge with blackberry compote (V) 33
    see also granola; muesli
obesity 10, 291, 308, 309, 327, 3426, 355, 364, 367
oestrogen 304, 306, 312, 367, 368, 369, 372, 373
oils 11, 288, 290, 294, 306, 315
okra 319
    Okra & ginger rice 213
    Stir-fried okra, cauliflower & tomato (V)(G) 145
oleic acid 294
olive oil 11, 161, 288, 290, 294, 306, 315
olives
    Tapenade (V)(G) 67
omega 3 fatty acids 11, 16, 81, 82, 101, 179, 199, 222,
    238, 250, 253, 288, 294, 306, 315, 323, 324, 331, 335,
    336, 337, 338, 340, 349, 350, 351, 355, 364, 370, 372,
    375, 378, 380
    alpha-linolenic acid (ALA) 294
    EPA and DHA 294
omega 6 fatty acids 11, 294, 315, 336, 337, 380
omelettes *see* eggs
onions 297
    Onion, cucumber & cashew nut salad (V)(G) 167
    Tomato & onion salad (V)(G) 195
orange foods 296
oranges
    Mini carrot & orange muffins (G) 256
    Orange & cranberry drops (G) 256
osteoarthritis 314
osteoporosis 312–13, 331, 367, 373
    For an index of recipes that may help with,
      see p408
Ottolenghi, Yotam: *Plenty* 140
overweight *see* obesity
oxalates 312

P

Pad Thai with brown rice noodles (G) 209
Pancakes, Raspberry 42
pantothenic acid *see* vitamin B5
papain 101
papayas 321, 330
    Green papaya salad (V)(G) 101
Parkinson's disease 296
pasta 10, 287, 289
    Griddled broccoli & pasta (V)(G) 179
    Pasta with broad beans & mint pesto (V)(G) 178
    Spicy prawn & tomato pasta (G) 232

vitamin B1 (thiamin) 19, 128, 146, 182, 209, 220, 233, 298, 330

vitamin B2 (riboflavin) 19, 142, 146, 182, 184, 209, 220, 233, 298, 330, 359

vitamin B3 (niacin) 19, 146, 182, 209, 220, 233, 298, 309, 330

vitamin B5 (pantothenic acid) 298

vitamin B6 19, 97, 116, 146, 182, 209, 212, 220, 222, 233, 298, 330, 350, 369–70

vitamin B12 19, 146, 182, 184, 185, 200, 209, 220, 222, 233, 237, 298, 330, 340, 341, 354, 378

vitamin C 33, 55, 95, 98, 164, 174, 188, 208, 220, 279, 280, 295, 296, 298, 314, 315, 328, 330, 354, 364, 369

vitamin D 39, 184, 222, 235, 293, 298, 310, 311, 312, 314, 328, 373, 375

vitamin E 16, 32, 38, 43, 55, 242, 261, 262, 275, 293, 295, 296, 298, 363, 373

vitamin K 293, 298, 312

vitamin supplements 295

W

walnut oil 11

walnuts 16, 294

   Candied walnuts (V)(G) 81

Watercress & turkey soup (G) 93

weight, gaining 346

weight, losing 113, 127, 236, 342–6; *see also* obesity

wheat 10, 287, 289, 290

wheatgrass powder 20, 48, 57

white foods 297

wholegrains 10, 146, 306

Wild rice, pepper & yogurt salad (V)(G) 252

Wild rice salad with jerusalem artichoke & heirloom tomatoes (V)(G) 154

women's health 366–7; *see also* menopausal problems; polycystic ovary syndrome; premenstrual syndrome; urinary tract infections

Y

yeast 320

yeast flakes 123, 148

yellow foods 296

yogurt 339

   coconut yogurt 17

   see also soya yogurt

Z

zeaxanthin 80, 297

zinc 15, 89, 104, 146, 222, 227, 232, 299, 309, 328, 335, 340, 341, 355, 362, 364, 365

INDEX OF RECIPES BY HEALTH ISSUE

Brown rice & mushroom risotto 182
Brown rice, pak choi & ginger broth 83
Butter beans with cherry tomatoes & salsa verde 160
Butternut squash & butter bean stew 138
Butternut steaks & roasted shallots 116
Cauliflower risotto with pistachios 130
Chicken & quinoa salad 205
Chickpea, pomegranate & pumpkin curry 164
Chickpeas & yogurt 157
Courgette spaghetti with king prawns 232
Courgette stuffed with beetroot & shallot 118
Creamy cauliflower & roasted garlic soup 90
Cucumber, pear, mint & wheatgrass juice 57
Dal with roasted fennel 163
Fresh pea & raw courgette salad 98
Griddled courgette & asparagus with rocket pesto 112
Halibut with chickpea stew & pesto 242
Kale, edamame & fennel frittata 199
King prawn, noodle & lemongrass broth 84
Lemongrass & coconut rice with edamame 181
Lentil bake 170
Lentil burgers with white cabbage & mange tout salad 171
Mexican bean soup 88
Mexican bean stew 139
Mung bean curry with onion, cucumber & cashew nut salad 167
Nettle & kale broth 92
Oven-baked asparagus & quail's eggs 187
Pad Thai with brown rice noodles 209
Pasta with broad beans & mint pesto 178
Pea & rocket soup 95
Pesto chicken with quinoa & peach salad 206
Pinto bean chilli 168
Pollock en papillote with brown lentils 249
Prawn, cashew & black rice salad 230
Quail's eggs, celery salt & cherry tomatoes 73
Quinoa & cashew salad 150
Quinoa, asparagus & almond salad 150
Quinoa pizza 148
Radish, edamame & lentil sprout salad 101
Raw cacao, avocado & raspberry cake 275
Red lentil soup 89
Roasted beetroot, fennel & apple salad 111
Roasted curried chickpeas 76
Roasted poussin with Brussels sprouts 217
Roasted pumpkin & tofu curry 135
Samphire, rocket & pea salad 104
Scotch broth 92
Shallot omelette 192
Shiitake mushroom & daikon stir-fry 142
Spring vegetable pie with courgette pastry 131
Sri Lankan butternut squash curry 134
Steamed salmon with pesto vegetables 236
Steamed sea bass with ginger & green chilli, with pak choi 244

Stir-fried cauliflower rice with shiitake mushrooms & tofu 143
Stir-fried okra, cauliflower & tomato 145
Sweet potato cakes with kale & green beans 113
Tenderstem & tahini 66
Tomato pesto with courgette spaghetti 127
Turkey & cashew curry 212
Turkey burgers and cabbage slaw 214
Vegetable lasagne 124
Warm quinoa, squash & spinach risotto 179
Watercress & turkey soup 93
Whole roasted cauliflower 174
Wild rice salad with jerusalem artichoke & heirloom tomatoes 154

ANXIETY
SEE PAGES 348, 349, 351, 356

Aubergine bake 123
Avocado smash with toasted nuts & seeds 36
Beetroot & apple Bircher muesli 25
Beetroot falafel 115
Butternut, coconut & chilli soup 87
Butternut squash & butter bean stew 138
Butternut squash & sage risotto 182
Butternut steaks & roasted shallots 116
Cacao milk 53
Cashew & goji berry flapjacks 80
Chicken & quinoa salad 205
Courgette spaghetti with king prawns 232
Courgette stuffed with beetroot & shallot 118
Cucumber, pear, mint & wheatgrass juice 57
Dal with roasted fennel 163
Edamame & seed salad 73
Flageolet bean salad with griddled sweetcorn 158
Fresh pea & raw courgette salad 98
Granola with pineapple & strawberries 30
Griddled broccoli & pasta 179
Griddled courgette & asparagus with rocket pesto 112
Grilled mackerel with ginger & saffron rice 253
Halibut with chickpea stew & pesto 242
King prawn & mango salad 227
King prawn stir-fry 230
Lemongrass & coconut rice with edamame 181
Lentil burgers with white cabbage & mange tout salad 171
Mango yogurt with dried apricots & banana 29
Mexican bean soup 88
Mexican bean stew 139
Nettle & kale broth 92
Pad Thai with brown rice noodles 209
Pasta with broad beans & mint pesto 178
Pesto chicken with quinoa & peach salad 206
Pinto bean chilli 168
Poached trout with fennel gratin 241

ARTHRITIS, RHEUMATOID
SEE PAGES 314–15

BLOATING
SEE PAGES 21, 30, 369

BLOOD PRESSURE, HIGH
SEE PAGES 307, 309

CHOLESTEROL, HIGH
SEE PAGES 293–4, 304–6, 379

Aduki bean stew 170
Apple & raspberry crumble 266
Apple, blueberry & cinnamon Bircher muesli 26
Aubergine bake 123
Avocado & broad bean smash on brown rice cakes 60
Avocado & quinoa salad 147
Avocado, apple, kiwi & spinach smoothie 55
Avocado salad 97
Avocado smash with toasted nuts & seeds 36
Baked apples 266
Baked aubergine with pomegranate 121
Baked sea bream with braised leeks 244
Banana bread 255
Beetroot & apple Bircher muesli 25
Beetroot & carrot tagine with cauliflower cous cous 132
Beetroot & cumin soup 89
Beetroot falafel 115
Beetroot hummus 65
Beetroot, tomato & coconut curry 137
Black pepper tofu 140
Blueberry & apple muffins 43
Borlotti bean, avocado, tomato & onion salad, with hard-boiled eggs 191
Broad bean & mint dip 70
Broccoli & ginger soup 84
Brown rice & mushroom risotto 182
Brown rice, pak choi & ginger broth 83
Butter beans with cherry tomatoes & salsa verde 160
Butternut, coconut & chilli soup 87
Butternut squash & butter bean stew 138
Butternut squash & sage risotto 182
Butternut steaks & roasted shallots 116
Cabbage, apple & tarragon salad 104
Cajun chicken with avocado salad & mango salsa 202
Candied walnuts 81
Carrot & cucumber ribbons 105
Cashew & goji berry flapjacks 80
Cauliflower, celeriac & paprika soup 90
Cauliflower risotto with pistachios 130
Chia seed pudding with blackberry & lime coulis 35
Chicken & quinoa salad 206
Chicken & vegetable pie 219
Chickpea, pomegranate & pumpkin curry 164
Chickpeas & yogurt 157
Courgette spaghetti with king prawns 232
Courgette stuffed with beetroot & shallot 118
Creamy cauliflower & roasted garlic soup 90
Cucumber, mint & yogurt dip 70
Dal with roasted fennel 163
Edamame & seed salad 73
Fennel, apple & butternut salad 208
Flageolet bean salad with griddled sweetcorn 158
Fresh pea & raw courgette salad 98
Gazpacho 95

Granola with pineapple & strawberries 30
Griddled broccoli & pasta 179
Griddled courgette & asparagus with rocket pesto 112
Grilled mackerel with ginger & saffron rice 253
Grilled salmon with ginger 238
Guacamole 59
Halibut with chickpea stew & pesto 242
King prawn & mango salad 227
King prawn stir-fry 230
Lavender poached pears 270
Lemongrass & coconut rice with edamame 181
Lentil bake 170
Lentil burgers with white cabbage & mange tout salad 171
Lentil sprout & celery salad 161
Mackerel & cucumber gazpacho 250
Mackerel with wild rice, pepper & yogurt salad 252
Mango cup with pomegranate 33
Mango yogurt with dried apricots & banana 29
Mexican bean soup 88
Mexican bean stew 139
Mixed seed crackers 77
Mung bean curry with onion, cucumber & cashew nut salad 167
Nettle & kale broth 92
Oat scones 259
Pasta with broad beans & mint pesto 178
Pea & rocket soup 95
Pearl barley, peas, spinach, broad beans & hazelnuts 176
Pearl barley with cantaloupe melon 151
Pecan & coconut granola 30
Pinto bean chilli 168
Pistachio oat bars 79
Pointed cabbage & mushroom stir-fry 142
Pollock en papillote with brown lentils 249
Prawn, cashew & black rice salad 230
Purple kale, broccoli, shallot & chilli salad 108
Puy lentils & roasted aubergine with basil pesto 161
Quinoa & cashew salad 150
Quinoa & oat porridge with blackberry compote 33
Quinoa, asparagus & almond salad 150
Quinoa bread 44
Quinoa, Brussels sprouts & cashews 175
Quinoa pizza 148
Radish, edamame & lentil sprout salad 101
Radishes & cauliflower with hummus 66
Raw cacao, avocado & raspberry cake 275
Raw cacao, ginger & avocado mousse 276
Raw vegetable & ginger salad 107
Red lentil soup 89
Red pepper & butter bean mash 68
Roasted baby aubergine with spinach salad 122
Roasted beetroot, fennel & apple salad 111
Roasted cauliflower, carrots & caraway with lemon yogurt 128
Roasted pumpkin & tofu curry 135

Salmon & brown rice noodles 237
Salmon & dill fishcakes 238
Salmon, green beans, orange & hazelnut salad 235
Samphire, rocket & pea salad 104
Scotch broth 92
Seared tuna & beetroot salad 253
Shiitake mushroom & daikon stir-fry 142
Soft-boiled eggs with avocado salad 38
Spicy nuts 76
Spring vegetable pie with courgette pastry 131
Sri Lankan butternut squash curry 134
Steamed salmon with pesto vegetables 236
Stir-fried cauliflower rice with shiitake mushrooms
    & tofu 143
Stir-fried okra, cauliflower & tomato 145
Strawberry & mango lassi 55
Strawberry soya yogurt 29
Sweet potato cakes with kale & green beans 113
Tapenade 67
Tenderstem & tahini 66
Thai green curry 137
Tomato pesto with courgette spaghetti 127
Turkey burgers with cabbage slaw 214
Vanilla almond milk 32
Vegetable lasagne 124
Watercress & turkey soup 93
Wild rice salad with jerusalem artichoke & heirloom
    tomatoes 154

CHRONIC FATIGUE SYNDROME (CFS)
SEE PAGES 355

Candied walnuts 81
Chia seed pudding with blackberry & lime coulis 35
Grilled mackerel with ginger & saffron rice 253
Mackerel & cucumber gazpacho 250
Mackerel with wild rice, pepper & yogurt salad 252
Mini frittatas 41
Quinoa bread 44
Salmon & brown rice noodles 237
Salmon & dill fishcakes 238
Salmon, green beans, orange & hazelnut salad 235
Seared tuna & beetroot salad 253

COMMON COLD
SEE PAGES 328–9

Avocado salad 97
Aduki bean stew 170
Apple & lychee granita 280
Apple, blueberry & cinnamon Bircher muesli 26
Aubergine bake 123
Avocado & broad bean smash on brown rice cakes 60

Avocado, apple, kiwi & spinach smoothie 55
Baked aubergine with pomegranate 121
Baked eggs with spinach & tomato 38
Baked sea bream with braised leeks 244
Beetroot & apple Bircher muesli 25
Beetroot & carrot tagine with cauliflower cous cous 132
Beetroot & cumin soup 89
Beetroot, tomato & coconut curry 137
Black pepper tofu 140
Borlotti bean, avocado, tomato & onion salad with
    hard-boiled eggs 191
Braised lettuce, mushrooms & prawns 233
Broad bean & mint dip 70
Broccoli & ginger soup 84
Broccoli stalk & cashew spread 63
Brown rice & mushroom risotto 182
Butter bean & spinach mash with crudités 68
Butter beans with cherry tomatoes & salsa verde 160
Butternut, coconut & chilli soup 87
Butternut squash & butter bean stew 138
Butternut squash & sage risotto 182
Butternut steaks & roasted shallots 116
Cabbage, apple & tarragon salad 104
Cabbage stuffed with chicken 208
Cajun chicken with avocado salad & mango salsa 202
Carrot & cucumber ribbons 105
Carrot, beetroot, apple & celery juice 57
Cashew & goji berry flapjacks 80
Cauliflower, celeriac & paprika soup 90
Cauliflower risotto with pistachios 130
Chia seed, coconut & pineapple smoothie 52
Chia seed pudding with blackberry & lime coulis 35
Chicken & quinoa salad 205
Chicken & vegetable pie 219
Chicken burgers with beetroot relish 216
Chickpea, pomegranate & pumpkin curry 164
Courgette spaghetti with king prawns 232
Courgette stuffed with beetroot & shallot 118
Creamy cauliflower & roasted garlic soup 90
Cucumber, pear, mint & wheatgrass juice 57
Dal with roasted fennel 163
Egg white & broccoli omelette 192
Fennel, apple & butternut salad 208
Fresh pea & raw courgette salad 98
Fresh sweetcorn soup 87
Gazpacho 95
Granola with pineapple & strawberries 30
Green papaya salad 101
Griddled courgette & asparagus with rocket pesto 112
Grilled mackerel with ginger & saffron rice 253
Grilled peaches, hazelnuts & raspberries 273
Halibut with chickpea stew & pesto 242
Hot apple smoothie 56
Kale crisps with cashew nuts & paprika 74
King prawn & mango salad 227
King prawn, kohlrabi & pear salad 224
King prawn, noodle & lemongrass broth 84

King prawn stir-fry 230

Lemon chicken 220

Lemongrass & coconut rice with edamame 181

Lentil bake 170

Lentil burgers with white cabbage & mange tout salad 171

Lentil sprout & celery salad 161

Mackerel & cucumber gazpacho 250

Mackerel with wild rice, pepper & yogurt salad 252

Mango & raspberry sorbet 280

Mango cup with pomegranate 33

Mango yogurt with dried apricots & banana 29

Mexican bean soup 88

Mini frittatas 41

Mung bean curry with onion, cucumber & cashew nut salad 167

Nettle & kale broth 92

Oven-baked asparagus & quail's eggs 187

Pad Thai with brown rice noodles 209

Pasta with broad beans & mint pesto 178

Pearl barley, peas, spinach, broad beans & hazelnuts 176

Pearl barley with cantaloupe melon 151

Pecan & coconut granola 30

Pesto chicken with quinoa & peach salad 206

Pinto bean chilli 168

Pistachio oat bars 79

Poached eggs & sweet potato hash 39

Poached trout with fennel gratin 241

Pointed cabbage & mushroom stir-fry 142

Pollock & prawn fishcakes with courgette spaghetti 247

Pollock with tempura green bean chips 246

Prawn, cashew & black rice salad 230

Purple kale, broccoli, shallot & chilli salad 108

Puy lentils & roasted aubergine with basil pesto 161

Quinoa & cashew salad 150

Quinoa & oat porridge with blackberry compote 33

Quinoa, asparagus & almond salad 150

Quinoa, Brussels sprouts & cashews 175

Quinoa, cauliflower & pistachio burgers 173

Quinoa pizza 148

Radish, cucumber & dill salad 102

Radish, edamame & lentil sprout salad 101

Radishes & cauliflower with hummus 66

Raspberry, blueberry & coconut water smoothie 49

Raw vegetable & ginger salad 107

Red lentil soup 89

Roasted baby aubergine with spinach salad 122

Roasted beetroot, fennel & apple salad 111

Roasted cauliflower, carrots & caraway with lemon yogurt 128

Roasted poussin with Brussels sprouts 217

Roasted pumpkin & tofu curry 135

Salmon & brown rice noodles 237

Salmon, green beans, orange & hazelnut salad 235

Samphire, rocket & pea salad 104

Scotch broth 92

Seared tuna & beetroot salad 253

Shiitake mushroom & daikon stir-fry 142

Soft-boiled eggs with avocado salad 38

Spicy nuts 76

Spicy prawn & tomato pasta 232

Spring vegetable pie with courgette pastry 131

Sri Lankan butternut squash curry 134

Steamed salmon with pesto vegetables 236

Steamed sea bass with ginger & green chilli, with pak choi 244

Stir-fried cauliflower rice with shiitake mushrooms & tofu 143

Stir-fried okra, cauliflower & tomato 145

Strawberry & banana ice cream 279

Strawberry cheesecake 279

Strawberry soya yogurt 29

Sweetcorn fritters with tomato & onion salad 195

Sweet potato & turkey Massaman curry 213

Tabouleh with pistachio 153

Tandoori chicken with pineapple salad 201

Tenderstem & tahini 66

Thai green curry 137

Tomato pesto with courgette spaghetti 127

Turkey & cashew curry 212

Turkey burgers and cabbage slaw 214

Vegetable lasagne 124

Whole roasted cauliflower 174

Watercress & turkey soup 93

CONSTIPATION
SEE PAGES 292, 318–19, 320

Aduki bean stew 170

Apple & raspberry crumble 266

Apple, blueberry & cinnamon Bircher muesli 26

Aubergine bake 123

Avocado & broad bean smash on brown rice cakes 60

Avocado salad 97

Avocado smash with toasted nuts & seeds 36

Baked aubergine with pomegranate 121

Beans on toast 47

Beetroot & apple Bircher muesli 25

Beetroot & carrot tagine with cauliflower cous cous 132

Beetroot & cumin soup 89

Beetroot hummus 65

Beetroot, tomato & coconut curry 137

Black pepper tofu 140

Borlotti bean, avocado, tomato & onion salad with hard-boiled eggs 191

Broad bean & mint dip 70

Broccoli & ginger soup 84

Brown rice & mushroom risotto 182

Brown rice, pak choi & ginger broth 83

Butter bean & spinach mash with crudités 68

Butter beans with cherry tomatoes & salsa verde 160

DEPRESSION
SEE PAGES 348, 349, 350, 355, 356

Thai green curry 137
Tomato pesto with courgette spaghetti 127
Turkey & cashew curry 212
Turkey burgers & cabbage slaw 214
Vegetable lasagne 124
Watercress & turkey soup 93
Whole roasted cauliflower 174
Wild rice salad with jerusalem artichoke & heirloom
    tomatoes 154

DIABETES, TYPE 2
SEE PAGES 290, 308–9, 365

Aduki bean stew 170
Apple, blueberry & cinnamon Bircher muesli 26
Avocado & quinoa salad 147
Avocado salad 97
Avocado smash with toasted nuts & seeds 36
Baked eggs with spinach & tomato 38
Beetroot falafel 115
Beetroot & apple Bircher muesli 25
Black pepper tofu 140
Brown rice, pak choi & ginger broth 83
Butternut, coconut & chilli soup 87
Butternut squash & sage risotto 182
Butternut steaks & roasted shallots 116
Cabbage stuffed with chicken 208
Cacao milk 53
Cajun chicken with avocado salad & mango
    salsa 202
Carrot & cucumber ribbons 105
Cashew & goji berry flapjacks 80
Cauliflower risotto with pistachios 130
Cherry & almond tart 269
Chia seed pudding with blackberry & lime coulis 35
Chicken & quinoa salad 205
Chicken & vegetable pie 219
Chicken burgers with beetroot relish 216
Chicken, cashew & tarragon wraps 211
Courgette spaghetti with king prawns 232
Dal with roasted fennel 163
Edamame & seed salad 73
Egg-fried brown rice 191
Flageolet bean salad with griddled sweetcorn 158
Fresh pea & raw courgette salad 98
Granola with pineapple & strawberries 30
Green papaya salad 101
Griddled broccoli & pasta 179
Griddled courgette & asparagus with rocket pesto 112
Grilled mackerel with ginger & saffron rice 253
Halibut with chickpea stew & pesto 242
King prawn & mango salad 227
King prawn stir-fry 230
Lemon chicken 220
Lemongrass & coconut rice with edamame 181

Lentil bake 170
Mackerel & cucumber gazpacho 250
Mackerel with wild rice, pepper & yogurt salad 252
Mexican bean soup 88
Mexican bean stew 139
Minced chicken in lettuce wraps 211
Oven-baked asparagus & quail's eggs 187
Pad Thai with brown rice noodles 209
Pasta with broad beans & mint pesto 178
Pinto bean chilli 168
Poached trout with fennel gratin 241
Pollock & prawn fishcakes with courgette spaghetti
    247
Pollock en papillote with brown lentils 249
Prawn, cashew & black rice salad 230
Purple kale, broccoli, shallot & chilli salad 108
Quinoa & oat porridge with blackberry compote 33
Quinoa, asparagus & almond salad 150
Quinoa, Brussels sprouts & cashews 175
Quinoa, cauliflower & pistachio burgers 173
Quinoa pizza 148
Raw vegetable & ginger salad 107
Roasted pumpkin & tofu curry 135
Salmon & brown rice noodles 237
Salmon & dill fishcakes 238
Samphire, rocket & pea salad 104
Scotch broth 92
Shiitake mushroom & daikon stir-fry 142
Spicy nuts 76
Spicy prawn & tomato pasta 232
Sri Lankan butternut squash curry 134
Steamed salmon with pesto vegetables 236
Stir-fried cauliflower rice with shiitake mushrooms
    & tofu 143
Stir-fried okra, cauliflower & tomato 145
Tandoori chicken with pineapple salad 201
Tenderstem & tahini 66
Tomato pesto with courgette spaghetti 127
Turkey & cashew curry 212
Turkey burgers & cabbage slaw 214
Vegetable lasagne 124
Warm quinoa, squash & spinach risotto 179
Watercress & turkey soup 93
Wild rice salad with jerusalem artichoke & heirloom
    tomatoes 154

ECZEMA
SEE PAGES 338–9

Beetroot & carrot tagine with cauliflower cous cous 132
Beetroot & cumin soup 89
Beetroot falafel 115
Broccoli & ginger soup 84
Brown rice & mushroom risotto 182
Butter bean & spinach mash with crudités 68

HAIR & SCALP PROBLEMS
SEE PAGES 340

INDIGESTION & HEARTBURN
SEE PAGES 10, 324

INSOMNIA
SEE PAGES 356

IRRITABLE BOWEL SYNDROME (IBS)
SEE PAGES 320, 322–3, 325

MALE FERTILITY
SEE PAGES 364

MENOPAUSAL PROBLEMS
SEE PAGES 312, 372–3

Roasted poussin with Brussels sprouts 217
Roasted pumpkin & tofu curry 135
Salmon & brown rice noodles 237
Salmon & dill fishcakes 238
Salmon, green beans, orange & hazelnut salad 235
Seared tuna & beetroot salad 253
Soft-boiled eggs with avocado salad 38
Spiced muffins 261
Spicy nuts 76
Steamed salmon with pesto vegetables 236
Stir-fried cauliflower rice with shiitake mushrooms
& tofu 143
Stir-fried okra, cauliflower & tomato 145
Strawberry & mango lassi 55
Strawberry cheesecake 279
Strawberry soya yogurt 29
Tabouleh with pistachio 153
Tomato pesto with courgette spaghetti 127
Vanilla almond milk 32

MIGRAINE
SEE PAGES 358–9

Aduki bean stew 170
Apple, blueberry & cinnamon Bircher muesli 26
Asparagus & egg smash 185
Aubergine bake 123
Avocado & quinoa salad 147
Avocado smash with toasted nuts & seeds 36
Beetroot & apple Bircher muesli 25
Beetroot falafel 115
Brown rice & mushroom risotto 182
Brown rice, pak choi & ginger broth 83
Butternut, coconut & chilli soup 87
Butternut squash & butter bean stew 138
Butternut squash & sage risotto 182
Butternut steaks & roasted shallots 116
Cacao milk 53
Cajun chicken with avocado salad & mango salsa 202
Cashew & goji berry flapjacks 80
Cherry & almond tart 269
Chia seed pudding with blackberry & lime coulis 35
Chicken & quinoa salad 205
Chicken, cashew & tarragon wraps 211
Courgette spaghetti with king prawns 232
Courgette stuffed with beetroot & shallot 118
Crab & chilli with cucumber salad 223
Cucumber, pear, mint & wheatgrass juice 57
Dal with roasted fennel 163
Edamame & seed salad 73
Egg-fried brown rice 191
Flageolet bean salad with griddled sweetcorn 158
Fresh pea & raw courgette salad 98
Granola with pineapple & strawberries 30
Griddled broccoli & pasta 179

Griddled courgette & asparagus with rocket pesto 112
Grilled mackerel with ginger & saffron rice 253
Halibut with chickpea stew & pesto 242
Kale, edamame & fennel frittata 199
King prawn & mango salad 227
King prawn stir-fry 230
Lemongrass & coconut rice with edamame 181
Lentil burgers with white cabbage & mange tout salad 171
Mango yogurt with dried apricots & banana 29
Mexican bean soup 88
Mexican bean stew 139
Pad Thai with brown rice noodles 209
Pasta with broad beans & mint pesto 178
Pesto chicken with quinoa & peach salad 206
Pinto bean chilli 168
Poached trout with fennel gratin 241
Pointed cabbage & mushroom stir-fry 142
Pollock & prawn fishcakes with courgette spaghetti 247
Pollock en papillote with brown lentils 249
Pollock with tempura green bean chips 246
Purple kale, broccoli, shallot & chilli salad 108
Quinoa & cashew salad 150
Quinoa & oat porridge with blackberry compote 33
Quinoa, asparagus & almond salad 150
Quinoa, Brussels sprouts & cashews 175
Quinoa, cauliflower & pistachio burgers 173
Quinoa pizza 148
Raw cacao, avocado & raspberry cake 275
Raw cacao, ginger & avocado mousse 276
Roasted poussin with Brussels sprouts 217
Roasted pumpkin & tofu curry 135
Shallot omelette 192
Shiitake mushroom & daikon stir-fry 142
Spicy nuts 76
Spicy prawn & tomato pasta 232
Sri Lankan butternut squash curry 134
Stir-fried cauliflower rice with shiitake mushrooms
& tofu 143
Stir-fried okra, cauliflower & tomato 145
Sweet potato & turkey Massaman curry 213
Sweet potato frittata 196
Tomato pesto with courgette spaghetti 127
Turkey & cashew curry 212
Vegetable lasagne 124
Wild rice salad with jerusalem artichoke & heirloom
tomatoes 154

OSTEOPOROSIS
SEE PAGES 10, 312–13, 331, 367, 373

Aduki bean stew 170
Apple, blueberry & cinnamon Bircher muesli 26
Asparagus & egg smash 185
Avocado & quinoa salad 147
Avocado smash with toasted nuts & seeds 36

POLYCYSTIC OVARY SYNDROME (PCOS)
SEE PAGES 334, 367, 374–5

PREMENSTRUAL SYNDROME (PMS)
SEE PAGES 268–70, 350

PROSTATE HEALTH
SEE PAGES 362–3

PSORIASIS
SEE PAGES 336–7

SUPPLIERS

Eat the Seasons
eattheseasons.co.uk
For finding out which fresh ingredients are in season.

Whole Foods
buywholefoodsonline.co.uk
Stocks wheatgrass and spirulina powder as well as other ingredients that are difficult to get hold of, such as raw cacao powder and goji berries.

Goodness Direct
goodnessdirect.co.uk
Online ordering and delivery of health foods.

Coyo
coyo.co.uk
For dairy-free yogurt made from coconut milk.

The Spice Shop
thespiceshop.co.uk
Online site for the Portobello Road shop specialising in herbs, spices and speciality ingredients.

Clifton Greens
16 Clifton Road, London W9 1SS
The best grocers in West London.

INFORMATION RESOURCES

British Dietetic Association
bda.uk.com
Trusted source of information about nutrition and health.

NHS Choices
nhs.uk
Contains information from the UK's National Health Service on health conditions, treatment and healthy living.

British Heart Foundation
bhf.org.uk
Charity that funds research, education and campaigns aimed at preventing heart disease.

Diabetes UK
diabetes.org.uk
Charity providing information, advice and support for people with diabetes.

National Osteoporosis Society
nos.org.uk
British charity dedicated to improving diagnosis, prevention and treatment of osteoporosis; the website is a reliable source of information.

Arthritis Care
arthritiscare.org.uk
UK charity that provides a source of information and support for people suffering from arthritis.

Coeliac UK
coeliac.org.uk
Charity that provides a source of expert advice and information for people with coeliac disease and dermatitis herpetiformis.

Mind
mind.org.uk
UK charity that provides advice and support for anyone experiencing a mental health problem.

Vegetarian Society
vegsoc.org
Offers support, advice and free resources for vegetarians.

Vegan Society
vegansociety.com
Provides support, advice and free resources for vegans.

The Soil Association
soilassociation.org
UK organisation that campaigns for organic food and farming.

Marine Conservation Society
fishonline.org
Gives up-to-date sustainability ratings for the different types of fish, so you know which ones are best to buy.

ABOUT THE AUTHORS

LILY SIMPSON is a chef who takes her ideas from travels in France, Spain, Italy, Thailand, Morocco and India. In 2012 she founded the Detox Kitchen, a unique detox food delivery service, which launched to dazzling success. Having attracted a loyal following of clients, the Detox Kitchen now serves a range of delicious, healthy dishes from delis across London.

ROB HOBSON is one of Britain's most talented nutritionists. An obsessed foodie and skilled cook, his food and nutrition features have appeared in a wide range of publications. He runs two food and nutrition consultancies in London, and has worked with private clients, government agencies and the NHS.

ACKNOWLEDGEMENTS

Thank you to our lovely agent Dorie Simmonds, whose positivity is contagious. To our clever editors at Bloomsbury, Natalie Bellos and Xa Shaw Stewart, you have such grace and elegance and this is totally reflected in the book. To the incredible and patient Norma MacMillan for her charming attention to detail. To the brilliant Polly Webb-Wilson and Keiko Oikawa, you are a dream team. Also to Spaniards Marian Alonso and Marina Asenjo for the author photograph and for the production expertise. To Peter Dawson and Namkwan Cho at Grade Design for being so calm and creative in equal measures.

Lily would like to thank

Thanks to all our Detox Kitchen customers – your loyalty has enabled us to continue making the food we love. I would also like to thank our head chef Claire Herrick, Sous Chef Lucy Cheyne and all of our talented chefs for continuing to create food that inspires me. Thank you to Harriet Jenkins for your day-to-day support, level head and general amazingness. Thanks to Jules Miller, Jayne Robinson and our entire team of office and deli staff, for believing in our brand as much as I do. To my dad for showing me how to cook with the holy grail of ingredients, onion, ginger and garlic. To my mum, for absolutely everything. To my husband for always telling me everything I cook is delicious and being my 'stone'!

Rob would like to thank

All of my (very patient) family and friends.

Lily *For Mum and Dad*
Rob *For Adie and my sister Claire*

First published in Great Britain 2016

Text © Lily Simpson and Rob Hobson 2015
Recipes © Lily Simpson 2015
Photography © Keiko Oikawa 2015
except photographs on front cover and p6 © Issy Croker 2016

The moral right of the authors has been asserted

No part of this book may be used or reproduced in any manner whatsoever without
written permission from the publisher except in the case of brief quotations embedded
in critical articles or reviews

Bloomsbury Publishing
An imprint of Bloomsbury Publishing Plc

50 Bedford Square   1385 Broadway
London   New York
WC1B 3DP   NY 10018
UK   USA

bloomsbury.com

BLOOMSBURY and the Diana logo are trademarks of Bloomsbury Publishing Plc

Bloomsbury Publishing, London, Oxford, New York, New Delhi and Sydney

A CIP catalogue record for this book is available from the British Library

ISBN HB: 978 1 4088 5285 9
ISBN TPB: 978 1 4088 5292 7

10 9 8 7 6 5 4 3 2 1

Project editing: Norma MacMillan
Design: Peter Dawson, Namkwan Cho gradedesign.com
Photography: Keiko Oikawa
Styling: Polly Webb-Wilson
Index: Vicki Robinson

Printed and bound in China by C&C Offset Printing Co., Ltd

The concepts, procedures and suggestions mentioned within this book are not intended
to be a substitute for consulting with your physician. All health matters personal to you
should be considered under medical supervision and neither the publisher or authors
are responsible for your specific health or allergy needs. The publisher or authors are
not responsible for any adverse reactions to the recipes contained within this book.
The menu plans contained within this book are intended to be used by healthy adults
and pregnant women should consult their physician before following any of the advice
or menu plans found in this book.